Hematology, Immunology and Infectious Disease: Neonatology Questions and Controversies

Hematology, Immunology and Infectious Disease

Neonatology Questions and Controversies

Series Editor

Richard A. Polin, MD
Professor of Pediatrics
College of Physicians and Surgeons
Columbia University
Director, Division of Neonatology
Morgan Stanley Children's Hospital of New York - Presbyterian
Columbia University Medical Center
New York, New York

Other Volumes in the Neonatology Questions and Controversies Series

Cardiology
Gastroenterology and Nutrition
Nephrology and Fluid/Electrolyte Physiology
Neurology
The Newborn Lung

Her

anc

Neor   rsies

Robin K

Professor
University
Associate
Clinical Tr
University
Albuquerq

Mervin

Richard an
Professor
Professor
Indiana Ur
Herman B
Attending
James Whi
Indianapol

Consultir

Richard A

Professor of Pediatrics
College of Physicians and Surgeons
Columbia University
Director, Division of Neonatology
Morgan Stanley Children's Hospital of New York - Presbyterian
Columbia University Medical Center
New York, New York

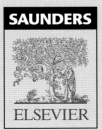

SAUNDERS

ELSEVIER

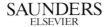

1600 John F. Kennedy Blvd.
Suite 1800
Philadelphia, PA 19103-2899

HEMATOLOGY, IMMUNOLOGY AND INFECTIOUS DISEASE:
Neonatology Questions and Controversies   ISBN: 978-1-4160-3158-1
Copyright © 2008 by Saunders, an imprint of Elsevier Inc.

Notice

Knowledge and best practice in this field are constantly changing. As new research and experience broaden our knowledge, changes in practice, treatment and drug therapy may become necessary or appropriate. Readers are advised to check the most current information provided (i) on procedures featured or (ii) by the manufacturer of each product to be administered, to verify the recommended dose or formula, the method and duration of administration, and contraindications. It is the responsibility of the practitioner, relying on their own experience and knowledge of the patient, to make diagnoses, to determine dosages and the best treatment for each individual patient, and to take all appropriate safety precautions. To the fullest extent of the law, neither the Publisher nor the Authors assumes any liability for any injury and/or damage to persons or property arising out of or related to any use of the material contained in this book.

The Publisher

Library of Congress Cataloging-in-Publication Data

Hematology, immunology, and infectious disease: neonatology questions and controversies/[edited by]
Robin Kjerstin Ohls, Mervin C. Yoder; consulting editior,
Richard A. Polin.—1st ed.
    p. ; cm.
  Includes bibliographical references.
  ISBN 978-1-4160-3158-1
  1. Neonatal hematology. 2. Newborn infants—Immunology. 3. Communicable diseases in newborn infants.
I. Ohls, Robin Kjerstin. II. Yoder, Mervin C. III. Polin, Richard A,
(Richard Alan), 1945-
  [DNLM: 1. Neonatology—methods. 2. Communicable Diseases. 3. Hematologic Diseases. 4. Immune System Diseases. 5. Infant, Newborn. WS 420 H487 2008]
RJ269.5.H52 2008
618.92′01—dc22

                                                                              2007043875

Acquisitions Editor: Judith Fletcher
Developmental Editor: Lisa Barnes
Associate Developmental Editor: Bernard Buckholz
Senior Project Manager: David Saltzberg
Design Direction: Karen O'Keefe-Owens

Working together to grow
libraries in developing countries

www.elsevier.com | www.bookaid.org | www.sabre.org

ELSEVIER   BOOK AID International   Sabre Foundation

Printed in China
Last digit is the print number: 9   8   7   6   5   4   3   2   1

Contents

Contributors

Ezra Aksoy, PhD
Post Doctoral Fellow
Centre for Cell Signalling
Institute of Cancer
Barts and The London
Queen Mary University of London
London, United Kingdom
> *Toll-like Receptor Responses in Neonatal Dendritic Cells*

Subbarao Bondada, PhD
Professor
Department of Microbiology, Immunology, and Molecular Genetics
Sanders Brown Center on Aging
Chandler Medical Center
University of Kentucky
Lexington, Kentucky
> *What Insights Into Human Cord Blood Lymphocyte Function Can Be Gleaned From Studying Newborn Mice?*

Robert D. Christensen, MD
Director, Neonatology Research
Intermountain Healthcare
Medical Director, Neonatology
Urban North Region
Intermountain Healthcare
Ogden, Utah
> *The Role of Recombinant Leukocyte Colony-Stimulating Factors in the Neonatal Intensive Care Unit*

Dominique De Wit, PhD
Senior Researcher
Institute for Medical Immunology
Charleroi-Gosselies, Belgium
> *Toll-like Receptor Responses in Neonatal Dendritic Cells*

Björn Fischler, MD, PhD
Associate Professor
Department of Pediatrics
Karolinska University Hospital, Huddinge
Stockholm, Sweden
> *Breast Milk and Viral Infection*

Marianne Forsgren MD, PhD

Associate Professor of Virology
Department of Laboratory Medicine
Karolinska University Hospital, Huddinge
Stockholm, Sweden
> *Breast Milk and Viral Infection*

W. Paul Glezen, MD

Professor
Departments of Molecular Virology and Immunology, and Pediatrics
Baylor College of Medicine
Adjunct Professor of Epidemiology
School of Public Health
The University of Texas Health Science Center
Houston, Texas
> *Influence of Passive Antibodies on the Immune Response of Young Infants*

Michel Goldman, MD, PhD

Director
The Institute for Medical Immunology
University Libre de Bruxelles
Charleroi-Gosselies, Belgium
> *Toll-like Receptor Responses in Neonatal Dendritic Cells*

Stanislas Goriely, MD, PhD, FNRS

Research Associate
Institute for Medical Immunology
Université Libre de Bruxelles
Charleroi-Gosselies, Belgium
> *Toll-like Receptor Responses in Neonatal Dendritic Cells*

Cheri D. Landers, MD

Associate Professor of Pediatrics
University of Kentucky
Chief, Heinrich A. Werner Division of Pediatric Critical Care
Director, Pediatric Sedation Service
Pediatric Critical Care
Lexington, Kentucky
> *What Insights Into Human Cord Blood Lymphocyte Function Can Be Gleaned From Studying Newborn Mice?*

David B. Lewis, MD

Professor of Pediatric
Stanford University School of Medicine
Attending Physician
Lucile Salter Packard Children's Hospital
Stanford, California
> *Neonatal T-cell Immunity and its Regulation by Innate Immunity and Dendritic Cells*

Akhil Maheshwari, MD

Assistant Professor of Pediatrics
Divisions of Neonatology and Pediatric Gastroenterology and Cell Biology
University of Alabama at Birmingham
Birmingham, Alabama
Practical Approaches to the Neutropenic Neonate

Marilyn J. Manco-Johnson, MD

Director
Mountain States Regional Hemophilia and Thrombosis Center
Aurora, Colorado
Controversies in Neonatal Thrombotic Disorders

Neelufar Mozaffarian, MD, PhD

Instructor
Seattle Children's Hospital Research Institute
Children's Hospital and Regional Medical Center
University of Washington
Seattle, Washington
Maternally Mediated Neonatal Autoimmunity

Lars Navér, MD, PhD

Consultant Pediatrician and Neonatologist
Department of Neonatology
Karolinska University Hospital Huddinge
Stockholm, Sweden
Breast Milk and Viral Infection

Robin K. Ohls, MD

Professor of Pediatrics
University of New Mexico
Associate Director-Pediatrics
Clinical Translational Sciences Center
University of New Mexico Health Sciences Center
Albuquerque, New Mexico
Why, When and How Should We Provide Red Cell Transfusions To Neonates?

David A. Osborn, MBBS, MMed (Clin Epi), FRACP, PhD

Clinical Associate Professor
Neonatologist
RPA Newborn Care
Royal Prince Alfred Hospital
Camperdown, Australia
What Evidence Supports Dietary Interventions to Prevent Infant Food Hypersensitivity and Allergy?

Luis Ostrosky-Zeichner, MD, FACP
Associate Professor
The University of Texas Health Science Center at Houston
Houston, Texas
Neonatal Fungal Infections

Gary D. Overturf, MD
Professor of Pediatrics and Pathology
University of New Mexico – School of Medicine
Albuquerque, New Mexico
Effects of Chemoprophylaxis for Neonatal Group B Streptococcal Infections on the Incidence of Gram-negative Infections and Antibiotic Resistance in Neonatal Pathogens

Matthew A. Saxonhouse, MD
Assistant Professor
Division of Neonatology
Department of Pediatrics
University of Florida College of Medicine
Gainesville, Florida
Current Issues in the Pathogenesis, Diagnosis, and Treatment of Neonatal Thrombocytopenia

Charles R. Sims, MD
Fellow
Division of Infectious Diseases
The University of Texas Health Science Center at Houston
Laboratory of Mycology Research
Houston, Texas
Neonatal Fungal Infections

John Sinn, MBBS (Syd), DCH, Dip Paed, MMed (Clin Epi), FRACP
Senior Lecturer
University of Sydney
Senior Staff Neonatologist
Royal North Shore Hospital
St. Leonards, Australia
What Evidence Supports Dietary Interventions to Prevent Infant Food Hypersensitivity and Allergy?

Martha C. Sola-Visner, MD
Associate Professor of Pediatrics
Drexel University College of Medicine
Philadelphia, Pennsylvania
Current Issues in the Pathogenesis, Diagnosis, and Treatment of Neonatal Thrombocytopenia

Anne M. Stevens, MD, PhD

Assistant Professor
Pediatric Rheumatology
Department of Pediatrics
University of Washington
Attending Physician
Children's Hospital and Regional Medical Center
Seattle, Washington
> *Maternally Mediated Neonatal Autoimmunity*

Philip Toltzis, MD

Division of Pharmacology and Critical Care
Rainbow Babies and Children's Hospital
Associate Professor
Case Western Reserve University School of Medicine
Cleveland, Ohio
> *Control of Antibiotic-Resistant Bacteria in the Neonatal Intensive Care Unit*

Fabienne Willems, PhD

Senior Scientist,
Institute for Medical Immunology
Charleroi-Gosselies, Belgium
> *Toll-like Receptor Responses in Neonatal Dendritic Cells*

Mervin C. Yoder, MD

Richard and Pauline Klinger Professor of Pediatrics
Professor of Biochemistry and Molecular Biology and
Professor of Cellular and Integrative Physiology
Indiana University School of Medicine
Herman B Wells Center for Pediatric Research
Attending Physician
James Whitcomb Riley Hospital for Children
Indianapolis, Indiana
> *Stem Cell Facts for the Neonatologist*

Series Foreword

Learn from yesterday, live for today, hope for tomorrow. The important thing is not to stop questioning.
ALBERT EINSTEIN

The art and science of asking questions is the source of all knowledge.
THOMAS BERGER

In the mid 1960s W.B. Saunders began publishing a series of books focused on the care of newborn infants. The series was entitled *Major Problems in Clinical Pediatrics*. The original series (1964–1979) consisted of ten titles dealing with problems of the newborn infant (*The Lung and its Disorders in the Newborn Infant* edited by Mary Ellen Avery, *Disorders of Carbohydrate Metabolism in Infancy* edited by Marvin Cornblath and Robert Schwartz, *Hematologic Problems in the Newborn* edited by Frank A. Oski and J. Lawrence Naiman, *The Neonate with Congenital Heart Disease* edited by Richard D. Rowe and Ali Mehrizi, *Recognizable Patterns of Human Malformation* edited by David W. Smith, *Neonatal Dermatology* edited by Lawrence M. Solomon and Nancy B. Esterly, *Amino Acid Metabolism and its Disorders* edited by Charles L. Scriver and Leon E. Rosenberg, *The High Risk Infant* edited by Lula O Lubchenco, *Gastrointestinal Problems in the Infant* edited by Joyce Gryboski and *Viral Diseases of the Fetus and Newborn* edited by James B Hanshaw and John A. Dudgeon). Dr. Alexander J. Schaffer was asked to be the consulting editor for the entire series. Dr. Schaffer coined the term "neonatology" and edited the first clinical textbook of neonatology entitled *Diseases of the Newborn*. For those of us training in the 1970s, this series and Dr. Schaffer's textbook of neonatology provided exciting, up-to-date information that attracted many of us into the subspecialty. Dr. Schaffer's role as "consulting editor" allowed him to select leading scientists and practitioners to serve as editors for each individual volume. As the "consulting editor" for *Neonatology Questions and Controversies*, I had the challenge of identifying the topics and editors for each volume in this series. The six volumes encompass the major issues encountered in the neonatal intensive care unit (newborn lung, fluid and electrolytes, neonatal cardiology and hemodynamics, hematology, immunology and infectious disease, gastroenterology and neurology). The editors for each volume were challenged to combine discussions of fetal and neonatal physiology with disease pathophysiology and selected controversial topics in clinical care. It is my hope that this series (like *Major Problems in Clinical Pediatrics*) will excite a new generation of trainees to question existing dogma (from my own generation) and seek new information through scientific investigation. I wish to congratulate and thank each of the volume editors (Drs. Bancalari, Oh, Guignard, Baumgart, Kleinman, Seri, Ohls, Yoder, Neu and Perlman) for their extraordinary effort and finished products. I also wish to acknowledge Judy Fletcher at Elsevier who conceived the idea for the series and who has been my "editor and friend" throughout my academic career.

Richard A. Polin, MD

Preface

Modern advances in the care of the high-risk pregnancy and the prematurely born neonate have led to steadily advancing improvement in the growth and long-term development of these infants. One of the major lingering areas of morbidity and mortality that continues to plague the preterm, and in particular the extremely low birthweight neonate, is acute infectious diseases. Over the past century, numerous strides have been made to attempt to prevent or aggressively treat infants at risk for sepsis including, advances in the discovery and use of a variety of parenteral antibiotics, safe and nutritious formulas, fresh or banked breast milk, recognition of the importance of hand washing, improvements in the design and use of equipment in the newborn intensive care unit, and rigorous protocols to identify and treat laboring mothers with high risk factors for delivering an infant that is infected. Despite these advances, many significant impediments remain that keep us from eradicating infections in the most vulnerable neonatal populations.

In this volume of the series *Neonatology Questions and Controversies*, we have attempted to update physicians, nurse practitioners, nurses, residents, and students in three ways: (1) provide overviews of the developmental physiology of some selected aspects of the immune response in the human fetus and neonate that are not typically highlighted, (2) discuss several areas of controversy with respect to cellular or cytokine replacement therapies to treat human neonates suffering from either hematologic or infectious maladies, and (3) discuss some controversies in immune modulation that may play a role in preventing allergic disorders in the developing infant. All of the chapters contribute to provide a glimpse of how the neonate must utilize cells of the hematologic and immune systems to thwart the onslaught of microbial challenges, how the caretaker of the neonate can quickly diagnose and intervene to augment neonatal hematologic or immunologic defenses, and how the caretaker can prospectively utilize nutritional and in some cases immunologic strategies to better equip the infant to be more prepared for further infectious challenges as the infant grows and develops. We further provide information as to how the immune system may go awry and result in the development of allergic disorders.

We wish to thank Judith Fletcher, Publishing Director at Elsevier and Dr. Richard Polin, Chairman of the Department of Pediatrics at the Morgan Stanley Children's Hospital of New York-Presbyterian, for their encouragement to write this volume. We of course are indebted and grateful to the authors of each chapter whose contributions from around the world will be fully appreciated by the readers.

Robin K. Ohls, MD
Mervin C. Yoder, MD

Chapter 1

Stem Cell Facts for the Neonatologist

Mervin C. Yoder, MD

Isolation of Embryonic Stem Cells

Isolation of Human Embryonic Stem Cells

Cloning via Nuclear Transfer in Domestic and Laboratory Animals

Therapeutic Cloning

Stem Cell Plasticity

Somatic Stem Cells

Pancreatic β-islet Cell Replacement Therapy

Cardiomyocyte Replacement Therapy

Umbilical Cord Hematopoietic Stem Cell Replacement Therapy

Summary

As a normal process of human growth and development, many organs and tissues display a need for continued replacement of the mature cells that are lost with aging or injury. For example, billions of red blood cells, white blood cells, and platelets are produced per kilogram of body weight daily. The principal site of blood cell production, the bone marrow, harbors the critically important stem cells that serve as the regenerating source for all the blood cells manufactured. These hematopoietic stem cells share several common features with all other kinds of stem cells. Stem cells display the ability to self-renew (to divide and give rise to other stem cells) and to produce offspring that mature along distinct differentiation pathways to form cells with specialized functions. Stem cells have classically been divided into two groups: embryonic stem cells (ESC) and non-embryonic stem cells, also called somatic or adult stem cells. The purpose of this review is to introduce several important stem cell facts that should be familiar to all clinicians and to update the reader on selected aspects of ESC and adult stem cell research.

The fertilized oocyte (zygote) is the 'mother' of all stem cells. All the potential for forming all the cells and tissues of the body including the placenta and extra-embryonic membranes is derived from this cell (reviewed in ref. 1). Furthermore, the zygote possesses the unique information leading to the establishment of the overall body plan and organogenesis. Thus, the zygote is a totipotent cell. The first few cleavage-stage divisions also produce blastomere cells retaining totipotent potential. However, by the blastocyst stage, many of the cells have adopted specific developmental pathways. One portion of the blastocyst is called the epiblast and this region contains cells (inner cell mass cells) that will go on to form the embryo proper. Trophectoderm cells comprise the cells at the opposite pole of the blastocyst and these cells will differentiate to form the placenta. Cells within in the inner cell mass of the blastocyst are pluripotent; that is, each cell possesses the potential to give rise to types of cells that develop from the three embryonic germ layers (mesoderm, endoderm, and ectoderm). ESC do not technically exist in the developing blastocyst, but are derived upon ex vivo culture of the inner cell mass cells from the epiblast using specific methods and reagents discussed below.

ISOLATION OF EMBRYONIC STEM CELLS

Mouse ESC were isolated more than 20 years ago in an extension of basic studies that had been conducted on how embryonic teratocarcinoma cells could be maintained in tissue culture (2, 3). Inner cell mass cells were recovered from murine blastocysts and plated over an adherent layer of mouse embryonic fibroblasts in the presence of culture medium containing fetal calf serum and in some instances conditioned medium from murine teratocarcinoma cells. Over a period of several weeks, colonies of rapidly growing cells emerged. These colonies of tightly adherent but proliferating cells could be recovered from the culture dishes, disaggregated with enzymes to form a single-cell suspension, and the cells replated on fresh embryonic fibroblasts. Within days, the individually plated cells had formed new colonies that could in like manner be isolated and recultured with no apparent restriction on proliferative potential. The cells comprising the colonies were eventually defined as ESC.

Murine (m) ESC display several unique properties. The cells are small, with a high nuclear to cytoplasmic ratio and prominent nucleoli. When plated in the presence of murine embryonic fibroblasts, with great care taken to keep the cells from clumping at each passage (the clumps can result in some of the mESC differentiating), mESC proliferate indefinitely as pluripotent cells (4). In fact, one can manipulate the genome of the mESC using homologous recombination to insert or remove specific genetic sequences and maintain mESC pluripotency (5). Injection of normal mESC into recipient murine blastocysts permits ESC-derived contribution to essentially all tissues of the embryo including germ cells. By injecting mutant mESC into donor blastocysts, one is able to generate genetically altered strains of mice (commonly referred to as knockout mice) (6).

While the molecular regulation of mESC self-renewal divisions remains unclear, the growth factor leukemia inhibitory factor (LIF) has been determined to be sufficient to maintain mESC in a self-renewing state in vitro, even in the absence of the mouse fibroblast feeder cells. More recently, addition of the growth factor bone morphogenetic protein-4 (BMP-4) to mESC cultures (with LIF) permits maintenance of the pluripotent state in serum-free conditions (7, 8). Several transcription factors including Oct-4 and nanog are required to maintain mESC self-renewal divisions (9, 10). Increasing MAP kinase activity and decreasing STAT2 activity results in loss of mESC self-renewal divisions and differentiation of the mESC into multiple cell lineages (7). Whether this pattern of molecular regulation will also dictate the fate of human ESC remains to be determined.

The strict culture conditions that are required to result in the in vitro differentiation of mESC into a wide variety of specific somatic cell types, such as neurons, hematopoietic cells, pancreatic cells, hepatocytes, muscle cells, cardiomyocytes, and endothelial cells, are now well described (11–14). In most differentiation protocols, mESC are first deprived of LIF, followed by addition of other growth factors, vitamins, morphogens, extracellular matrix molecules, or drugs to stimulate the ESC to differentiate along specific pathways. It is also usual for the ESC differentiation protocol to give rise to a predominant but not a pure population of differentiated cells. Obtaining highly purified differentiated cell populations generally requires some form of cell selection to either enhance the survival of a selected population or to preferentially eliminate a non-desired population (15). The ability to isolate enriched populations of differentiated cells has encouraged many investigators to postulate that ESC may be a desirable source of cells for replacement of aged, injured, or diseased tissues in human subjects if pluripotent human (h) ESC were readily available (16, 17).

ISOLATION OF HUMAN EMBRYONIC STEM CELLS

The growth conditions that have permitted isolation and characterization of hESC have only become available in the last decade (18). Left-over cleavage-stage human embryos originally produced by in vitro fertilization for clinical purposes are one prominent source for hESC derivation. Embryos are grown to the blastocyst stage, the inner cell mass cells isolated, and the isolated cells plated on irradiated mouse embryonic fibroblast feeder layers in vitro. After growing in culture for several cell divisions, colonies of hESC emerge, similar to mESC. These hESC are very small cells with minimal cytoplasm and prominent nucleoli and, like the mouse cells, grow very rapidly without evidence of developing senescence and possess high telomerase activity. Unlike mESC, LIF is not sufficient to maintain hESC in a self-renewing state in the absence of the mouse fibroblast feeder cells. However, hESC can be grown on extracellular matrix coated plates in the presence of murine embryonic fibroblast conditioned medium without the presence of the mouse feeder cells. Relatively high doses of fibroblast growth factor-2 (FGF-2) also serve to help maintain hESC in an undifferentiated state even in the absence of feeder cells (19, 20).

The pluripotent nature of hESC has been demonstrated by injecting the cells into the hind leg musculature of an immunodeficient mouse (18). A tumor emerges from the site of the injected cells (specifically called a teratoma) and histologically contains numerous cell types, including gastric and intestinal epithelium, renal tubular cells, and neurons; descendants of the endoderm, mesoderm, and ectoderm germ cell layers, respectively. At present, teratoma formation in immunodeficient mice continues to serve as the only method to document hESC pluripotency. Oct-4 and alkaline phosphatase expression, as biomarkers of ESC pluripotency, help to support but are inadequate alone as evidence of hESC pluripotency (20).

CLONING VIA NUCLEAR TRANSFER IN DOMESTIC AND LABORATORY ANIMALS

The successful cloning of a variety of domestic animals and laboratory rodents has also been widely reported (21). This technology is largely based on nuclear transfer techniques, where the nucleus is removed from an oocyte, and a donor somatic cell nucleus is electrically fused with the enucleated oocyte. The created zygote is grown to the blastocyst stage, where the embryo is disaggregated and cells from the inner cell mass are harvested for creation of ES cells in vitro or the blastocyst is implanted into a recipient female. Such a procedure is technically challenging but possible and multiple cloned examples of several species have been reported.

Some of the challenges to overcome when using nuclear transfer technology to create viable cloned animals include the great inefficiency of the process (hundreds to thousands of oocytes are often injected with only a few viable animals surviving beyond birth as an outcome). Much of this inefficiency may be a result of poor epigenetic reprogramming of the donor somatic nucleus in the oocyte (22). In adult somatic tissues, epigenetic modifications of DNA and chromatin are stably maintained and characteristic of each specialized tissue or organ. During nuclear transfer, epigenetic reprogramming of the somatic nucleus must occur similar to the epigenetic reprogramming that normally occurs during oocyte activation following fertilization (23). Epigenetic reprogramming deficiencies during animal cloning may lead to a host of problems, including epigenetic mutations and altered epigenetic inheritance patterns causing altered gene expression and resulting in embryonic lethality or maldeveloped fetuses with poor postnatal survival. While great strides in identifying the molecules involved in chromatin remodeling and epigenetic programming have been made, considerable work remains to identify strategies to facilitate this process during nuclear transfer for animal cloning. It is interesting that hESC have recently been used to reprogram human somatic cells and may serve as an alternative to the use of oocytes (24).

THERAPEUTIC CLONING

Combining the techniques of nuclear transfer and ESC generation could be applied to human therapeutic organ or tissue repair. In this strategy, a donor oocyte is enucleated and the nucleus of a somatic cell from the patient is isolated and transferred into the oocyte. A blastocyst is created, disaggregated, and hESC isolated. These ESC cells would be immunologically nearly identical to the donor with the exception of antigens expressed by mitochondria originally derived from the donor oocyte. Once cloned hESC have been generated, then use of specific differentiation protocols designed to derive the specific cells for creation of a replacement organ or tissue could be employed. Since the differentiated cells generated from the ESC would be formed as a monolayer of cells, and most tissues and organs for replacement purposes may need to be synthesized in three dimensions with an accessible vascular supply, a composite synthetic matrix with suspended differentiated cells may need to be engineered in vitro. While this hypothetical scheme may appear too complicated for any practical near-term application, a recent proof-of-principle experiment has demonstrated that an engineered tissue with functioning nephrons can be produced from domestic cattle (25).

Great excitement followed the announcement by Hwang and colleagues that an hESC line had been generated via somatic cell nuclear transfer in 2004 (26). Even greater excitement ensued a year later with a subsequent publication from the same group, reporting that 11 hESC lines had been generated by nuclear transfer technology from patients with several common clinical disorders (27). However, this enthusiasm rapidly changed to great disappointment and alarm when it was learned that these studies had been fabricated and there was no evidence to support these claims. Several important lessons were learned from that scientific debacle, including support for a strong educational program for all student scientists in the responsible conduct of research, improvements in the peer-review of articles for journal publication, and new dialog on how the raw scientific data supporting research publications may one day be required for a detailed review of support for the submitted manuscript. Other investigators continue to attempt to derive hESC lines from patients with specific clinical disorders both in the United States and abroad (28, 29).

Transfer of human nuclei into donor oocytes presents many ethical and practical challenges. Where will the donor oocytes come from? In fact, the concern about coerced oocyte donation by some of the scientists participating in the work of Hwang and colleagues was one of the early concerns that led to the uncovering of the fabricated work reported by that group (30). How much money should donors be paid for their oocyte donation? Over-compensation could serve to coerce some donors to participate. Such issues have been discussed in some detail elsewhere (31–33).

Technically, while hESC can be created, no protocols for differentiation of specific lineages of cells with documented therapeutic benefit to human subjects have been reported. Several excellent research protocols for differentiation of hESC into human blood cells, neurons, chondrocytes, and endothelial cells have been reported (34–38). Furthermore, while use of artificial matrices as scaffolds for transplantable cells is currently feasible (engineered blood vessels, bladder, skin, and cartilage), there have been no reports of using undifferentiated hESC to repopulate artificial matrices.

STEM CELL PLASTICITY

A number of studies have reported that adult stem cells isolated from one organ possess the ability to differentiate into cells normally found in completely different organs following transplantation. For example, bone marrow cells have been demonstrated to contribute to muscle, lung, gastric, intestinal, lung, and liver cells following adoptive transfer, while neuronal stem cells can contribute to blood, muscle, and neuronal tissues. More recent studies suggest that stem cell plasticity is an extremely rare event and that, in most study subjects, the apparent donor stem cell differentiation event was in fact a monocyte-macrophage fusion event with epithelial cells of the recipient tissues (39–41). At present, enthusiasm for therapeutic multi-tissue repair in ill patients from infusion of a single population of multipotent stem cells has waned considerably (42).

SOMATIC STEM CELLS

Adult (also called somatic, postnatal, or non-embryonic) stem cells are multipotent cells that reside in specialized tissues and organs and retain the ability to self-renew and to develop into progeny that yield all the differentiated cells that comprise the tissue or organ of residence. For example, intestinal stem cells replenish the intestinal villus epithelium several times a week and skin stem cells give rise to cells that replace the epidermis in 3-week cycles. Other sources of self-renewing adult stem cells include the cornea, bone marrow, retina, brain, skeletal muscle, dental pulp, pancreas, and liver (reviewed in ref. 1). Though numerous examples of adult stem cell replacement strategies may be discussed, this review will highlight three areas of current interest in which some pre-clinical or clinical data have been acquired. In each area, both animal and human studies will be reviewed. Consensus approaches will be discussed where identified.

PANCREATIC β-ISLET CELL REPLACEMENT THERAPY

Diabetes mellitus is a chronic debilitating disease in which elevated blood glucose concentrations and deficient insulin production or intracellular responses to insulin lead to an increased risk of affected patients developing hypertension, vascular disease, stroke, and kidney failure. Oral hypoglycemic medications in some patients and insulin injections for most severely affected patients can be effective in lowering blood glucose concentrations. However, no permanent cure for insulin-dependent diabetes is currently available.

Some success has recently been reported in the transplantation of donor pancreatic islets into diabetic recipients; however, these patients require lifelong immunosuppressive medications to suppress tissue rejection, and the lack of available donor material will undoubtedly limit this treatment strategy (43, 44). Development of methods to expand differentiated donor β-islets are being sought but this approach is not currently effective in improving the number of islets for transplantation. Alternative approaches include finding stem cell sources that could be used to generate β-islet cells in vitro in sufficient quantities for transplantation.

Insulin-producing cells have been generated from both murine and human ESC in vitro (45–47). Implantation of mESC-derived insulin-producing cells into the spleen of recipient mice rendered hyperglycemic via streptozotocin (STZ) injection led to euglycemia in nearly all of the transplanted but none of the sham-operated animals. Some of the treated animals remained euglycemic for months after the transplant, while hyperglycemia returned in other transplant recipients; no mechanisms have yet been determined to explain the persistent beneficial effect in only a subpopulation of the diabetic recipient mice. Nevertheless, the in vivo regulation of blood glucose concentrations by the implanted ESC-derived cells was an encouraging outcome (45).

Insulin-producing cells have also been generated from pancreatic ductal tissue, liver stem cells (oval cells), and liver cells transduced with an adenoviral vector expressing a transcription factor known to be necessary for pancreatic formation (reviewed in (48)). In some cases, not only did the cells secrete insulin in vitro, but the cells responded with accelerated differentiation when exposed to molecules known to stimulate β-islet cell growth and differentiation in vivo. Implantation of the insulin-producing cells also ameliorated the hyperglycemia in STZ-treated recipient mice in some instances.

These data suggest that cells synthesizing and releasing insulin may be derived from either ESC or adult stem cell populations. It remains unclear whether there is de novo β-islet cell production from a stem cell population in vivo or if the limited replicative potential of β-islet cells observed in situ is derived from the endogenous β-islet pool of cells directly. Whether implanting β-islet cells produced from stem cells ex vivo will function as well as donor pancreatic β-islet transplantation (which may contain other pancreatic cell types) and whether immunosuppressive regimens will be necessary to accept and maintain the implanted cells remains unknown. Further work will also be required to determine whether either ESC or adult stem cells can be produced in mass to accommodate the number of β-islet cells required for clinically relevant protocols and whether stem-cell-generated pancreatic cells will be effective in establishing euglycemic outcomes in large animal models of diabetes mellitus (48).

CARDIOMYOCYTE REPLACEMENT THERAPY

Chronic heart failure is another disease entity affecting a large population worldwide. Nearly 5 million patients in the United States alone suffer from persistent and worsening heart failure. Mortality is high (up to 40%) and there is morbidity to society greater than the $40 billion attributed annually to patient hospitalization, medication, and medical follow-up costs. Of greater concern is the knowledge that these costs will increase considerably with the advancing age of the United States population.

Unlike many organs of the body that can replace aged or injured cells, cardiomyocyte loss in the adult heart is thought to be irreversible (49). Some controversial recent data suggest that the heart may contain a population of cells that can proliferate and replace injured or aged cardiomyocytes (50). However, most strategies to repair injured cardiac tissue are focused on methods to recruit stem cells to the site of injury or to inject stem cells into the injured areas (49).

Numerous laboratories have attempted some form of cell-based therapy for cardiac repair. A variety of cell sources and different types of myocytes have been demonstrated to engraft in infarcted hearts; however, little evidence of these cells vigorously interacting with the host cardiomyocytes to establish functional electophysiological interactions has been demonstrated (51). Fetal cardiomyocytes have been demonstrated to functionally connect with injured adult cardiomyocytes and improve heart function; however, fetal cardiomyocytes are limited in number and difficult to isolate and transplant with high efficiency. Some recent data suggest that bone marrow-derived cells, including mesenchymal stem cells, may possess the potential to improve the outcome of patients with myocardial injury (52–54). Some evidence has been presented that non-cardiac-derived cardiomyocytes have been detected in sex-mismatched transplanted human hearts. However, the majority of evidence to date suggests that any improvements in cardiac function following cellular adoptive transfer strategies may occur via paracrine secretion of unknown molecules, with little or no evidence of donor cell engraftment and long-term replacement of cardiomyocytes (49, 51).

Cardiomyocytes have also been produced in vitro from murine and human ESCs (55, 56). Specific culture conditions, including transfection of cells with genes to confer a selective survival advantage, have been used to generate nearly pure populations of cardiomyocytes (49). These cells spontaneously beat in culture and respond in appropriate fashion to pharmacologic agents that normally increase or decrease cardiomyocyte beating in vivo. ESC-derived cardiomyocytes express proteins known to be restricted to cardiomyocytes in vivo, display normal sacromeric structures, and can engraft into injured murine hearts in vivo (57–59).

In summary, the in vitro differentiation of cardiomyocytes from murine ESCs has been accomplished. Results to date suggest that the cells display morphological, electrophysiological, and molecular expression patterns similar to cardiomyocytes developing during embryogenesis. Human ESC-derived cardiomyocytes have also been isolated and characterized. It is not yet known whether these cells will engraft and facilitate recovery of damaged human heart tissue. In contrast, the current experimental approach of transplanting marrow-derived cells may provide some short-term paracrine support leading to improved recovery for some patients. These clinical studies have moved into the realm of experimental therapy more quickly than the basic scientific understanding of which stem cell population or combination of populations may be best.

UMBILICAL CORD HEMATOPOIETIC STEM CELL REPLACEMENT THERAPY

Transplantation of bone marrow cells to alleviate marrow failure in human subjects has been practiced since 1959 and patient outcomes have improved greatly over the past decade (60). One very interesting and exciting area of research has been the use of umbilical cord blood as an alternative source of hematopoietic stem cells for transplantation (61, 62). Cord blood is an essentially renewable resource of available stem cells. Several large clinical studies have documented the efficacy of using these cells to engraft not only pediatric but adult subjects as well (61). One remarkable outcome of these studies was the recognition that the graft-versus-host disease is ameliorated when using donor allogeneic (non-self) cord blood cells compared to adult marrow or mobilized peripheral blood stem cells.

One limitation of the use of cord blood stem cells for transplantation into adult subjects is the limitation in the quantity of stem cells present in some cord blood aliquots. Current estimates suggest that at least 3×10^5 CD34+ cells/kg are required for effective engraftment of donor cord blood cells in a recipient patient. Attempts to increase the number of cord blood CD34+ cells by expanding the cells in vitro with recombinant growth factor stimulation have been largely unsuccessful (63). It is apparent that the total number of hematopoietic progenitor cells is increased under these expansion conditions but at the expense of the number of stem cells in the starting population (63). Recent experiments in mice to expand the number of engrafting and repopulating stem cells via overexpression of certain transcription and survival factors, growth factors, and via interaction with certain non-hematopoietic cells have been encouraging, including some studies in non-human primates (64–67).

One immediate approach that appears to be clinically efficacious is to transplant cord blood cells from more than one donor aliquot into a single recipient. Increasing the number of donor cells leads to a more rapid recovery of donor-derived granulocytes and platelets in the recipient patients (68). One fascinating realization is that, over time, the donor repopulating cells from only one of the multiple donor units appear to predominate. Further studies will be required to understand the cellular mechanisms of donor stem cell competitive expansion in vivo to permit the induction of a more strategic advantage of the donor cord blood unit with the least predilection to the development of graft-versus-host disease in the recipient (69).

Private cord blood banking is feasible and actively practiced worldwide. A strategy to form a national program of public cord blood banking has been developed in the USA and the Department of Health and Human Services has recently announced a competitive program for the formation of the organizing center for such a program. It is anticipated that such a program will provide education to increase cord blood donation from underrepresented minority populations, thereby permitting acquisition of a larger pool of tissue-matched stem cells for patients in need of transplantation, and enlarge the stored inventory and enhance management of the stored units to facilitate physician discovery of the most suitable donor cord blood stem cell unit for their patient.

SUMMARY

Stem cells may be derived in vitro from preimplantation mammalian blastocysts (ESC) or from somatic tissues and organs (adult stem cells). ESCs display certain unique properties that generate enthusiasm for these cells as a source of differentiated cells for future applications of cell-based therapies for human disease. Adult stem cell populations are also being investigated as potential sources for clinical cell-based therapies. While ESC approaches may offer many theoretical advantages over current adult stem cell approaches, the use of adult stem cells to treat patients with certain ailments is the current treatment of choice. Investigators will continue to focus on improvements in cell isolation, in vitro stem cell expansion, regulating stem cell commitment to specific cell lineages, facilitating in vitro cellular differentiation, tissue engineering using synthetic matrices and stem cell progeny, optimizing transplantation protocols, and in vivo stem cell or stem-cell-derived tissue testing for safety and efficacy in appropriate animal models of human disease. Many challenges lie ahead but successful outcomes of this work may lead to new patient treatment paradigms.

REFERENCES

1. National Institutes of Health, Stem Cells: Scientific Progress and Future Research Directions. 2001, www.nih.gov.news/stemcell.scireport.htm.
2. Evans M, Kaufman M. Establishment in culture of pluripotential cells from mouse embryos. Nature 292:145–147, 1981.
3. Martin G. Isolation of a pluripotent cell line from early mouse embryos cultured in medium conditioned by teratocarcinoma stem cells. Proc Natl Acad Sci USA 78:7634–7638, 1981.
4. Roach ML, McNeish JD. Methods for the isolation and maintenance of murine embryonic stem cells. Methods Mol Biol 185:1–16, 2002.
5. Capecchi M. The new mouse genetics: altering the genome by gene targeting. Trends in Genetics 5:70–76, 1989.
6. Robertson E. Using embryonic stem cells to introduce mutations into the mouse germ line. Biol Reprod 44:238–245, 1991.
7. Keller G. Embryonic stem cell differentiation: emergence of a new era in biology and medicine. Genes Dev 19(10):1129–1155, 2005.
8. Bouhon IA, et al. Neural differentiation of mouse embryonic stem cells in chemically defined medium. Brain Res Bull 68(1–2):62–75, 2005.
9. Buehr M, et al. Rapid loss of Oct-4 and pluripotency in cultured rodent blastocysts and derivative cell lines. Biol Reprod 68(1):222–229, 2003.
10. Mitsui K, et al. The homeoprotein Nanog is required for maintenance of pluripotency in mouse epiblast and ES cells. Cell 113(5):631–642, 2003.
11. Fraser S, et al. Embryonic Stem Call Differentiation as a model to study hematopoietic and endothelial cell development. Methods Mol Biol 185:71–81, 2002.
12. Li M. Lineage selection for generation and amplification of neural precursor cells. Methods Mol Biol 185:205–215, 2002.
13. Wobus AM, et al. Embryonic stem cells as a model to study cardiac, skeletal muscle, and vascular smooth muscle cell differentiation. Methods Mol Biol 185:127–156, 2002.
14. Bautch VL. Embryonic stem cell differentiation and the vascular lineage. Methods Mol Biol 185:117–125, 2002.
15. Pasumarthi KB, Field LJ. Cardiomyocyte enrichment in differentiating ES cell cultures: strategies and applications. Methods Mol Biol 185:157–168, 2002.
16. Srivastava D, Ivey KN. Potential of stem-cell-based therapies for heart disease. Nature 441(7097):1097–1099, 2006.
17. Kassem M. Stem cells: potential therapy for age-related diseases. Ann NY Acad Sci 1067:436–442, 2006.
18. Thomson JA, et al. Embryonic stem cell lines derived from human blastocysts. Science 282:1145–1147, 1998.
19. Levenstein ME, et al. Basic fibroblast growth factor support of human embryonic stem cell self-renewal. Stem Cells 24(3):568–574, 2006.
20. Ludwig TE, et al. Feeder-independent culture of human embryonic stem cells. Nat Methods 3(8):637–646, 2006.
21. Hochedlinger K, Jaenisch R. Nuclear reprogramming and pluripotency. Nature 441(7097):1061–1067, 2006.
22. Jouneau A, Renard JP. Reprogramming in nuclear transfer. Curr Opin Genet Dev 13(5):486–491, 2003.
23. Armstrong L, et al. Epigenetic modification is central to genome reprogramming in somatic cell nuclear transfer. Stem Cells 24(4):805–814, 2006.
24. Cowan CA, et al. Nuclear reprogramming of somatic cells after fusion with human embryonic stem cells. Science 309(5739):1369–1373, 2005.
25. Lanza R, et al. Generation of histocompatible tissues using nuclear transplantation. Nat Biotechnol 20:689–696, 2002.
26. Hwang WS, et al. Evidence of a pluripotent human embryonic stem cell line derived from a cloned blastocyst. Science 303(5664):1669–1674, 2004.
27. Hwang WS, et al. Patient-specific embryonic stem cells derived from human SCNT blastocysts. Science 308(5729):1777–1783, 2005.
28. Wilmut I. Recent stem cell research poses several challenges. Cloning Stem Cells 8(2):67–8, 2006.
29. Holden C. Stem cell research. Harvard cloners Get OK to proceed with caution. Science 312(5780):1584, 2006.
30. Aldhous P. Hwang's forgotten crime: the exploitation of women is a far worse offence than data fabrication. New Sci 189(2437):22, 2006.
31. Kamm FM. Moral status and personal identity: clones, embryos, and future generations. Soc Philos Policy 22(2):283–307, 2005.
32. Cameron NM. Pandora's progeny: ethical issues in assisted human reproduction. Fam Law Q 39(3):745–779, 2005.
33. Hall VJ, Stojkovic P, Stojkovic M. Using therapeutic cloning to fight human disease: a conundrum or reality? Stem Cells 24(7):1628–1637, 2006.
34. Olsen AL, Stachura DL, Weiss MJ. Designer blood: creating hematopoietic lineages from embryonic stem cells. Blood 107(4):1265–1275, 2006.

35. Tian X, Kaufman DS. Hematopoietic development of human embryonic stem cells in culture. Methods Mol Med 105:425–436, 2005.
36. Lowell S, et al. Notch promotes neural lineage entry by pluripotent embryonic stem cells. PLoS Biol 4(5):e121, 2006.
37. Khillan JS. Generation of chondrocytes from embryonic stem cells. Methods Mol Biol 330:161–170, 2006.
38. Wiese C, et al. Pluripotency: capacity for in vitro differentiation of undifferentiated embryonic stem cells. Methods Mol Biol 325:181–205, 2006.
39. Vassilopoulos G, Wang P, Russel D. Transplanted bone marrow regenerates liver by cell fusion. Nature 422:901–904, 2003.
40. Rizvi AZ, et al. Bone marrow-derived cells fuse with normal and transformed intestinal stem cells. Proc Natl Acad Sci USA 103(16):6321–6325, 2006.
41. Willenbring H, et al. Myelomonocytic cells are sufficient for therapeutic cell fusion in liver. Nat Med 10(7):744–748, 2004.
42. Anderson D, Gage F, Weissman I. Can stem cells cross lineage boundaries? Nat Med 7(4):393–395, 2001.
43. Rother KI, Harlan DM. Challenges facing islet transplantation for the treatment of type 1 diabetes mellitus. J Clin Invest 114(7):877–883, 2004.
44. Robertson RP, et al. Pancreas and islet transplantation in type 1 diabetes. Diabetes Care 29(4):935, 2006.
45. Soria B, et al. Insulin-secreting cells derived from embryonic stem cells normalize glycemia in streptozotocin-induced diabetic mice. Diabetes 49:1–6, 2000.
46. Brolen GK, et al. Signals from the embryonic mouse pancreas induce differentiation of human embryonic stem cells into insulin-producing beta-cell-like cells. Diabetes 54(10):2867–2874, 2005.
47. Segev H, et al. Differentiation of human embryonic stem cells into insulin-producing clusters. Stem Cells 22(3):265–274, 2004.
48. Meier JJ, Bhushan A, Butler PC. The potential for stem cell therapy in diabetes. Pediatr Res 59(4 Pt 2):65R–73R, 2006.
49. Rubart M, Field LJ. Cardiac regeneration: repopulating the heart. Annu Rev Physiol 68:29–49, 2006.
50. Linke A, et al. Stem cells in the dog heart are self-renewing, clonogenic, and multipotent and regenerate infarcted myocardium, improving cardiac function. Proc Natl Acad Sci USA 102(25):8966–8971, 2005.
51. Stamm C, et al. Stem cell therapy for ischemic heart disease: beginning or end of the road? Cell Transplant 15(Suppl 1):S47–56, 2006.
52. Chien K. Making a play at regrowing hearts. Scientist 35–39, 2006.
53. Yang ZJ, et al. Experimental study of bone marrow-derived mesenchymal stem cells combined with hepatocyte growth factor transplantation via noninfarct-relative artery in acute myocardial infarction. Gene Ther 13:1564–1568, 2006.
54. van Veen TA, de Bakker JM, van der Heyden MA. Mesenchymal stem cells repair conduction block. J Am Coll Cardiol 48(1):219–220, 2006; author reply 220.
55. Boheler K, et al. Differentiation of pluripotent embryonic stem cells into cardiomyocytes. Circ Res 91(3):189–201, 2002.
56. Xu C, et al. Characterization and enrichment of cardiomyocytes derived from human embryonic stem cells. Circ Res 91(6):501–508, 2002.
57. Rubart M, Field LJ. Cardiac repair by embryonic stem-derived cells. Handb Exp Pharmacol 174:73–100, 2006.
58. Fukuda K, Yuasa S. Stem cells as a source of regenerative cardiomyocytes. Circ Res 98(8):1002–1013, 2006.
59. Wei H, et al. Embryonic stem cells and cardiomyocyte differentiation: phenotypic and molecular analyses. J Cell Mol Med 9(4):804–817, 2005.
60. Clift RA, Thomas ED. Follow-up 26 years after treatment for acute myelogenous leukemia. N Engl J Med 351(23):2456–2457, 2004.
61. Rocha V, Gluckman E. Clinical use of umbilical cord blood hematopoietic stem cells. Biol Blood Marrow Transplant 12(1 Suppl 1):34–41, 2006.
62. Goldstein G, Toren A, Nagler A. Human umbilical cord blood biology, transplantation and plasticity. Curr Med Chem 13(11):1249–1259, 2006.
63. Wagner JE, Verfaillie CM. Ex vivo expansion of umbilical cord blood hemopoietic stem and progenitor cells. Exp Hematol 32(5):412–413, 2004.
64. Mohamed AA, et al. Ex vivo expansion of stem cells: defining optimum conditions using various cytokines. Lab Hematol 12(2):86–93, 2006.
65. Araki H, et al. Expansion of human umbilical cord blood SCID-repopulating cells using chromatin-modifying agents. Exp Hematol 34(2):140–149, 2006.
66. Zhang CC, et al. Angiopoietin-like proteins stimulate ex vivo expansion of hematopoietic stem cells. Nat Med 12(2):240–245, 2006.
67. Zhang XB, et al. Differential effects of HOXB4 on nonhuman primate short- and long-term repopulating cells. PLoS Med 3(5):e173, 2006.
68. Barker JN, et al. Transplantation of 2 partially HLA-matched umbilical cord blood units to enhance engraftment in adults with hematologic malignancy. Blood 105(3):1343–1347, 2005.
69. Brunstein CG, Wagner JE. Umbilical cord blood transplantation and banking. Annu Rev Med 57:403–417, 2006.

Chapter 2

Current Issues in the Pathogenesis, Diagnosis, and Treatment of Neonatal Thrombocytopenia

Matthew A. Saxonhouse, MD • Martha C. Sola-Visner, MD

Platelet Production in Neonates

Neonatal Platelet Function

Approach to the Neonate with Thrombocytopenia

Treatment/Management of Neonatal Thrombocytopenia

The evaluation and management of the thrombocytopenic neonate (platelet count $<150 \times 10^9/L$) is a frequent challenge for neonatologists, as 22–35% of infants admitted to the neonatal intensive care unit (NICU) are affected by thrombocytopenia at some point during their hospital stay (1–5). Of these neonates, 25% (approximately 35 000 neonates per year in the USA) develop platelet counts low enough that their risk of hemorrhage is thought to be significantly increased (6). Treatment of these patients with platelet transfusions is provided in an attempt to diminish the occurrence, or severity, of hemorrhage. However, there is considerable debate on what constitutes an "at risk" platelet count, particularly because a number of other variables (such as mechanism of thrombocytopenia and platelet function) also significantly influence the bleeding risk. Unfortunately, there are currently no reliable and/or rapid methods for assessing the mechanisms of thrombocytopenia, and how different disease processes affect the platelet function is poorly understood. Thus, we have very limited data to guide our decisions of when to administer platelet transfusions to decrease an infant's presumed risk for hemorrhage. In this chapter, we will review the current concepts on normal and abnormal neonatal thrombopoiesis and the existing methods of evaluating platelet production and function. We will then provide a stepwise approach to the evaluation of the thrombocytopenic neonate, and will finally review current controversies regarding neonatal platelet transfusions and potential use of thrombopoietic growth factors.

PLATELET PRODUCTION IN NEONATES

The rather complex process of platelet production can be schematically represented as consisting of four main steps (Fig. 2-1). The first is the thrombopoietic stimulus that drives the production of megakaryocytes and ultimately platelets. Although a number of cytokines (i.e. IL-3, IL-6, IL-11, and GM-CSF) contribute to this process,

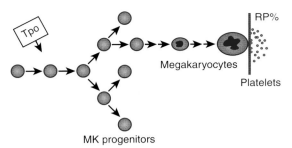

Figure 2-1 Schematic representation of neonatal megakaryocytopoiesis. Tpo acts by promoting the proliferation of megakaryocyte progenitors and the maturation of the megakaryocytes. Through a poorly understood process, mature megakaryocytes release new platelets into the circulation. These new platelets represent the reticulated platelet percentage. Adapted from Sola MC, Fetal megakaryocytopoiesis. In: Christensen RD (ed). Hematologic Problems of the Neonate. Philadelphia, PA: W.B. Saunders; 2000:43–59, with permission. Tpo, thrombopoietin; MK, megakaryocyte; RP%, reticulated platelet percentage.

thrombopoietin (Tpo) is now widely recognized as the most potent known stimulator of platelet production (7). Tpo mostly acts by promoting the next two steps of the process: the proliferation of megakaryocyte progenitors (the cells that multiply and give rise to megakaryocytes), and the maturation of the megakaryocytes, characterized by a progressive increase in nuclear ploidy and cytoplasmic maturity that leads to the generation of large polyploid (8N–64N) megakaryocytes (7, 8). Through a poorly understood process, these mature megakaryocytes then generate and release new platelets into the circulation.

Although in general the process of platelet production follows the same steps in neonates and adults, there are important developmental differences that need to be taken into consideration when evaluating neonates with platelet disorders. For example, plasma Tpo concentrations are higher in normal neonates than in healthy adults, but neonates with thrombocytopenia have in general lower Tpo concentrations than adults with similar degrees and mechanisms of thrombocytopenia (9–11). Megakaryocyte progenitors of neonates have a higher proliferative potential than those of adults, giving rise to significantly larger megakaryocyte colonies when cultured in vitro (11–13). Furthermore, neonatal megakaryocyte progenitors are more sensitive to Tpo in vitro and in vivo than adult progenitors, and are present in both the bone marrow and the peripheral blood (as opposed to adult progenitors, which reside almost exclusively in the bone marrow) (7, 12, 14). Finally, neonatal megakaryocytes are smaller and of lower ploidy than adult megakaryocytes (15–20). Since smaller megakaryocytes produce fewer platelets than larger megakaryocytes (21), it has been postulated that neonates maintain normal platelet counts on the basis of the increased proliferative rate of their progenitors.

An important question that has remained unanswered has been how these developmental differences impact the ability of neonates to respond to thrombocytopenia, particularly secondary to increased platelet consumption. Specifically, it is unknown whether neonates can increase the number and/or size of their megakaryocytes, as adult patients with platelet consumptive disorders do. Finding the answer to this question has been challenging, mostly due to the limited availability of bone marrow specimens from living neonates, the rarity of megakaryocytes in the fetal marrow, the fragility of these cells, and the inability to accurately differentiate small megakaryocytes from cells of other lineages. A recent study using state-of-the-art techniques to evaluate megakaryocytes in neonatal bone marrow biopsies (combining immunohistochemistry and image analysis) suggests that thrombocytopenic neonates do not increase the size of their megakaryocytes

(15, 22). In fact, most thrombocytopenic neonates evaluated in that study had a lower megakaryocyte mass than their non-thrombocytopenic counterparts (15).

Since bone marrow studies remain technically difficult in neonates (particularly in those born prematurely), significant efforts have been aimed at developing blood tests to evaluate platelet production that would be suitable for neonates. Among those tests, Tpo concentrations (9–11, 23), circulating megakaryocyte progenitors (11, 13, 24–26), reticulated platelet percentages (RP%) (27–30), and glycocalicin concentrations (31–33) have been used most recently, and have shown promising results. As shown in Fig. 2–1, circulating Tpo concentrations are a measure of the thrombopoietic stimulus. Because serum Tpo levels are a reflection of both the level of Tpo production and the availability of Tpo receptor (on progenitor cells, megakaryocytes, and platelets), elevated Tpo levels in the presence of thrombocytopenia usually suggest inflammatory conditions leading to upregulated gene expression (i.e. during infections) (34), or hyporegenerative thrombocytopenias characterized by a decreased megakaryocyte mass (such as aplastic anemia or chemotherapy-induced thrombocytopenia). In addition, several investigators have published Tpo concentrations in healthy neonates of different gestational and post-conceptional ages, as well as in neonates with thrombocytopenia secondary to different etiologies (9–11, 35–39). However, Tpo concentrations are not yet routinely available in the clinical setting.

As previously stated, megakaryocyte progenitors (the precursors for megakaryocytes) are present both in the blood and in the bone marrow of neonates. Investigators have capitalized on this observation, and have used the concentration of circulating progenitors as an indirect marker of marrow megakaryocytopoiesis, although the correlation between blood and marrow progenitors has never been clearly established (11, 25, 26). In normal neonates, the concentration of circulating megakaryocyte progenitors decreases with increasing post-conceptional age, a finding that has been thought to reflect the migration of megakaryocyte progenitor from the liver to the bone marrow (26). When applied to thrombocytopenic neonates, Murray et al. showed that preterm neonates with early-onset thrombocytopenia (secondary to placental insufficiency in most cases) had decreased concentrations of circulating megakaryocyte progenitors compared to their non-thrombocytopenic counterparts (25). Furthermore, the number of progenitors increased during the period of platelet recovery, thus suggesting that the thrombocytopenia observed in these neonates was secondary to decreased platelet production. Again, however, it is unlikely that this relatively labor-intensive test (which requires culturing of the megakaryocyte progenitors for 10 days) will ever become clinically available.

A test that could potentially become available to clinicians for the evaluation of neonatal thrombocytopenia is the reticulated platelet percentage (RP%). RPs are newly released platelets (<24 h old), which contain residual RNA, thus allowing their detection and quantification in the blood by flow cytometry (40–43). In adults and children, the reticulated platelet percentage (RP%) has been evaluated as a way of classifying thrombocytopenia kinetically, similar to the way the reticulocyte count is used to evaluate anemia, so that a low RP% would signify diminished platelet production while an elevated RP% would signify increased platelet production (27). Most importantly, RP% in adults correlated well with marrow megakaryocytes. Unfortunately, RP% values reported for adults and children have varied significantly, mostly because of the lack of standardized methodology. Two prior studies measured RP% in non-thrombocytopenic term and preterm neonates, and (similar to adult studies) the methods used and RP% values varied significantly (28, 29). Our group recently modified a whole blood method to determine RP% in preterm neonates admitted to the NICU over the first 28 days of life, and found that the RP% in preterm neonates increased over the first 2–5 days of life and then decreased to a stable level of 2.6 ± 1.4 over the first 28 days. In addition, RP% values were higher in neonates than adults, and inversely related to gestational age (30).

Glycocalicin concentrations have also been used as a marker of platelet turnover. Glycocalicin is a soluble proteolytic fragment of the α-subunit of glycoprotein Ib (GPIb), which is normally expressed on mature megakaryocytes and platelets (44). Its levels are increased in patients with increased platelet consumption, and decreased in patients with defective platelet formation (31–33).

Although none of these tests has yet been adequately validated with concomitant bone marrow or platelet kinetic studies in neonates, recent reports in adults and children have suggested that the use of several of these tests in combination can help differentiate between disorders of increased platelet destruction and those of decreased production, and sometimes can provide important diagnostic clues (31–33, 45, 46). In an ongoing study, the simultaneous measurement of Tpo concentrations, circulating megakaryocyte progenitors, and RP% in neonates with severe thrombocytopenia, coupled with bone marrow studies in some of them, is being evaluated (47). Although preliminary, data from this study have shown that very specific patterns can be recognized by using these tests in combination, such as ineffective platelet production in congenital HIV infection (48), and unresponsiveness to thrombopoietin in congenital amegakaryocytic thrombocytopenia (47).

In summary, the use of these tests in combination has the potential to make the mechanistic evaluation of thrombocytopenia more accurate than ever before. Particularly in neonates with severe and unexplained thrombocytopenia, this type of evaluation is likely to offer useful information leading to the diagnosis, although a single test that is useful and suitable for wide clinical use is yet to emerge. Bone marrow studies still provide information that cannot be obtained through any indirect measures of platelet production (such as marrow cellularity, megakaryocyte morphology, or evidence of hemophagocytosis), and should be performed in selected patients (22).

NEONATAL PLATELET FUNCTION

Although platelet transfusions are routinely provided to neonates with the goal of decreasing their risk of catastrophic hemorrhage, it is known that not only the platelet count but also the disease process and the platelet function at that time significantly influence an infant's risk of bleeding. Therefore, it has been postulated that the concomitant use of tests to assess platelet function and primary hemostasis might offer more insight into an infant's bleeding risk than the platelet count alone. The limitation to this approach, however, has been the lack of simple, rapid, and reproducible techniques for determining neonatal platelet function.

To evaluate the contribution of platelet function to hemostasis, investigators have used two different approaches. The first consists of measuring specific platelet functions, such as adhesion, activation, or aggregation. The second approach consists of evaluating primary hemostasis in whole blood samples. Although platelet number and function are critical to primary hemostasis, the latter tests also evaluate the contribution of many other factors in the blood, and thus represent a more global and physiological measure.

In the evaluation of platelet function alone, researchers have used aggregometry to assess platelet aggregation and flow cytometry to assess platelet activation. Initial platelet aggregation studies were performed using platelet-rich plasma, and demonstrated that platelets from neonatal cord blood (preterm greater than term) (49) were hyporesponsive to the agonists adenosine diphosphate (ADP), epinephrine, collagen, thrombin, and thromboxane analogues (e.g., U46619), when compared with adult platelets (50–55). The hyporesponsiveness of neonatal platelets to epinephrine is probably due to the decreased numbers of α2-adrenergic receptors, binding sites for epinephrine, found on neonatal platelets (56). The reduced response to collagen is probably due to the impairment of calcium mobilization (57, 58), and the decreased response to thromboxane may be the result of signaling differences downstream from the receptor (49). In contrast to these findings, the ristocetin-induced agglutination of neonatal platelets was enhanced compared with adults, most likely reflecting the higher levels and enhanced activity of circulating von Willebrand factor (vWF) in neonates (54, 59–65). The main limitation of platelet-rich plasma aggregometry was that large volumes of blood were needed, thus limiting its application in neonatology to cord blood samples. New platelet aggregometers, however, can accommodate whole blood samples and require smaller volumes, thus opening the door to whole blood aggregometry studies in preterm neonates (66).

When platelets become activated, they undergo a series of changes in the presence or conformation of several surface proteins. These changes are known as "activation markers". Using specific monoclonal antibodies to detect platelet activation markers, flow cytometry studies of cord blood and postnatal (term and preterm) samples demonstrated decreased platelet activation in response to platelet agonists such as thrombin, ADP, and epinephrine (concordant with aggregometry studies) (58, 67–74). This platelet hyporesponsiveness appeared to resolve by day ten of life (67). Flow cytometry is particularly appealing because very small volumes of blood (5–100 μl) are needed, and because it allows evaluation of both the basal status of platelet activation as well as the reactivity of the platelets in response to various agonists. However, there are limited data applying this technique to neonates with thrombocytopenia, sepsis, liver failure, DIC, and other disorders (67).

The second approach to evaluating platelet function involved methods to determine whole blood primary hemostasis, a more global and physiologic measure of platelet function in the context of whole blood. Historically, the bleeding time has been considered the gold standard test of in vivo primary hemostasis. Bleeding-time studies performed on healthy term neonates demonstrated shorter times than those from adults, suggesting enhanced primary hemostasis (75). This finding was in contrast to the platelet hyporesponsiveness observed in aggregometry and flow cytometry studies. It has been suggested that the shorter bleeding times were a result of higher hematocrits (76), higher mean corpuscular volumes (77), higher vWF concentrations (61, 62, 78), and predominance of longer vWF polymers in neonates (63, 64). When bleeding times were measured in preterm neonates, they were found to be longer that those from healthy term neonates. (79) A single study attempted to determine the relationship between bleeding times and platelet counts in thrombocytopenic neonates. This study revealed prolonged bleeding times in patients with platelet counts below 100×10^9/L, but no correlation between the degree of thrombocytopenia and the prolongation in the bleeding time (80). However, since bleeding times are highly operator-dependent and the existing evidence suggests that bleeding times do not correlate well with bleeding tendency or predict the likelihood of bleeding (81–83), it was unclear whether this finding was more a reflection of the limitations of the test, or a true lack of correlation.

The cone and platelet analyzer tests whole blood platelet adhesion and aggregation on an extracellular matrix-coated plate, under physiological arterial flow conditions (84). When a modified technique was applied to healthy full-term neonatal platelets, they demonstrated more extensive adhesion properties than adult platelets with similar aggregate formation (60). However, healthy preterm platelets had decreased platelet adhesion compared with term infants, but still greater than those from adults (85, 86). Adherence in preterm infants correlated with gestational age in the first 48 h of life, but did not increase with increasing post-conceptional age, even up to 10 weeks of life (85). Interestingly, using the cone and platelet analyzer, septic preterm infants displayed lower adherence than healthy preterm infants, suggesting a mechanism for the bleeding tendencies in this population (86). Unfortunately, the cone and platelet analyzer is not available for clinical use in most institutions, thus limiting its use to research purposes.

More recently, a highly reproducible, automated measure of primary hemostasis was developed and commercialized as a substitute for the bleeding time. The platelet function analyzer (PFA-100) measures primary hemostasis by simulating an in vivo quantitative measurement of platelet adhesion, activation, and aggregation. Specifically, anticoagulated blood is aspirated under high shear rates through an aperture cut into a membrane coated with collagen and either ADP or epinephrine, which mimics exposed subendothelium. Platelets are activated in response to the shear stress plus the physiologic agonists of platelet activation (collagen + ADP or epinephrine), adhere to the membrane, and aggregate until a stable platelet plug occludes the blood flow through the aperture (87). The time to reach occlusion is recorded by the instrument as the closure time. Two closure times are measured with each instrument run, one obtained with collagen and epinephrine and the other with collagen and ADP (88, 89). Four studies so far have applied this method to neonates, and have demonstrated shorter closure times in term neonates compared with adults, in concordance with previous bleeding time studies (87, 90–92). However, these studies were all performed on term cord blood samples, thus making the interpretation of this diagnostic test in neonates of different gestational and post-conceptional ages very difficult (in the absence of reference values). Furthermore, recent evidence has suggested that cord blood values may be different from peripheral blood values obtained from non-thrombocytopenic neonates during the first few days of life (93). Preliminary data evaluating closure times from thrombocytopenic neonates have shown a prolongation of closure times compared with cord blood and peripheral blood values from non-thrombocytopenic neonates, but no direct correlation between degree of thrombocytopenia and prolongation of closure times (94). The PFA-100 has the advantage of being rapid, accurate, reproducible, and only requiring 1.8 ml of citrated blood. However, until accurate reference ranges are available for non-thrombocytopenic neonates, taking into account gestational age and days of life, this test will have limited screening value in the NICU.

APPROACH TO THE NEONATE WITH THROMBOCYTOPENIA

The fetal platelet count reaches a level of 150×10^9/L by the end of the first trimester of pregnancy (95). Thus, any neonate with a platelet count $<150 \times 10^9$/L, regardless of gestational age (23–42 weeks), is defined as having thrombocytopenia. Platelet counts in the $100–150 \times 10^9$/L range are somewhat more common among healthy neonates than among healthy adults. For that reason, careful follow-up and expectant management in an otherwise healthy-appearing neonate with transient thrombocytopenia in this range is acceptable, although lack of resolution or worsening should prompt further evaluation.

For practicing neonatologists, the first step in the approach to the thrombocytopenic neonate is to attempt to recognize patterns that have been associated with specific illnesses. Table 2-1 lists the most common diagnoses reported in the literature as potential causes of neonatal thrombocytopenia, as well as their presentations. If the pattern of thrombocytopenia fits any of the listed categories, then confirmatory testing is indicated. There is obviously some overlap in these processes, such as sepsis and necrotizing enterocolitis (NEC), or birth asphyxia and disseminated intravascular coagulation (DIC).

Figures 2-2 and 2-3 provide algorithms for the evaluation of a neonate with either severe (platelet count $<50 \times 10^9$/L) or mild ($100–150 \times 10^9$/L) to moderate

Table 2-1   Specific Illnesses and Patterns Associated with Neonatal Thrombocytopenia

Categories	Subtypes	Differential diagnoses (where applicable)	Severity	Onset
Immune	Alloimmune	Neonatal Alloimmune	Severe	Early
	Autoimmune	Thrombocytopenia	Severe-moderate	Early
		Maternal ITP, Lupus, other collagen vascular disorder		
Infectious	Bacterial	GBS, *E. coli, Klebsiella, Serratia, Enterobacter,* H. flu, *Staph aureus, Staph epi, Enterococcus*	Variable	Variable
	Viral	CMV, HSV, HIV, parvovirus, coxsackie, EBV	Variable	Usually early
	Fungal	Candida, other	Severe	Usually late
	Parasite	Toxoplasmosis	Variable	Early
Placental insufficiency		Preeclampsia, eclampsia, chronic hypertension	Mild-moderate	Early
Medication-induced*	Antibiotic		Variable	Late
	Heparin		Variable	Late
	Anticonvulsants		Variable	Late
	NSAIDs		Variable	Late
	Histamine H$_2$-receptor antagonists		Variable	Late
DIC		Asphyxia	Severe	Early
		Sepsis	Severe	Variable
		Congenital TTP (rare)	Severe	Variable
Genetic disorders**	Chromosomal	Trisomy 13, trisomy 18, trisomy 21, Turner syndrome, Jacobsen syndrome	Variable	Early
	Familial	Macrothrombocytopenias, Wiskott-Aldrich syndrome, X-linked thrombocytopenias, Amegakaryocytic thrombocytopenia, TAR, Fanconi anemia***, Noonan syndrome	Variable	Early***
	Metabolic	Proprionic acidemia, methylmalonic acidemia, hyperthyroidism, infant of diabetic mother	Mild-moderate	Variable
Miscellaneous	Thrombosis	RVT, line-associated thrombosis, sagittal sinus thrombosis	Moderate	Variable
	Tumor	Kasabach Merritt, hepatic hemangioendothelioma	Moderate	Variable
	NEC		Severe-moderate	Usually Late
	Polycythemia		Mild-moderate	Early
	ECMO		Variable	Variable

Adapted from Sola MC. Evaluation and treatment of severe and prolonged thrombocytopenia in neonates. In: Christensen RD (ed). Hematopoietic Growth Factors in Neonatal Medicine. Philadelphia, PA: W.B. Saunders; 2004:1–14, with permission.

ITP, Immune thrombocytopenic purpura; CMV, cytomegalovirus; HSV, herpes simplex virus I and II; HIV, human immunodeficiency virus; EBV, Epstein Barr virus; IUGR, intrauterine growth retardation; TTP, thrombotic thrombocytopenic purpura; TAR, thrombocytopenia absent-radii syndrome; RVT, renal vein thrombosis; NEC, necrotizing enterocolitis; ECMO, extra-corporeal membrane oxygenation; NSAIDs, non-steroidal anti-inflammatory medications.

*Refer to Table 2-3 for further description.

**Refer to Table 2-2 for further description.

***Most familial thrombocytopenias are present at birth except for Fanconi anemia, which usually does not appear until childhood.

$(50-100 \times 10^9/L)$ thrombocytopenia, respectively. In addition to severity, this approach uses time of presentation to classify the different causes of thrombocytopenia as early (onset at <72 h of life) vs. late (>72 h of life) thrombocytopenia. When faced with severe, early thrombocytopenia (Fig. 2-2) in a term or preterm neonate, infection (usually bacterial) should be suspected and evaluated for.

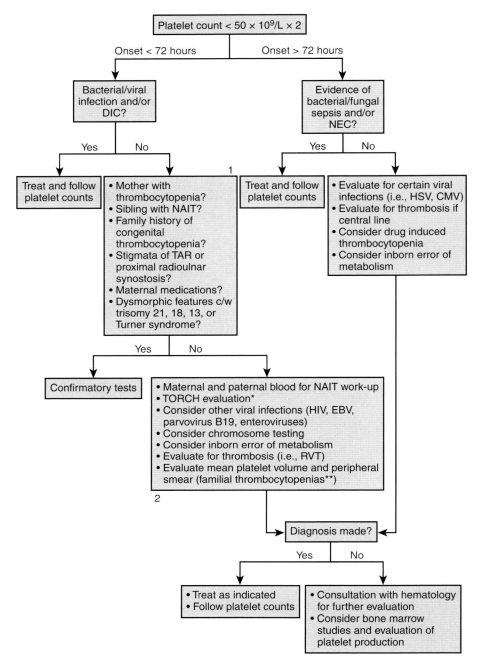

Figure 2-2 Evaluation of the neonate with severe thrombocytopenia ($< 50 \times 10^9$/L) of early (<72 h of life) vs. late (>72 h of life) onset. DIC, disseminated intravascular coagulation; NEC, necrotizing enterocolitis; ITP, immune thrombocytopenic purpura; NAIT, neonatal alloimmune thrombocytopenia; TAR, thrombocytopenia absent-radii syndrome; EBV, Epstein Barr virus; RVT, renal vein thrombosis. *TORCH evaluation consisting of diagnostic work-up for toxoplasmosis, rubella, CMV, HSV, and syphilis. **Refer to Table 2-2 for listing of disorders.

If the neonate is well-appearing and infection has been ruled out, then a careful family history and physical exam can provide critical clues to the diagnosis. For example, a prior sibling with a history of neonatal alloimmune thrombocytopenia (NAIT) strongly supports this diagnosis, prompting immediate evaluation and treatment (see next section). A family history of any form of congenital

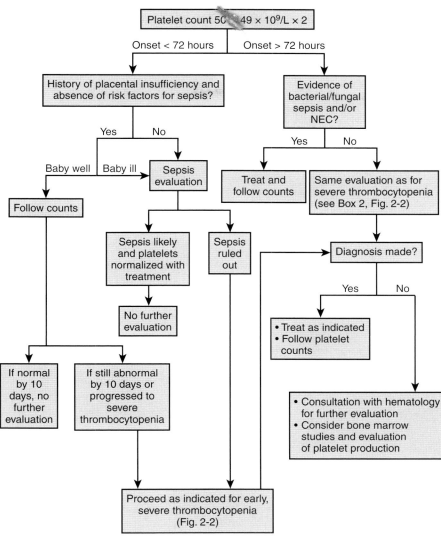

Figure 2-3 Evaluation of the neonate with mild-moderate thrombocytopenia (50–149 $\times$ 10^9/L) of early (<72 h of life) vs. late (>72 h of life) onset. NEC, necrotizing enterocolitis.

thrombocytopenia warrants further investigation in that direction (Table 2-2). Presence of physical findings of trisomy 13 (i.e. cutis aplasia, cleft-lip-and-palate), 18 (i.e. clinodactyly, IUGR, rocker-bottom feet), 21 (i.e. macroglossia, single palmar crease, AV canal, hypotonia), or Turner syndrome (edema, growth retardation, congenital heart defects) dictates chromosomal evaluation. Decreased ability to pronate/supinate the forearm in an otherwise normal-appearing neonate suggests congenital amegakaryocytic thrombocytopenia with proximal radio-ulnar synostosis (96). The presence of hepatosplenomegaly suggests the possibility of viral infection, and an abdominal mass should prompt an abdominal ultrasound to evaluate for renal vein thrombosis.

In the absence of any obvious diagnostic clues, in an otherwise well-appearing infant, the most common cause is immune (allo- or auto-) thrombocytopenia, caused by the passage of anti-platelet antibodies from the mother to the fetus. If the anti-platelet antibody work-up is negative, then a more detailed evaluation is indicated. This should consist of TORCH evaluation, including HIV testing and parvovirus evaluation. Rarer diagnoses such as thrombosis (renal vein thrombosis,

Table 2-2 Familial Thrombocytopenias, Including Platelet Size, Mode of Inheritance, and Associated Physical Findings

Syndrome	Platelet size	Mode of inheritance	Associated clinical findings
Wiskott-Aldrich syndrome	Small	X-linked	Immunodeficiency, eczema
X-linked thrombocytopenia	Small	X-linked	None
Congenital amegakaryocytic thrombocytopenia	Normal	AR	None
Congenital amegakaryocytic thrombocytopenia and radio-ulnar synostosis	Normal	AR	Restricted forearm pronation, proximal radio-ulnar synostosis in forearm X-ray (96)
Fanconi anemia	Normal	AR	Hypopigmented and hyperpigmented skin lesions, urinary tract abnormalities, microcephaly, upper extremity radial-side abnormalities involving the thumb, pancytopenia (rarely present in the neonatal period) (107,108)
Chromosome 10/THC2*	Normal	AD	None
Thrombocytopenia and absent radii	Normal	AR	Shortened/absent radii bilaterally, normal thumbs, ulnar and hand abnormalities, abnormalities of the humerus, cardiac defects (TOF, ASD, VSD), eosinophilia, leukemoid reaction (182-184)
May-Hegglin anomaly	Large/giant	AD	Neutrophilic inclusions
Fechtner syndrome	Large/giant	AD	Sensorineural hearing loss, cataracts, nephritis, neutrophilic inclusions
Epstein syndrome	Large/giant	AD	Sensorineural hearing loss, nephritis
Sebastian syndrome	Large/giant	AD	Neutrophilic inclusions
Mediterranean thrombocytopenia	Large/giant	AD	None
Bernard-Soulier syndrome	Large/giant	AR	None
GATA1 mutation	Large/giant or Normal	X-linked	Anemia, Genitourinary abnormalities (cryptorchidism) (167,185,186)
Gray platelet syndrome	Large/giant	AD	None
11q Terminal deletion disorder (Jacobsen syndrome)	Large/giant	AD	Congenital heart defects, genitourinary abnormalities, growth retardation, mild facial anomalies, limb anomalies, abnormal brain imaging (97,98)

Adapted from Drachman JG. Inherited thrombocytopenia: when a low platelet count does not mean ITP. Blood 13(2)390–398, 2004; with permission.

AR, autosomal recessive; AD, autosomal dominant; TOF, tetralogy of Fallot; ASD, atrial septal defect; VSD, ventricular septal defect.

*Mild-moderate thrombocytopenia associated with genetic linkage to the short arm of chromosome 10, 10p11-12 (187, 188).

sagittal sinus thrombosis), Kasabach-Merritt syndrome, and inborn errors of metabolism (mainly proprionic acidemia and methylmalonic acidemia) should be considered and evaluated for if clinically indicated. Platelet counts in these disorders may range from severe to mild depending on the particular presentation. It is also important to recognize that some chromosomal disorders have very subtle phenotypic features, such as can be the case in the 11q terminal deletion disorder (previously referred to as Jacobsen syndrome) (97), which has a wide range of phenotypes (including any combination of growth retardation, genitourinary anomalies, limb anomalies, mild facial anomalies, abnormal brain imaging, heart defects, and ophthalmologic problems) (97, 98). Therefore, a growth-restricted neonate without an obvious reason for the growth restriction or an infant with subtle dysmorphic features and thrombocytopenia warrants chromosomal analysis. Severe and persistent isolated thrombocytopenia in an otherwise normal neonate can also represent congenital amegakaryocytic thrombocytopenia. If the

Table 2-3   Medications frequently used in Neonates that may cause Thrombocytopenia

Medication Class	Examples
Antibiotics	Penicillin and derivatives
	Ciprofloxacin
	Cephalosporin
	Metronizadole
	Vancomycin
	Rifampin
Nonsteroidals	Indomethacin
Anticoagulants	Heparin
Histamine H$_2$-receptor antagonists	Famotidine, cimetidine
Anticonvulsants	Phenobarbital, phenytoin

The majority of the medications listed have been reported to cause neonatal thrombocytopenia in isolated case reports (99-106).

thrombocytopenia is part of a pancytopenia, osteopetrosis should be considered. After following this algorithm, if the diagnosis is still unknown, consultation with a pediatric hematologist is warranted, especially if the platelet count has not improved by 10 days of life.

When a neonate presents with severe thrombocytopenia after 72 h of life (Fig. 2-2), then prompt evaluation and treatment for bacterial/fungal sepsis and/or NEC must be initiated. If all cultures are negative and there is no clinical evidence of NEC, but the platelet count is still severely low, then the evaluation must be expanded. Appropriate testing should include evaluations for (i) DIC and liver dysfunction; (ii) certain viral infections (i.e. HSV, CMV, EBV); (iii) thrombosis, especially with a history of a central line; (iv) drug-induced thrombocytopenia (Table 2-3) (99–106); (v) inborn errors of metabolism; and (vi) Fanconi anemia (rare) (107, 108). If a diagnosis is still not made, then consultation with a hematologist and potential bone marrow studies and evaluation of platelet production are warranted.

The presentation of mild-moderate thrombocytopenia (Fig. 2-3) within the first 72 h of life in a well-appearing preterm infant without risk factors for infection and with a maternal history of preeclampsia or chronic hypertension is most likely related to placental insufficiency (9, 25). If the platelet count normalizes within 10 days, no further evaluation is necessary. However, if the thrombocytopenia becomes severe or the platelet count does not return to normal, then further evaluation (especially for infection or immune thrombocytopenia) is required. Mild-moderate thrombocytopenia within the first 72 h of life in an ill-appearing term or preterm neonate warrants an immediate evaluation for sepsis. If sepsis is ruled out, then the evaluation should be very similar to the one described for early, severe thrombocytopenia in a non-septic neonate (Fig. 2-2). If the thrombocytopenia is persistent, the differential diagnosis should be expanded to include familial thrombocytopenias, which frequently (but not always) are in the mild-moderate range. Many of these familial thrombocytopenias can be identified based on platelet size, mode of inheritance, and associated clinical findings (Table 2-2). The platelet size can be evaluated using the mean platelet volume (MPV; normal 7–11 fL) (98), which is frequently reported on routine complete blood counts, or reviewing the blood smear and looking for large or small platelets. For example, Jacobsen syndrome, May-Hegglin anomaly, Fechtner syndrome, and Epstein syndrome present with large platelets (MPV>11 fL) (98), as well as other associated clinical findings that may be identified during the neonatal period (98). In contrast, Wiskott-Aldrich syndrome and X-linked thrombocytopenia present with abnormally small platelets (MPV<7 fL) (98). Certain physical findings on exam may also provide key diagnostic clues to the underlying diagnosis (Table 2-2). The inability to supinate/pronate the forearm may be a sign of congenital amegakaryocytic thrombocytopenia with proximal radio-ulnar synostosis, which can be easily confirmed by forearm X-rays (96).

If the presentation of thrombocytopenia is at >72 h of life, the most likely diagnosis is bacterial or fungal sepsis with or without NEC. Late-onset thrombocytopenia associated with sepsis has been reported to occur in 6% of all admissions to the NICU in some institutions (6). However, if these are ruled out, then an approach similar to that outlined for late-onset severe thrombocytopenia should be followed (Fig. 2-2). If a diagnosis is still not found, then consultation with a pediatric hematologist is warranted.

In neonates with thrombocytopenia of unclear etiology, identifying the mechanisms responsible (increased destruction, decreased production, sequestration, or a combination) may aid in narrowing the differential diagnosis. Neonatal alloimmune or autoimmune thrombocytopenias are examples of increased destruction, whereas infants born to mothers with placental insufficiency or who have inherited bone marrow failure syndromes are examples of decreased platelet production (11, 25, 109, 110). However, the exact mechanism remains unknown for a large percentage of neonates with thrombocytopenia (111, 112). In adults, bone marrow studies and radiolabeled platelet survival studies provide a thorough mechanistic evaluation (113, 114). Unfortunately, these studies are cumbersome and technically difficult in neonates (115). For that reason, the use of the tests described in the first section may prove to be of particular value in the evaluation of neonates with thrombocytopenia of unknown etiology, as evidenced by some recent publications (47, 48, 96).

TREATMENT/MANAGEMENT OF NEONATAL THROMBOCYTOPENIA

Despite the frequency of thrombocytopenia in the NICU, and the severity of its potential consequences, there has only been one prospective, randomized trial evaluating different thresholds for platelet transfusions in neonates (116). In that study, performed by Andrew et al. in 1993 (116), thrombocytopenic premature infants were randomly assigned to maintain a platelet count $>150 \times 10^9$/L at all times, or to only receive platelet transfusions for clinical indications or for a platelet count $<50 \times 10^9$/L. Overall, these investigators found no differences in the frequency or severity of intracranial hemorrhages between the two groups, suggesting that non-bleeding premature infants with platelet counts $>50 \times 10^9$/L did not benefit from prophylactic platelet transfusions. Since that study only evaluated neonates with a platelet count $>50 \times 10^9$/L, it remained unclear whether lower platelet counts could be safely tolerated in otherwise stable neonates. To answer that question, Murray et al. (6) performed a retrospective review of their use of platelet transfusions among neonates with platelet counts $<50 \times 10^9$/L ($n = 53$ of the 901 admissions over a 3-year period). They reported that 51% of these neonates (27/53) received at least one platelet transfusion (all infants with a platelet count $<30 \times 10^9$/L and those with platelet counts between 30 and 50×10^9/L who had a previous hemorrhage or were clinically unstable). They also did not observe any major hemorrhage in this group of severely thrombocytopenic neonates, and therefore concluded that a prophylactic platelet transfusion trigger threshold of $<30 \times 10^9$/L probably represents a safe practice for clinically stable ICU patients (6). As the authors themselves recognized, however, this was a relatively small retrospective study, which should be interpreted with caution.

In the absence of good evidence to guide our transfusion decisions, numerous experts and consensus groups have published guidelines for the administration of

Table 2-4   Summary of Recent Guidelines for Platelet Transfusions in Term and Preterm Neonates (platelet counts $\times 10^9$/L)

Source	Non-bleeding sick preterm	Non-bleeding stable preterm	Non-bleeding term	Before invasive procedure	Active bleeding
Calhoun et al. 2000 (145)	<50	<25	Same as preterm	<50	Not addressed
Strauss 2000 (121)	<100	<20	<20	<50	<100
Murray et al. 2002 (6)	<50	<30	<30	<50	<100
Roseff et al. 2002 (189)	Not addressed	<30 with failure of production	<30 with failure of production	<100 if sick preterm with DIC;<50 if stable preterm with failure of production	<100 if sick preterm; <50 if stable preterm
Gibson et al. 2004* (119)	<50	<30	Same as preterm	<50	<50

*Guidelines from the British Committee for Standards in Haematology Transfusion Task Force.
Adapted from Saxonhouse M, Slayton W, Sola MC. Platelet transfusions in the infant and child. In: Hillyer CD, Strauss RG, Luban NLC (eds). Handbook of Pediatric Transfusion Medicine. San Diego, CA: Elsevier Academic Press; 2004:253–269.

platelet transfusions to neonates. The most recent guidelines are summarized in Table 2-4, although it is important to recognize that these only represent educated opinions based on the limited existing evidence. This lack of evidence is clearly reflected in the variability of neonatal platelet transfusion practices world-wide, as exposed by recent papers describing platelet transfusion usage in different NICUs (6, 116–119). Three recent reports have retrospectively documented platelet transfusion practice in NICUs from the USA, UK and Mexico (6, 117, 118). In summary, these reports highlighted that approximately 2–9% of neonates admitted to the NICU receive at least one platelet transfusion, that most platelet transfusions are given to non-bleeding patients with platelet counts $<50 \times 10^9$/L, and that more than 50% of neonates who receive a transfusion will receive more than one.

While when to administer a platelet transfusion is relatively controversial, what to administer is less unclear. In this regard, experts agree that neonates should receive 10–15 ml/kg of a CMV-safe standard platelet suspension. Whole blood-derived platelet concentrates (or random-donor platelets) are prepared from a single donated unit of whole blood that contains approximately 50 ml of volume. Each concentrate contains approximately 10×10^9 platelets per 10 ml. A single random-donor platelet unit is usually sufficient to provide a platelet transfusion to a neonate. This exposes them to only one donor, and they receive approximately 10×10^9 platelets/kg body weight, a dose expected to increase the blood platelet count to $>100 \times 10^9$/L. Volume reduction is not routinely recommended.

Due to concerns of CMV infection, most institutions transfuse infants with blood products obtained from donors without detectable antibodies to CMV (120). However, the incidence of CMV infection following transfusion with CMV-negative platelets is still 1–4% due to an intrinsic false negative rate of the test for antibody to CMV, a low antibody titer, or transient viremia quenching the circulating antibody (121–123). A major limitation to the use of CMV-negative blood is that <50% of the blood donor population is CMV-antibody negative. An alternative to CMV-negative blood is leukocyte reduction, although whether this offers comparable safety is controversial (124–128).

There is also the concern of transfusion-associated graft-versus-host disease (TA-GVHD), the result of contaminating T lymphocytes that are present in platelet concentrates. TA-GVD presents between 8–10 days following a transfusion and it is characterized by a rash, diarrhea, elevated hepatic transaminases, hyperbilirubinemia, and pancytopenia. TA-GVHD is a condition characterized by an extremely high mortality rate (>90%) (129). Exposure of platelets to 2500 cGy of gamma irradiation before transfusion effectively prevents GVHD, and irradiated cellular products are definitely indicated in cases of suspected or confirmed underlying immunodeficiency (e.g., DiGeorge, Wiskott-Aldrich syndrome), intrauterine or exchange transfusions, or blood transfusions from a first- or second-degree relative or a HLA-matched donor (119, 130–132). However, because an underlying primary immunodeficiency disorder may not be apparent in the neonatal period, some groups choose to irradiate all cellular blood products administered to neonates.

When a full-term, well-appearing neonate presents with severe thrombocytopenia at birth, a diagnosis of neonatal alloimmune thrombocytopenia (NAIT) must be considered. NAIT is caused by the fetomaternal mismatch for human platelet alloantigens, and the pathogenesis resembles that of erythroblastosis fetalis. Platelets exhibit a large number of antigens on their membranes, including ABO, HLA antigens, and platelet-specific antigens, named human platelet antigens (HPAs). If incompatibility between parental platelet antigens exists, the mother can become sensitized to an antigen expressed on the fetal platelets. These maternal antibodies may then cross the placenta, bind to fetal platelets, and induce platelet removal by the reticuloendothelial system, resulting in severe thrombocytopenia as early as 24 weeks gestation (133). This diagnosis is further supported if a random-donor platelet transfusion is given and the neonate does not respond. Intracranial hemorrhage has been reported in 10–15% of cases of NAIT (134), and it is therefore important to provide effective therapy as soon as possible. A recent large study evaluating human platelet antigen-specific antibodies showed that in approximately 31% of the cases where NAIT is suspected, a specific anti-platelet antibody was identified (135). In these cases, maternal HPA-1 alloimmunization accounted for the majority (79%) (135), but many other specific platelet alloantigens have been implicated in the pathogenesis of NAIT and should be considered, particularly when maternal serum is shown to react with paternal platelets (135–141). When the platelet count is $<30 \times 10^9$/L, transfusion with maternal platelets is recommended, although HPA-1a negative/HPA-5b negative platelets are suitable the majority of the time (4). If maternal platelets are used, they must be irradiated and washed or plasma-depleted prior to transfusion (44). In cases where there is a long wait for compatible platelets or they are not available, high-dose IVIG or a trial of random-donor platelets is indicated. A small percentage of neonates will have a response to random-donor platelets, which can be due to receiving HPA-1a negative platelets, the presence of weak HPA-1a antibodies, or NAIT caused by platelet antibodies against antigens other than HPA-1a (140, 142). When using IVIG (143, 144), the usual recommended dose is 1–2 g/kg administered as 0.4 g/kg daily for 3–5 days or 1 g/kg daily for 1 or 2 days (142, 145). Steroids have also been used in cases of severe thrombocytopenia not responsive to IVIG (44).

Because of the risks associated with blood products, the potential use of thrombopoietic growth factors has been explored as an appealing therapeutic alternative for thrombocytopenia. IL-3, IL-6, IL-11, stem cell factor (SCF), and thrombopoietin (Tpo) all support megakaryocyte development in vitro, and have been touted for their preclinical thrombopoietic activity, but have led to limited platelet recovery in the adult patient care setting (146). No trials in neonates have been conducted. There still remains hope that certain types of patients may respond to one or a combination of these factors, and thus their modes of action and potential use in the NICU will be briefly discussed.

Clinical studies using IL-3 and IL-6 alone or in combination for adult bone marrow failure, HIV-associated cytopenias, and congenital amegakaryocytic thrombocytopenia have demonstrated limited efficacy and/or significant toxicity, thus making their therapeutic use impractical (147–160).

Recombinant IL-11 is the only thrombopoietic growth factor that has been approved by the FDA for the prevention of severe thrombocytopenia after myelosuppressive chemotherapy for nonmyeloid malignancies (161), although significant side-effects such as fluid retention and atrial arrhythmias may limit its use (162, 163). Reports of experimental benefits for NEC (164, 165) and sepsis (166) in animal models have made the thought of using this cytokine in neonates somewhat appealing. However, safety and efficacy in neonates have never been investigated, and its use should therefore be restricted to well-controlled clinical trials.

The cloning of Tpo (the most potent known stimulator of platelet production) led to a flurry of studies that quickly progressed from bench research to clinical trials. Unfortunately, a few of the subjects treated with a truncated form of recombinant Tpo (PEG-rHMGDG) (167) developed neutralizing antibodies against endogenous Tpo, resulting in severe thrombocytopenia and aplastic anemia. This led pharmaceutical companies to discontinue all clinical trials involving Tpo. As an alternative, much interest has recently been devoted to the development of thrombopoietin-mimetic molecules. These are mostly small peptides that have no molecular homology to Tpo, but bind to the Tpo receptor and have biologically comparable effects. Among the significant number of thrombopoietin receptor agonists that have been described, two (AMG-531 and SB-497115) are currently undergoing phase I and II clinical trials (168–171).

In general, the use of thrombopoietic growth factors in adults has been associated with modest or somewhat disappointing results (172). Significant side-effect profiles and development of cross-reactive antibodies may further limit their use. Prolonged administration of these compounds may also be required to see a response, which may apply to the adult or child with bone marrow failure, but very few neonates exhibit this pathophysiology. However, certain neonatal conditions predisposing them to prolonged and severe thrombocytopenia may make them candidates for one or a combination of these factors. Appropriately designed clinical trials are certainly necessary before this can be entertained.

Recombinant Factor VIIa (rFVIIa) is produced by biotechnology and approved for use in severe, life-threatening bleeding episodes in patients with hemophilia A and B with and without inhibitors (173, 174). The use of rFVIIa in thrombocytopenia-associated conditions has been debated. High-dose rFVIIa has been found to shorten the bleeding time in thrombocytopenic adult patients, and recent studies have explored the use of rFVIIa in the treatment and prevention of bleeding in patients with inherited and acquired platelet function disorders (175–177). Whether rFVIIa has potential in the NICU as a treatment to improve platelet function in thrombocytopenic neonates remains to be determined. However, several case reports using rFVIIa in bleeding preterm neonates as a desperate measure have been published, most of them with at least some success (178–181). Until further studies improving our understanding of the physiology of rFVIIa in neonates and its effects in well-designed randomized clinical trials are available, its use should be reserved for only select circumstances.

In conclusion, although the majority of cases of neonatal thrombocytopenia are mild to moderate and do not warrant aggressive treatment, this constitutes a significant problem in the NICU and may be the presenting sign of a serious diagnosis. It appears from recent studies that neonates have a relative inability to increase platelet production when faced with thrombocytopenia. Improved indirect tests of thrombopoiesis are currently being applied to neonates with prolonged and severe thrombocytopenia in an attempt to better understand the pathophysiology of the different varieties of thrombocytopenia. In addition, the application of the PFA-100 to neonates may eventually provide a better screening mechanism for evaluating platelet function, thus allowing neonatologists to determine an infant's risk of bleeding when faced with a low platelet count. Platelet transfusions remain the only current treatment for thrombocytopenia, and although most agree that platelet counts $<30 \times 10^9/L$ in a sick neonate would justify a transfusion, there is no solid evidence to guide our decisions of when to administer transfusions in other situations. Future studies are required to determine what constitutes a safe count and to better balance the risks of significant hemorrhage vs. additional donor exposures in individual situations.

Acknowledgments

This work was supported by grant No. HL69990 from the National Institutes of Health and a grant from the American Heart Association, Florida/Puerto Rico Affiliate.

REFERENCES

1. Mehta P, Vasa R, Neumann L, et al. Thrombocytopenia in the high-risk infant. J Pediatr 97:791–794, 1980.
2. Castle V, Andrew M, Kelton J, et al. Frequency and mechanism of neonatal thrombocytopenia. J Pediatr 108:749–755, 1986.
3. de Moerloose P, Boehlen F, Extermann P, et al. Neonatal thrombocytopenia: incidence and characterization of maternal antiplatelet antibodies by MAIPA assay. Br J Haematol 100:735–740, 1998.
4. Chakravorty S, Murray N, Roberts I. Neonatal thrombocytopenia. Early Hum Dev 81:35–41, 2005. Epub 2004 Nov 2019.
5. Sainio S, Jarvenpaa AL, Renlund M, et al. Thrombocytopenia in term infants: a population-based study. Obstet Gynecol 95:441–446, 2000.
6. Murray NA, Howarth LJ, McCloy MP, et al. Platelet transfusion in the management of severe thrombocytopenia in neonatal intensive care unit patients. Transfus Med 12:35–41, 2002.
7. Kaushansky K, Broudy VC, Lin N, et al. Thrombopoietin, the Mpl ligand, is essential for full megakaryocyte development. Proc Natl Acad Sci USA 92:3234–3238, 1995.
8. Kaushansky K. Thrombopoietin: the primary regulator of platelet production. Blood 86:419–431, 1995.
9. Sola MC, Calhoun DA, Hutson AD, et al. Plasma thrombopoietin concentrations in thrombocytopenic and non-thrombocytopenic patients in a neonatal intensive care unit. Br J Haematol 104:90–92, 1999.
10. Sola MC, Juul SE, Meng YG, et al. Thrombopoietin (Tpo) in the fetus and neonate: Tpo concentrations in preterm and term neonates, and organ distribution of Tpo and its receptor (c-mpl) during human fetal development. Early Hum Dev 53:239–250, 1999.
11. Murray NA, Watts TL, Roberts IA. Endogenous thrombopoietin levels and effect of recombinant human thrombopoietin on megakaryocyte precursors in term and preterm babies. Pediatr Res 43:148–151, 1998.
12. Sola MC, Du Y, Hutson AD, et al. Dose-response relationship of megakaryocyte progenitors from the bone marrow of thrombocytopenic and non-thrombocytopenic neonates to recombinant thrombopoietin. Br J Haematol 110:449–453, 2000.
13. Nishihira H, Toyoda Y, Miyazaki H, et al. Growth of macroscopic human megakaryocyte colonies from cord blood in culture with recombinant human thrombopoietin (c-mpl ligand) and the effects of gestational age on frequency of colonies. Br J Haematol 92:23–28, 1996.
14. Sola MC, Christensen RD, Hutson AD, et al. Pharmacokinetics, pharmacodynamics, and safety of administering pegylated recombinant megakaryocyte growth and development factor to newborn rhesus monkeys. Pediatr Res 47:208–214, 2000.
15. Sola MC, CR, Du Y, Hutson AD, et al. Neonates fail to increase their marrow megakaryocyte mass in response to thrombocytopenia. Pediatr Res 51:242A, 2002.
16. Olson TA, Levine RF, Mazur EM, et al. Megakaryocytes and megakaryocyte progenitors in human cord blood. Am J Pediatr Hematol Oncol 14:241–247, 1992.
17. Levine RF, Olson TA, Shoff PK, et al. Mature micromegakaryocytes: an unusual developmental pattern in term infants. Br J Haematol 94:391–399, 1996.
18. Hegyi E, Nakazawa M, Debili N, et al. Developmental changes in human megakaryocyte ploidy. Exp Hematol 19:87–94, 1991.
19. de Alarcon PA, Graeve JL. Analysis of megakaryocyte ploidy in fetal bone marrow biopsies using a new adaptation of the feulgen technique to measure DNA content and estimate megakaryocyte ploidy from biopsy specimens. Pediatr Res 39:166–170, 1996.
20. Ma DC, Sun YH, Chang KZ, et al. Developmental change of megakaryocyte maturation and DNA ploidy in human fetus. Eur J Haematol 57:121–127, 1996.

21. Mattia G, Vulcano F, Milazzo L, et al. Different ploidy levels of megakaryocytes generated from peripheral or cord blood CD34+ cells are correlated with different levels of platelet release. Blood 99:888–897, 2002.

22. Sola MC, Rimsza LM, Christensen RD. A bone marrow biopsy technique suitable for use in neonates. Br J Haematol 107:458–460, 1999.

23. Emmons RV, Reid DM, Cohen RL, et al. Human thrombopoietin levels are high when thrombocytopenia is due to megakaryocyte deficiency and low when due to increased platelet destruction. Blood 87:4068–4071, 1996.

24. Zauli G, Valvassori L, Capitani S. Presence and characteristics of circulating megakaryocyte progenitor cells in human fetal blood. Blood 81:385–390, 1993.

25. Murray NA, Roberts IA. Circulating megakaryocytes and their progenitors in early thrombocytopenia in preterm neonates. Pediatr Res 40:112–119, 1996.

26. Saxonhouse MA, Christensen RD, Walker DM, et al. The concentration of circulating megakaryocyte progenitors in preterm neonates is a function of post-conceptional age. Early Hum Dev 78:119–124, 2004.

27. Kienast J, Schmitz G. Flow cytometric analysis of thiazole orange uptake by platelets: a diagnostic aid in the evaluation of thrombocytopenic disorders. Blood 75:116–121, 1990.

28. Joseph MA, Adams D, Maragos J, et al. Flow cytometry of neonatal platelet RNA. J Pediatr Hematol Oncol 18:277–281, 1996.

29. Peterec SM, Brennan SA, Rinder HM, et al. Reticulated platelet values in normal and thrombocytopenic neonates. J Pediatr 129:269–274, 1996.

30. Saxonhouse MA, Sola MC, Pastos KM, et al. Reticulated platelet percentages in term and preterm neonates. J Pediatr Hematol Oncol 26:797–802, 2004.

31. Robinson M, Machin S, Mackie I, et al. Comparison of glycocalicin, thrombopoietin and reticulated platelet measurement as markers of platelet turnover in HIV+ samples. Platelets 12:108–113, 2001.

32. van den Oudenrijn S, Bruin M, Folman CC, et al. Three parameters, plasma thrombopoietin levels, plasma glycocalicin levels and megakaryocyte culture, distinguish between different causes of congenital thrombocytopenia. Br J Haematol 117:390–398, 2002.

33. Fabris F, Cordiano I, Steffan A, et al. Indirect study of thrombopoiesis (TPO, reticulated platelets, glycocalicin) in patients with hereditary macrothrombocytopenia. Eur J Haematol 64:151–156, 2000.

34. Kaser A, Brandacher G, Steurer W, et al. Interleukin-6 stimulates thrombopoiesis through thrombopoietin: role in inflammatory thrombocytosis. Blood 98:2720–2725, 2001.

35. Dame C, Cremer M, Ballmaier M, et al. Concentrations of thrombopoietin and interleukin-11 in the umbilical cord blood of patients with fetal alloimmune thrombocytopenia. Am J Perinatol 18:335–344, 2001.

36. Dame C. Thrombopoietin in thrombocytopenias of childhood. Semin Thromb Hemost 27:215–228, 2001.

37. Dame C. Developmental biology of thrombopoietin in the human fetus and neonate. Acta Paediatr Suppl 91:54–65, 2002.

38. Sola MC, Dame C, Christensen RD. Toward a rational use of recombinant thrombopoietin in the neonatal intensive care unit. J Pediatr Hematol Oncol 23:179–184, 2001.

39. Dame C, Sutor AH. Primary and secondary thrombocytosis in childhood. Br J Haematol 129:165–177, 2005.

40. Bonan JL, Rinder HM, Smith BR. Determination of the percentage of thiazole orange (TO)-positive, "reticulated" platelets using autologous erythrocyte TO fluorescence as an internal standard. Cytometry 14:690–694, 1993.

41. Ault KA, Rinder HM, Mitchell J, et al. The significance of platelets with increased RNA content (reticulated platelets). A measure of the rate of thrombopoiesis. Am J Clin Pathol 98:637–646, 1992.

42. Matic GB, Chapman ES, Zaiss M, et al. Whole blood analysis of reticulated platelets: improvements of detection and assay stability. Cytometry 34:229–234, 1998.

43. Richards EM, Baglin TP. Quantitation of reticulated platelets: methodology and clinical application. Br J Haematol 91:445–451, 1995.

44. Sola M. Evaluation and treatment of severe and prolonged thrombocytopenia in neonates. In: Christensen RD, ed. Hematopoietic growth factors in neonatal medicine, Vol. 31. Philadelphia: W.B. Saunders Company; 2004: 1–14.

45. Koike Y, Yoneyama A, Shirai J, et al. Evaluation of thrombopoiesis in thrombocytopenic disorders by simultaneous measurement of reticulated platelets of whole blood and serum thrombopoietin concentrations. Thromb Haemost 79:1106–1110, 1998.

46. Kurata Y, Hayashi S, Kiyoi T, et al. Diagnostic value of tests for reticulated platelets, plasma glycocalicin, and thrombopoietin levels for discriminating between hyperdestructive and hypoplastic thrombocytopenia. Am J Clin Pathol 115:656–664, 2001.

47. Sola MC, Christensen RD, Pastos K, et al. Mechansims underlying severe and prolonged thrombocytopenia in neonates. Pediatr Res 55:291A, 2004.

48. Tighe P, Rimsza LM, Christensen RD, et al. Severe thrombocytopenia in a neonate with congenital HIV infection. J Pediatr 146:408–413, 2005.

49. Israels SJ, Odaibo FS, Robertson C, et al. Deficient thromboxane synthesis and response in platelets from premature infants. Pediatr Res 41:218–223, 1997.

50. Corby DG, Schulman I. The effects of antenatal drug administration on aggregation of platelets of newborn infants. J Pediatr 79:307–313, 1971.

51. Corby DG, O'Barr TP. Neonatal platelet function: a membrane-related phenomenon? Haemostasis 10:177–185, 1981.

52. Louden KA, Broughton Pipkin F, Heptinstall S, et al. Neonatal platelet reactivity and serum thromboxane B2 production in whole blood: the effect of maternal low dose aspirin. Br J Obstet Gynaecol 101:203–208, 1994.

53. Mull MM, Hathaway WE. Altered platelet function in newborns. Pediatr Res 4:229–237, 1970.

54. Ts'ao CH, Green D, Schultz K. Function and ultrastructure of platelets of neonates: enhanced ristocetin aggregation of neonatal platelets. Br J Haematol 32:225–233, 1976.

55. Israels SJ, Daniels M, McMillan EM. Deficient collagen-induced activation in the newborn platelet. Pediatr Res 27:337–343, 1990.

56. Corby DG, O'Barr TP. Decreased alpha-adrenergic receptors in newborn platelets: cause of abnormal response to epinephrine. Dev Pharmacol Ther 2:215–225, 1981.

57. Gelman B, Setty BN, Chen D, et al. Impaired mobilization of intracellular calcium in neonatal platelets. Pediatr Res 39:692–696, 1996.

58. Israels SJ, Rand ML, Michelson AD. Neonatal platelet function. Semin Thromb Hemost 29:363–372, 2003.

59. Israels SJ, Andrew M. Haemostasis and thrombosis (3rd edn). Edinburgh (UK); 1994.

60. Shenkman B, Linder N, Savion N, et al. Increased neonatal platelet deposition on subendothelium under flow conditions: the role of plasma von Willebrand factor. Pediatr Res 45:270–275, 1999.

61. Andrew M, Paes B, Milner R, et al. Development of the human coagulation system in the full-term infant. Blood 70:165–172, 1987.

62. Andrew M, Paes B, Milner R, et al. Development of the human coagulation system in the healthy premature infant. Blood 72:1651–1657, 1988.

63. Katz JA, Moake JL, McPherson PD, et al. Relationship between human development and disappearance of unusually large von Willebrand factor multimers from plasma. Blood 73:1851–1858, 1989.

64. Weinstein MJ, Blanchard R, Moake JL, et al. Fetal and neonatal von Willebrand factor (vWF) is unusually large and similar to the vWF in patients with thrombotic thrombocytopenic purpura. Br J Haematol 72:68–72, 1989.

65. Johnson SS, Montgomery RR, Hathaway WE. Newborn factor VIII complex: elevated activities in term infants and alterations in electrophoretic mobility related to illness and activated coagulation. Br J Haematol 47:597–606, 1981.

66. Watala C, Golanski J, Rozalski M, et al. Is platelet aggregation a more important contributor than platelet adhesion to the overall platelet-related primary haemostasis measured by PFA-100? Thromb Res 109:299–306, 2003.

67. Gatti L, Guarneri D, Caccamo ML, et al. Platelet activation in newborns detected by flow-cytometry. Biol Neonate 70:322–327, 1996.

68. Pietrucha T, Wojciechowski T, Greger J, et al. Differentiated reactivity of whole blood neonatal platelets to various agonists. Platelets 12:99–107, 2001.

69. Kuhne T, Imbach P. Neonatal platelet physiology and pathophysiology. Eur J Pediatr 157:87–94, 1998.

70. Grosshaupt B, Muntean W, Sedlmayr P. Hyporeactivity of neonatal platelets is not caused by preactivation during birth. Eur J Pediatr 156:944–948, 1997.

71. Rajasekhar D, Kestin AS, Bednarek FJ, et al. Neonatal platelets are less reactive than adult platelets to physiological agonists in whole blood. Thromb Haemost 72:957–963, 1994.

72. Rajasekhar D, Barnard MR, Bednarek FJ, Michelson AD. Platelet hyporeactivity in very low birth weight neonates. Thromb Haemost 77:1002–1007, 1997.

73. Sitaru AG, Holzhauer S, Speer CP, et al. Neonatal platelets from cord blood and peripheral blood. Platelets 16:203–210, 2005.

74. Hezard N, Potron G, Schlegel N, et al. Unexpected persistence of platelet hyporeactivity beyond the neonatal period: a flow cytometric study in neonates, infants and older children. Thromb Haemost 90:116–123, 2003.

75. Andrew M, Paes B, Bowker J, et al. Evaluation of an automated bleeding time device in the newborn. Am J Hematol 35:275–277, 1990.

76. Fernandez F, Goudable C, Sie P, et al. Low haematocrit and prolonged bleeding time in uraemic patients: effect of red cell transfusions. Br J Haematol 59:139–148, 1985.

77. Aarts PA, Bolhuis PA, Sakariassen KS, et al. Red blood cell size is important for adherence of blood platelets to artery subendothelium. Blood 62:214–217, 1983.

78. Andrew M, Paes B, Johnston M. Development of the hemostatic system in the neonate and young infant. Am J Pediatr Hematol Oncol 12:95–104, 1990.

79. Sola MC, del Vecchio A, Edwards TJ, et al. The relationship between hematocrit and bleeding time in very low birth weight infants during the first week of life. J Perinatol 21:368–371, 2001.

80. Andrew M, Castle V, Saigal S, et al. Clinical impact of neonatal thrombocytopenia. J Pediatr 110:457–464, 1987.

81. Diamond LK, Porter FS. The inadequacies of routine bleeding and clotting times. N Engl J Med 259:1025–1027, 1958.

82. Peterson P, Hayes TE, Arkin CF, et al. The preoperative bleeding time test lacks clinical benefit: College of American Pathologists' and American Society of Clinical Pathologists' position article. Arch Surg 133:134–139, 1998.

83. Rodgers RP, Levin J. A critical reappraisal of the bleeding time. Semin Thromb Hemost 16:1–20, 1990.

84. Varon D, Dardik R, Shenkman B, et al. A new method for quantitative analysis of whole blood platelet interaction with extracellular matrix under flow conditions. Thromb Res 85:283–294, 1997.

85. Linder N, Shenkman B, Levin E, et al. Deposition of whole blood platelets on extracellular matrix under flow conditions in preterm infants. Arch Dis Child Fetal Neonatal Ed 86:F127–130, 2002.

86. Finkelstein Y, Shenkman B, Sirota L, et al. Whole blood platelet deposition on extracellular matrix under flow conditions in preterm neonatal sepsis. Eur J Pediatr 161:270–274, 2002. Epub 2002 Mar 2016.

87. Roschitz B, Sudi K, Kostenberger M, et al. Shorter PFA-100 closure times in neonates than in adults: role of red cells, white cells, platelets and von Willebrand factor. Acta Paediatr 90:664–670, 2001.

88. Mammen EF, Alshameeri RS, Comp PC. Preliminary data from a field trial of the PFA-100 system. Semin Thromb Hemost 21:113–121, 1995.

89. Kundu SK, Heilmann EJ, Sio R, et al. Description of an in vitro platelet function analyzer – PFA-100. Semin Thromb Hemost 21:106–112, 1995.

90. Boudewijns M, Raes M, Peeters V, et al. Evaluation of platelet function on cord blood in 80 healthy term neonates using the Platelet Function Analyzer (PFA-100); shorter in vitro bleeding times in neonates than adults. Eur J Pediatr 162:212–213, 2003.

91. Carcao MD, Blanchette VS, Dean JA, et al. The Platelet Function Analyzer (PFA-100): a novel in-vitro system for evaluation of primary haemostasis in children. Br J Haematol 101:70–73, 1998.

92. Israels SJ, Cheang T, McMillan-Ward EM, et al. Evaluation of primary hemostasis in neonates with a new in vitro platelet function analyzer. J Pediatr 138:116–119, 2001.

93. Saxonhouse MS, Rimsza LR, Christensen RD, et al. PFA-100 closure time in thrombocytopenic and non-thrombocytopenic neonates. Pediatr Res 55:289a, 2004.

94. Saxonhouse MA, Rimsza LR, Stevens G, et al. Neonatal thrombocytopenia and PFA-100 closure times. Pediatr Res. 2005.

95. Pahal GS, Jauniaux E, Kinnon C, Thrasher AJ, et al. Normal development of human fetal hematopoiesis between eight and seventeen weeks' gestation. Am J Obstet Gynecol 183:1029–1034, 2000.

96. Sola MC, Slayton WB, Rimsza LM, et al. A neonate with severe thrombocytopenia and radio-ulnar synostosis. J Perinatol 24:528–530, 2004.

97. Grossfeld PD, Mattina T, Lai Z, et al. The 11q terminal deletion disorder: a prospective study of 110 cases. Am J Med Genet A 129:51–61, 2004.

98. Drachman JG. Inherited thrombocytopenia: when a low platelet count does not mean ITP. Blood 103:390–398, 2004. Epub 2003 Sep 2022.

99. Pedersen-Bjergaard U, Andersen M, Hansen PB. Drug-specific characteristics of thrombocytopenia caused by non-cytotoxic drugs. Eur J Clin Pharmacol 54:701–706, 1998.

100. Dlott JS, Danielson CF, Blue-Hnidy DE, et al. Drug-induced thrombotic thrombocytopenic purpura/hemolytic uremic syndrome: a concise review. Ther Apher Dial 8:102–111, 2004.

101. Aster RH. Drug-induced immune cytopenias. Toxicology 209:149–153, 2005. Epub 2005 Jan 2027.

102. Aranda JV, Portuguez-Malavasi A, Collinge JM, et al. Epidemiology of adverse drug reactions in the newborn. Dev Pharmacol Ther 5:173–184, 1982.

103. Kumar P, Hoppensteadt DA, Prechel MM, et al. Prevalance of heparin-dependent platelet-activating antibodies in preterm newborns after exposure to unfractionated heparin. Clin Appl Thromb Hemost 10:335–339, 2004.

104. Nguyen TN, Gal P, Ransom JL, et al. Lepirudin use in a neonate with heparin-induced thrombocytopenia. Ann Pharmacother 37:229–233, 2003.

105. Schmugge M, Risch L, Huber AR, et al. Heparin-induced thrombocytopenia-associated thrombosis in pediatric intensive care patients. Pediatrics 109:E10, 2002.

106. Spadone D, Clark F, James E, et al. Heparin-induced thrombocytopenia in the newborn. J Vasc Surg 15:306–311, 1992; discussion 311–302.

107. Landmann E, Bluetters-Sawatzki R, Schindler D, et al. Fanconi anemia in a neonate with pancytopenia. J Pediatr 145:125–127, 2004.

108. Butturini A, Gale RP, Verlander PC, et al. Hematologic abnormalities in Fanconi anemia: an International Fanconi Anemia Registry study. Blood 84:1650–1655, 1994.

109. Bussel JB. Alloimmune thrombocytopenia in the fetus and newborn. Semin Thromb Hemost 27:245–252, 2001.

110. Blanchette VS, Rand ML. Platelet disorders in newborn infants: diagnosis and management. Semin Perinatol 21:53–62, 1997.

111. Saxonhouse MA, Rimsza LM, Stevens G, et al. Effects of hypoxia on megakaryocyte progenitors obtained from the umbilical cord blood of term and preterm neonates. Biol Neonate 89:104–108, 2005.

112. Saxonhouse MA, Rimsza LM, Christensen RD, et al. Effects of anoxia on megakaryocyte progenitors derived from cord blood CD34pos cells. Eur J Haematol 71:359–365, 2003.

113. Harker LA, Finch CA. Thrombokinetics in man. J Clin Invest 48:963–974, 1969.

114. Cole JL, Marzec UM, Gunthel CJ, et al. Ineffective platelet production in thrombocytopenic human immunodeficiency virus-infected patients. Blood 91:3239–3246, 1998.

115. Tate DY, Carlton GT, Johnson D, et al. Immune thrombocytopenia in severe neonatal infections. J Pediatr 98:449–453, 1981.

116. Andrew M, Vegh P, Caco C, et al. A randomized, controlled trial of platelet transfusions in thrombocytopenic premature infants. J Pediatr 123:285–291, 1993.

117. Garcia MG, Duenas E, Sola MC, et al. Epidemiologic and outcome studies of patients who received platelet transfusions in the neonatal intensive care unit. J Perinatol 21:415–420, 2001.

118. Del Vecchio A, Sola MC, Theriaque DW, et al. Platelet transfusions in the neonatal intensive care unit:factors predicting which patients will require multiple transfusions. Transfusion 41:803–808, 2001.

119. Gibson BE, Todd A, Roberts I, et al. Transfusion guidelines for neonates and older children. Br J Haematol 124:433–453, 2004.

120. Strauss RG, Levy GJ, Sotelo-Avila C, et al. National survey of neonatal transfusion practices: II. Blood component therapy. Pediatrics 91:530–536, 1993.

121. Strauss R. Blood banking and transfusion issues in perinatal medicine. In: Christensen R, ed. Hematologic problems of the neonate. Philadelphia: W.B. Saunders, 2000.

122. Miller WJ, McCullough J, Balfour HH, Jr., et al. Prevention of cytomegalovirus infection following bone marrow transplantation: a randomized trial of blood product screening. Bone Marrow Transplant 7:227–234, 1991.

123. Lang DJ, Ebert PA, Rodgers BM, et al. Reduction of postperfusion cytomegalovirus-infections following the use of leukocyte depleted blood. Transfusion 17:391–395, 1977.

124. Zwicky C, Tissot JD, Mazouni ZT, et al. [Prevention of post-transfusion cytomegalovirus infection: recommendations for clinical practice]. Schweiz Med Wochenschr 129:1061–1066, 1999.

125. Blajchman MA, Goldman M, Freedman JJ, et al. Proceedings of a consensus conference: prevention of post-transfusion CMV in the era of universal leukoreduction. Transfus Med Rev 15:1–20, 2001.

126. Eisenfeld L, Silver H, McLaughlin J, et al. Prevention of transfusion-associated cytomegalovirus infection in neonatal patients by the removal of white cells from blood. Transfusion 32:205–209, 1992.

127. Strauss RG. Selection of white cell-reduced blood components for transfusions during early infancy. Transfusion 33:352–357, 1993.

128. Gilbert GL, Hayes K, Hudson IL, et al. Prevention of transfusion-acquired cytomegalovirus infection in infants by blood filtration to remove leucocytes. Neonatal Cytomegalovirus Infection Study Group. Lancet 1:1228–1231, 1989.

129. Saxonhouse MA, Slayton W, Sola MC. Platelet transfusions in the infant and child. In: Hillyer CD, Strauss RG, Luban NLC, eds. Handbook of pediatric transfusion medicine. San Diego: Elsevier Academic Press; 2004: 253–269.

130. Strauss RG. Data-driven blood banking practices for neonatal RBC transfusions. Transfusion 40:1528–1540, 2000.

131. Sanders MR, Graeber JE. Posttransfusion graft-versus-host disease in infancy. J Pediatr 117:159–163, 1990.

132. Ohto H, Anderson KC. Posttransfusion graft-versus-host disease in Japanese newborns. Transfusion 36:117–123, 1996.

133. Bussel JB. Fetal neonatal thrombocytopenia. Thromb Haemost 74:426–428, 1995.

134. Blanchette VS. Neonatal alloimmune thrombocytopenia: a clinical perspective. Curr Stud Hematol Blood Transfus 54:112–126, 1988.

135. Davoren A, Curtis BR, Aster RH, et al. Human platelet antigen-specific alloantibodies implicated in 1162 cases of neonatal alloimmune thrombocytopenia. Transfusion 44:1220–1225, 2004.

136. Peterson JA, Balthazor SM, Curtis BR, et al. Maternal alloimmunization against the rare platelet-specific antigen HPA-9b (Max a) is an important cause of neonatal alloimmune thrombocytopenia. Transfusion 45:1487–1495, 2005.

137. Mandelbaum M, Koren D, Eichelberger B, et al. Frequencies of maternal platelet alloantibodies and autoantibodies in suspected fetal/neonatal alloimmune thrombocytopenia, with emphasis on human platelet antigen-15 alloimmunization. Vox Sang 89:39–43, 2005.

138. Ertel K, Al-Tawil M, Santoso S, et al. Relevance of the HPA-15 (Gov) polymorphism on CD109 in alloimmune thrombocytopenic syndromes. Transfusion 45:366–373, 2005.

139. Kroll H, Yates J, Santoso S. Immunization against a low-frequency human platelet alloantigen in fetal alloimmune thrombocytopenia is not a single event: characterization by the combined use of reference DNA and novel allele-specific cell lines expressing recombinant antigens. Transfusion 45:353–358, 2005.

140. Kaplan C. Immune thrombocytopenia in the foetus and the newborn: diagnosis and therapy. Transfus Clin Biol 8:311–314, 2001.

141. de Alarcon PA. Newborn platelet disorders. In: de Alarcon PA, Werner E, eds. Neonatal Hematology, Vol. 1. New York: Cambridge University Press; 2005:187-253.

142. Blanchette VS, Johnson J, Rand M. The management of alloimmune neonatal thrombocytopenia. Baillieres Best Pract Res Clin Haematol 13:365–390, 2000.

143. Massey GV, McWilliams NB, Mueller DG, et al. Intravenous immunoglobulin in treatment of neonatal isoimmune thrombocytopenia. J Pediatr 111:133–135, 1987.

144. Sidiropoulos D, Straume B. The treatment of neonatal isoimmune thrombocytopenia with intravenous immunoglobin (IgG i.v.). Blut 48:383–386, 1984.

145. Calhoun DA, Christensen RD, Edstrom CS, et al. Consistent approaches to procedures and practices in neonatal hematology. Clin Perinatol 27:733–753, 2000.

146. Kurzrock R. Thrombopoietic factors in chronic bone marrow failure states: the platelet problem revisited. Clin Cancer Res 11:1361–1367, 2005.
147. Kurzrock R, Talpaz M, Estrov Z, et al. Phase I study of recombinant human interleukin-3 in patients with bone marrow failure. J Clin Oncol 9:1241–1250, 1991.
148. Scadden DT, Levine JD, Bresnahan J, et al. In vivo effects of interleukin 3 in HIV type 1-infected patients with cytopenia. AIDS Res Hum Retroviruses 11:731–740, 1995.
149. Guinan EC, Lee YS, Lopez KD, et al. Effects of interleukin-3 and granulocyte-macrophage colony-stimulating factor on thrombopoiesis in congenital amegakaryocytic thrombocytopenia. Blood 81:1691–1698, 1993.
150. Nimer SD, Paquette RL, Ireland P, et al. A phase I/II study of interleukin-3 in patients with aplastic anemia and myelodysplasia. Exp Hematol 22:875–880, 1994.
151. Ganser A, Lindemann A, Seipelt G, et al. Effects of recombinant human interleukin-3 in aplastic anemia. Blood 76:1287–1292, 1990.
152. Wu HH, Talpaz M, Champlin RE, et al. Sequential interleukin 3 and granulocyte-macrophage-colony stimulating factor therapy in patients with bone marrow failure with long-term follow-up of responses. Cancer 98:2410–2419, 2003.
153. Asano S, Okano A, Ozawa K, et al. In vivo effects of recombinant human interleukin-6 in primates: stimulated production of platelets. Blood 75:1602–1605, 1990.
154. Bruno E, Hoffman R. Effect of interleukin 6 on in vitro human megakaryocytopoiesis: its interaction with other cytokines. Exp Hematol 17:1038–1043, 1989.
155. Hill RJ, Warren MK, Levin J. Stimulation of thrombopoiesis in mice by human recombinant interleukin 6. J Clin Invest 85:1242–1247, 1990.
156. Ishibashi T, Kimura H, Uchida T, et al. Human interleukin 6 is a direct promoter of maturation of megakaryocytes in vitro. Proc Natl Acad Sci USA 86:5953–5957, 1989.
157. Ishibashi T, Kimura H, Shikama Y, et al. Interleukin-6 is a potent thrombopoietic factor in vivo in mice. Blood 74:1241–1244, 1989.
158. Pojda Z, Tsuboi A. In vivo effects of human recombinant interleukin 6 on hemopoietic stem and progenitor cells and circulating blood cells in normal mice. Exp Hematol 18:1034–1037, 1990.
159. Stahl CP, Zucker-Franklin D, Evatt BL, et al. Effects of human interleukin-6 on megakaryocyte development and thrombocytopoiesis in primates. Blood 78:1467–1475, 1991.
160. Gordon MS, Nemunaitis J, Hoffman R, et al. A phase I trial of recombinant human interleukin-6 in patients with myelodysplastic syndromes and thrombocytopenia. Blood 85:3066–3076, 1995.
161. Isaacs C, Robert NJ, Bailey FA, et al. Randomized placebo-controlled study of recombinant human interleukin-11 to prevent chemotherapy-induced thrombocytopenia in patients with breast cancer receiving dose-intensive cyclophosphamide and doxorubicin. J Clin Oncol 15:3368–3377, 1997.
162. Smith JW, 2nd. Tolerability and side-effect profile of rhIL-11. Oncology (Williston Park) 14:41–47, 2000.
163. Bussel JB, Mukherjee R, Stone AJ. A pilot study of rhuIL-11 treatment of refractory ITP. Am J Hematol 66:172–177, 2001.
164. Dickinson EC, Tuncer R, Nadler EP, et al. Recombinant human interleukin-11 prevents mucosal atrophy and bowel shortening in the defunctionalized intestine. J Pediatr Surg 35:1079–1083, 2000.
165. Nadler EP, Stanford A, Zhang XR, et al. Intestinal cytokine gene expression in infants with acute necrotizing enterocolitis: interleukin-11 mRNA expression inversely correlates with extent of disease. J Pediatr Surg 36:1122–1129, 2001.
166. Chang M, Williams A, Ishizawa L, et al. Endogenous interleukin-11 (IL-11) expression is increased and prophylactic use of exogenous IL-11 enhances platelet recovery and improves survival during thrombocytopenia associated with experimental group B streptococcal sepsis in neonatal rats. Blood Cells Mol Dis 22:57–67, 1996.
167. Li Z, Godinho FJ, Klusmann JH, et al. Developmental stage-selective effect of somatically mutated leukemogenic transcription factor GATA1. Nat Genet 37:613–619, 2005. Epub 2005 May 2015.
168. Erickson MC, Delorme E, Giampa L, et al. Biological activity and selectivity for Tpo receptor agonist, SB-497115. Blood 104:796a, 2004.
169. Broudy VC, Lin NL. AMG531 stimulates megakaryopoiesis in vitro by binding to Mpl. Cytokine 25:52–60, 2004.
170. Li J, Yang C, Xia Y, et al. Thrombocytopenia caused by the development of antibodies to thrombopoietin. Blood 98:3241–3248, 2001.
171. Basser RL, O'Flaherty E, Green M, et al. Development of pancytopenia with neutralizing antibodies to thrombopoietin after multicycle chemotherapy supported by megakaryocyte growth and development factor. Blood 99:2599–2602, 2002.
172. Brown JR, Demetri GD. Challenges in the development of platelet growth factors: low expectations for low counts. Curr Hematol Rep 1:110–118, 2002.
173. Lusher JM, Roberts HR, Davignon G, et al. A randomized, double-blind comparison of two dosage levels of recombinant factor VIIa in the treatment of joint, muscle and mucocutaneous haemorrhages in persons with haemophilia A and B, with and without inhibitors. rFVIIa Study Group. rFVIIa Study Group. Haemophilia 4:790–798, 1998.
174. Lusher JM. Early treatment with recombinant factor VIIa results in greater efficacy with less product. Eur J Haematol Suppl 63:7–10, 1998.
175. Kristensen J, Killander A, Hippe E, et al. Clinical experience with recombinant factor VIIa in patients with thrombocytopenia. Haemostasis 26:159–164, 1996.

176. Laurian Y. Treatment of bleeding in patients with platelet disorders: is there a place for recombinant factor VIIa? Pathophysiol Haemost Thromb 32:37–40, 2002.
177. Almeida AM, Khair K, Hann I, et al. The use of recombinant factor VIIa in children with inherited platelet function disorders. Br J Haematol 121:477–481, 2003.
178. Chuansumrit A, Nuntnarumit P, Okascharoen C, et al. The use of recombinant activated factor VII to control bleeding in a preterm infant undergoing exploratory laparotomy. Pediatrics 110:169–171, 2002.
179. Chuansumrit A, Visanuyothin N, Puapunwattana S, et al. Outcome of intracranial hemorrhage in infants with congenital factor VII deficiency. J Med Assoc Thai 85 Suppl 4:S1059–1064, 2002.
180. Wong WY, Huang WC, Miller R, et al. Clinical efficacy and recovery levels of recombinant FVIIa (NovoSeven) in the treatment of intracranial haemorrhage in severe neonatal FVII deficiency. Haemophilia 6:50–54, 2000.
181. Olomu N, Kulkarni R, Manco-Johnson M. Treatment of severe pulmonary hemorrhage with activated recombinant factor VII (rFVIIa) in very low birth weight infants. J Perinatol 22:672–674, 2002.
182. Hedberg VA, Lipton JM. Thrombocytopenia with absent radii. A review of 100 cases. Am J Pediatr Hematol Oncol 10:51–64, 1988.
183. Hall JG, Levin J, Kuhn JP, et al. Thrombocytopenia with absent radius (TAR). Medicine (Baltimore) 48:411–439, 1969.
184. Fayen WT, Harris JW. Thrombocytopenia with absent radii (the TAR syndrome). Am J Med Sci 280:95–99, 1980.
185. Freson K, Devriendt K, Matthijs G, et al. Platelet characteristics in patients with X-linked macrothrombocytopenia because of a novel GATA1 mutation. Blood 98:85–92, 2001.
186. Del Vecchio GC, Giordani L, De Santis A, et al. Dyserythropoietic anemia and thrombocytopenia due to a novel mutation in GATA-1. Acta Haematol 114:113–116, 2005.
187. Savoia A, Del Vecchio M, Totaro A, et al. An autosomal dominant thrombocytopenia gene maps to chromosomal region 10p. Am J Hum Genet 65:1401–1405, 1999.
188. Drachman JG, Jarvik GP, Mehaffey MG. Autosomal dominant thrombocytopenia: incomplete megakaryocyte differentiation and linkage to human chromosome 10. Blood 96:118–125, 2000.
189. Roseff SD, Luban NL, Manno CS. Guidelines for assessing appropriateness of pediatric transfusion. ransfusion 42:1398–1413, 2002.

Chapter 3

The Role of Recombinant Leukocyte Colony-Stimulating Factors in the Neonatal Intensive Care Unit

Robert D. Christensen, MD

Neutrophils in Host Defense

Neutropenia in a Neonate

Severe Chronic Neutropenia in the Neonate

Neonatal Neutropenia Not Categorized as Severe Chronic Neutropenia

A Consistent Approach to the use of rG-CSF in the NICU

NEUTROPHILS IN HOST DEFENSE

Neutrophils are pivotal to the process of antibacterial host defense (1, 2). Individuals who lack neutrophils, whether by a congenital or acquired defect, will experience a natural history that includes repeated local and systemic infections and early death (3, 4). Severe chronic neutropenia (SCN) is a cluster of diagnoses bearing the common feature of very low circulating neutrophil concentrations, present from birth (5, 6). The advent of recombinant granulocyte colony-stimulating factor (rG-CSF) dramatically improved the lives of patients with SCN, elevating their circulating neutrophil concentrations, markedly reducing infectious illnesses, and extending their life expectancy (3, 7).

Rarely, patients with SCN are diagnosed as neonates, or even as patients in neonatal intensive care units (8, 9). However, the majority of patients with SCN are not diagnosed until several months of age, after many infectious episodes have prompted an evaluation into immunological deficiencies. When SCN is diagnosed in a neonate, that patient should receive the benefit of rG-CSF treatment (3, 7–10). Whether neonates who have other varieties of neutropenia, distinct from SCN, benefit from rG-CSF treatment is less clear (11–15). This chapter will review the biological plausibility and the clinical trials aimed at testing rG-CSF treatment for neonates with neutropenia of the SCN category and not of the SCN category. The chapter is divided into the diagnosis of neutropenia in a neonate, the use of rG-CSF in neonates with SCN, and the potential use of rG-CSF in neonates who have varieties of neutropenia other than SCN.

NEUTROPENIA IN A NEONATE

The definition of neutropenia in a neonate can be ambiguous. One method involves determining whether the blood neutrophil concentration is below an expected time post-birth standard. The Manroe chart (16) and the Mouzinho chart (17) are examples of this approach (Fig. 3-1). Applying these definition to neonates >1500 g (11) or <1500 g (12) in the first days of life requires consulting a figure or table to determine whether the patient's count is below the lower standard. For example, at 18 h after birth, a neonate >1500 g with a blood neutrophil concentration of 5000/µL would be labeled as neutropenic, but at 72 h the count must fall to <1500/µL to warrant the definition of neutropenia.

A simpler approach is to define neutropenia by a blood neutrophil concentration <1000/µL, and to define severe neutropenia by a count <500/µL (10). Although this approach lacks the accuracy, and the data-derivation, of the Manroe (16) and Mouzinho (17) approach, it has the advantages that it is easy to remember and that it is in keeping with the standard definition for neutropenia used in pediatric and adult medicine (18, 19). Furthermore, it is not clear whether blood neutrophil counts labeled as low by the Manroe and Mouzinho approach actually convey a host-defense deficiency, unless they are <1000/µL.

SEVERE CHRONIC NEUTROPENIA IN THE NEONATE

Kostmann Syndrome

Table 3-1 lists varieties of neutropenia that are generally considered as part of the SCN syndrome. The prototype for SCN is Kostmann syndrome, initially described

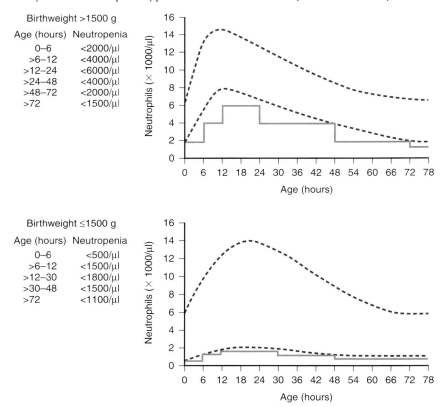

Figure 3-1 Definitions of neutropenia (16, 17). From Funke A, Berner R, Traichel B, et al. Frequency, natural course, and outcome of neonatal neutropenia. Pediatrics 106:45–51, 2000.

Table 3-1	Varieties of Neutropenia Among Neonates that are Generally Considered "Severe Chronic Neutropenia"

Kostmann syndrome
Shwachman-Diamond syndrome
Barth syndrome
Cartilage-hair hypoplasia
Cyclic neutropenia
Glycogen storage disease type 1b
Severe immune-mediated neonatal neutropenias

in 1956 within a kindred in northern Sweden (20–23). Patients with this variety of SCN generally have circulating neutrophil concentrations <200/μL, and a marrow aspirate or biopsy shows a "maturation arrest" where few neutrophilic cells are seen beyond the promyelocyte stage. The original family had what appeared to be an autosomal recessive disorder, but most kindreds subsequently reported seem to have an autosomal dominant inheritance. The condition is the result of mutations in the ELA2 (neutrophil elastase) gene (24–26). Although rG-CSF treatment is effective in increasing blood neutrophils and reducing febrile illnesses, it does not generally correct the gingivitis that is a prominent feature of this condition in some families. This is probably because rG-CSF does not increase the natural antimicrobial peptide (LL-37) deficiency in these patients (27, 28).

Shwachman-Diamond Syndrome

This variety of severe chronic neutropenia is generally diagnosed after manifestations of exocrine pancreatic insufficiency, with diarrhea and failure to thrive. It is generally an autosomal recessive condition. Some children with this syndrome respond favorably to rG-CSF, yet some progress to bone marrow failure and require bone marrow transplantation (29, 30).

Barth Syndrome

These patients are generally males (X- linked) with dilated cardiomyopathy, organic aciduria, growth failure, muscle weakness, and neutropenia (31). The underlying genetic abnormality has not yet been mapped. rG-CSF can be helpful in patients as an adjunct to treating infections, or as a preventive measure if their neutropenia is sufficiently severe (32, 33).

Cartilage-hair Hypoplasia

This is a form of short-limbed dwarfism associated with frequent infections. These patients have short pudgy hands, redundant skin, and hyperextensible joints in the hands and feet but flexor contractions at the elbow. Neutropenia occurs in some patients with cartilage-hair hypoplasia and these have been reported to benefit from rG-CSF administration (34).

Cyclic Neutropenia

This condition is caused by mutation in the ELA2 (neutrophil elastase) gene, and results in periodic drops in blood neutrophil concentration, generally on an every 3 to sometimes 4-week cycle (30, 31). Counts can drop to <500/μL or lower, and infections can be a periodic problem (35, 36). Because it generally takes several cycles before the diagnosis is considered, most cases are not diagnosed as neonates. rG-CSF administration is useful in preventing the very low nadir counts and in preventing infectious complications (7, 37).

Glycogen Storage Disease Type 1b

von Gierke disease is an autosomal recessive disorder caused by a deficiency of the enzyme glucose-6-phosphate translocase, which transports glucose-6-phosphate into the endoplasmic reticulum for further metabolism. In GSD-1b, glucose-6-phosphate accumulates intracellularly. Affected neonates present with hypoglycemia, hepatomegaly, growth failure, and neutropenia. Patients with GSD-1b have recurrent bacterial infections, oral ulcers, and inflammatory bowel disease. The gene causing GSD-1b is located on chromosome 11q23 (38). rG-CSF can help these patients avoid the recurrent bacterial infections that are otherwise a problematic part of this condition.

Severe Immune-Mediated Neonatal Neutropenia

Most of the very severe and prolonged immune-mediated neutropenias in the neonate are alloimmune (39–42). However, a few severe and prolonged cases of neonatal neutropenia have been found to be autoimmune neutropenia (maternal autoimmune disease) (42, 43), and a few have been found to be autoimmune neutropenia of infancy (a primary isolated autoimmune phenomenon in neonates) (42, 44).

Alloimmune neonatal neutropenia is a relatively common condition where the mother develops antibodies to antigens present on paternal and fetal neutrophils (39–43). Antineutrophil antibodies have been found in the serum of as many as 20% of randomly surveyed pregnant and postpartum women (42, 43). Most such antibodies cause little problem to the fetus and neonate, but up to 2% of consecutively sampled neonates have neutropenia on this basis. This variety of neutropenia can be severe and prolonged, with a median duration of neutropenia of about 7 weeks, but a range up to 6 months. Repeated infections can occur in these patients until their severe neutropenia remits. Delayed separation of the umbilical cord and skin infections are the most common infectious complications, but serious and life-threatening infections can occur. The mortality rate in this condition, due to overwhelming infection, is reported to be 5% (38). Severe cases have been successfully treated with rG-CSF (38). Unlike patients with other varieties of SCN, the neutropenia in this condition will remit spontaneously and the rG-CSF treatment can be stopped. Remission occurs when maternal antineutrophil antibody in the neonate has dropped significantly.

Neonatal autoimmune neutropenia occurs when mothers have autoimmune diseases, and their antineutrophil antibodies cross the placenta and bind to fetal neutrophils. Clinical features are generally much more mild than in alloimmune neonatal neutropenia and it is rare that a patient with this variety of neonatal neutropenia needs rG-CSF treatment (37, 38).

Autoimmune neutropenia of infancy is an unusual disorder where the fetus, and subsequently the neonate, has a primary isolated autoimmune phenomenon (45–49). Neutrophil-specific antibodies are found in the neonate's serum, reactive against his/her own neutrophils, but no antibodies are found in the mother's serum. Most cases occur in children between 3 and 30 months of age, with a reported incidence of 1:100 000 children. Affected children present with minor infections. Bux et al. reported 240 cases and reported that 12% presented with severe infections, including pneumonia, sepsis, or meningitis (47). The neutropenia in this condition generally persists much longer than in cases of alloimmune neutropenia, with a median duration of about 30 months and a range from 6 to 60 months (48, 49). This variety of neonatal neutropenia can be severe, with blood neutrophil concentrations often <500/µL. rG-CSF administration can increase the neutrophil count and reduce infections complications (47, 49).

Table 3-2   Varieties of Neutropenia Among Neonates that are NOT Classified as "Severe Chronic Neutropenia"

Pregnancy-induced hypertension
Severe intrauterine growth restriction
The twin-twin transfusion syndrome
Rh hemolytic disease
Bacterial infection
Fungal infection
Necrotizing enterocolitis
Chronic idiopathic neutropenia of prematurity

NEONATAL NEUTROPENIA NOT CATEGORIZED AS SEVERE CHRONIC NEUTROPENIA

Table 3-2 lists varieties of neutropenia that are not considered as part of the SCN syndrome.

Pregnancy-Induced Hypertension

This is the most common variety of neutropenia seen in the NICU (50–57). Perhaps 50% of neonates born to mothers with PIH have this variety of neutropenia. The ANC can be very low, frequently <500/μL, but the count generally rises spontaneously within the first days, and is almost always >1000/μL by day 2 or 3. Usually no leukocyte "left shift" is seen, and no toxic granulation, Dohle bodies, or vacuolization are present in the neutrophils. It is not clear whether this variety of neutropenia predisposes neonates to acquire bacterial infection. Usually the condition is so transient that such a predisposition is unlikely. The condition is probably caused by an inhibitor of neutrophil production of placental origin that might function mechanically by depressing natural G-CSF production (51–53).

Severe Intrauterine Growth Restriction

This variety of neonatal neutropenia seems to be identical to that associated with PIH. In a recent study, we observed no difference in the onset, duration, or severity of neutropenia in SGA neonates vs. neonates born after PIH (58). Obviously, some neonates born after PIH are also SGA, and it might be that the most severe neutropenias in this category are among those with both PIH and SGA. We assume that the neutropenias of PIH and SGA are mechanistically similar, and that both are transient with few clinical consequences, and no need of rG-CSF administration.

The Twin-Twin Transfusion Syndrome

The donor in a twin-twin transfusion is generally neutropenic, but the recipient can also have neutropenia, although usually not as severe (59). As with the varieties of neutropenia accompanying PIH and SGA, there is generally no leukocyte "left shift" nor are there neutrophil morphological abnormalities. This condition is also transient, with the ANC generally spontaneously rising to >1000/μL by 2 or 3 days, and thus no rG-CSF administration is warranted.

Rh Hemolytic Disease

Neonates with anemia from Rh hemolytic disease are almost always neutropenic on the first day of life (60). This variety of neutropenia is similar to that of PIH/SGA and donors in a twin-twin transfusion, and is probably due to reduced neutrophil production. The neutropenia is transient, generally resolving in a day or two, and thus no specific treatment is generally required.

Bacterial Infection

Two strategies have been proposed for rG-CSF usage during neonatal infections. Since neutropenia commonly accompanies overwhelming septic shock in neonates, perhaps rG-CSF might be a reasonable adjunct to antibiotics and intensive care treatment. Second, since neutrophil function, particularly chemotaxis, is immature among neonates, perhaps rG-CSF administration might be a reasonable way to prevent nosocomial infections among high-risk neonatal patients. Animal models for both potential uses of rG-CSF were established and supported these hypotheses. In a Cochrane review, Carr et al. examined both potential uses (61). They located seven studies (involving 257 neonates) where infected neonates were treated with rG-CSF vs. placebo (62–68). They located three studies (359 neonates) where rG-CSF vs. placebo was used as prophylaxis against infections (69–71). They found no evidence that the addition of rG-CSF or rGM-CSF to antibiotic therapy in preterm infants with suspected systemic infection reduces immediate all-causemortality. No significant survival advantage was seen at 14 days from the start of therapy (typical RR 0.71 (95% CI 0.38, 1.33); typical RD −0.05 (95% CI −0.14, 0.04)). They conducted a subgroup analysis of 97 infants from three of the studies who, in addition to systemic infection, had a low neutrophil count (<1700/ μL) at trial entry. This subgroup did show a significant reduction in mortality by day 14 (RR 0.34 (95% CI 0.12, 0.92); RD −0.18 (95% CI −0.33, −0.03); NNT 6 (95% CI 3–33)).

The three prophylaxis studies (69–71) did not show a significant reduction in mortality in neonates receiving rGM-CSF (RR 0.59 (95% CI 0.24, 1.44); RD −0.03 (95% CI −0.08, 0.02)). The identification of sepsis as the primary outcome of prophylaxis studies has been hampered by inadequately stringent definitions of systemic infection. However, data from one study suggest that prophylactic rGM-CSF may provide protection against infection when given to preterm infants who are neutropenic (71). Carr et al. concluded that there is currently insufficient evidence to support the introduction of either rG-CSF or rGM-CSF into neonatal practice, either as treatment of established systemic infection to reduce resulting mortality, or as prophylaxis to prevent systemic infection in high-risk neonates (61). This conclusion is consistent with other meta-analyses and reviews (71–82).

Fungal Infection

Thrombocytopenia is known to accompany fungal infection in the NICU, but neutropenia can also accompany such infections. No studies have specifically focused on using rG-CSF among neutropenic neonates with fungal infection (10).

Necrotizing Enterocolitis

Neutropenia is relatively common among severe cases of NEC. Some cases are transient and resemble the neutropenia following endotoxin (83, 84). No studies have focused on using rG-CSF among neutropenic neonates with NEC.

Chronic Idiopathic Neutropenia of Prematurity

Certain preterm neonates develop neutropenia when 4–10 weeks old. This variety of neutropenia is often associated with a patient's spontaneous recovery from the anemia of prematurity. Neutrophil counts are generally <1000/μL but rarely <500/μL (85–89). The condition is transient, lasting a few weeks to perhaps a month or more. It appears to be a hyporegenerative neutropenia, because it is not accompanied by a leukocyte "left shift" or morphological abnormalities of the neutrophils. Patients with this condition have a "rG-CSF mobalizable neutrophil reserve", meaning that if rG-CSF is given, their neutrophil count increases within hours. This fact has been taken as evidence that these patients do not have a significant host-defense deficiency, as in theory they can supply neutrophils to tissues when needed (86). Thus, although these patients are neutropenic, this condition is probably benign and needs no treatment.

A CONSISTENT APPROACH TO THE USE OF rG-CSF IN THE NICU

A few years ago we proposed a schema for making decisions regarding when to use rG-CSF in the NICU (89). Our proposal was intended as a rough guideline, to serve until sufficient data accumulated for conducting an evidence-based assessment of the risks and benefits of rG-CSF use in each of the various neutropenic conditions in the NICU. Few such data have accumulated in the intervening years and we have found no need to change the schema thus far.

Briefly (Fig. 3-2), we propose that if a neonatal patient has neutropenia, and that variety of neutropenia is known, and that it is a variety of SCN, the patient should be enrolled in the SCN International Registry and treatment with rG-CSF initiated. Enrollment in the SCN International Registry can be accomplished at the website http://depts.washington.edu/registry/, using the entry criteria and exclusion criteria given in Table 3-3.

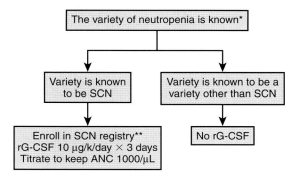

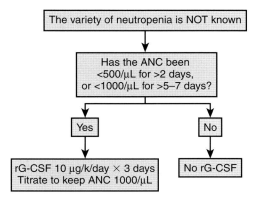

Figure 3-2 Guidelines for assisting in the decision as to which neutropenic NICU patients should be treated with rG-CSF, based on the variety of neutropenia. From Calhoun DA, Christenson RD, Edstrom CS, et al. Consistent approaches to procedures and practices in neonatal hematology. Clin Perinatol 27:733–753, 2000.

*The reason that the variety of neutropenia might be known (or highly suspected) might be on the basis of family history (Kostmann syndrome or cyclic neutropenia), or obstetrical circumstances (SGA/PIH), or neonatal circumstances (twin-twin transfusion, Rh hemolytic disease, NEC).

**The Severe Chronic Neutropenia International Registry. http://depts.washington.edu/registry/

Table 3-3	Screening for Severe Chronic Neutropenia: http://depts.washington.edu/registry/

Inclusion Questions:

1. Has a blood neutrophil count of <500/μL been documented on at least three occasions in the past 3 months?
2. Is there a history of recurrent infections? (specify)
3. Is the bone marrow evaluation consistent with severe chronic neutropenia? (date performed)
4. Has a cytogenetic evaluation been completed?
5. Is the patient now receiving Neupogen (rG-CSF)?

Exclusion Criteria

1. The neutropenia is known to be drug-induced
2. Thrombocytopenia is present (<50 000/μL) except in the case of Shwachman-Diamond syndrome of glycogen storage disease type 1b
3. Anemia is present (Hgb <8 g/dL) except in the case of Shwachman-Diamond syndrome of glycogen storage disease type 1b
4. The patient has a myelodysplastic syndrome, aplastic anemia, is HIV-positive, has some other hematological disease, has rheumatoid arthritis, or has had previous chemotherapy for cancer

We propose beginning treatment with a dose of 10 μg/kg subcutaneously, once per day for 3 consecutive days. Thereafter doses are given as needed to titrate the ANC to around 1000–1200/μL. We propose that if a neonatal patient has neutropenia, and the variety of neutropenia is known, and that variety is NOT one of the varieties of SCN, rG-CSF treatment should not be used. We propose that if a neonatal patient has neutropenia, and the variety of neutropenia is NOT known (and therefore might be an SCN variety), while evaluating the variety of neutropenia, rG-CSF treatment could be instituted if the ANC was <500/μL for 2 days or more, or <1000/μL for 5–7 days or more.

We did not include criteria for administering rGM-CSF, as we found insufficient evidence for its use in the NICU. If one follows this schema (Fig. 3-2) it will result in little use of rG-CSF in any given NICU. However, the schema should focus the rG-CSF usage on those patients with the most to gain and least to lose by its application. As additional pertinent investigative work is published, these guidelines should be modified accordingly.

REFERENCES

1. Hill HR. Biochemical, structural, and functional abnormalities of polymorphonuclear leukocytes in the neonate. Pediatr Res 22:375–382, 1987.
2. Cairo MS. Neutrophil storage pool depletion in neonates with sepsis. J Pediatr 114:1064–1065, 1989.
3. Morstyn G, Foote M, Nelson S. Clinical benefits of improving host defenses with rHuG-CSF. Ciba Found Symp 204:78–85, 1997.
4. Alter BP. Bone marrow failure syndromes in children. Pediatr Clin North Am 49:973–988, 2002.
5. Zeidler C, Schwinzer B, Welte K. Congenital neutropenias. Rev Clin Exp Hematol 7:72–83, 2003.
6. Stein SM, Dale DC. Molecular basis and therapy of disorders associated with chronic neutropenia. Curr Allergy Asthma Rep 3:385–388, 2003.
7. Zeidler C, Boxer L, Dale DC, et al. Management of Kostmann syndrome in the G-CSF era. Br J Haematol 109:490–495, 2000.
8. Calhoun DA, Christensen RD. The occurrence of Kostmann syndrome in preterm neonates. Pediatrics 99:259–261, 1997.
9. Fujiu T, Maruyama K, Koizumi T. Early-onset group B streptococcal sepsis in a preterm infant with Kostmann syndrome. Acta Paediatr 91:1397–1399, 2002.
10. Christensen RD, Calhoun DA. Congenital neutropenia. Clin Perinatol 31:29–38, 2004.
11. Engle WD, Rosenfeld CR. Neutropenia in high risk neonates. J Pediatr 105:982–986, 1984.

12. Gessler P, Luders R, Konig S, et al. Neonatal neutropenia in low birthweight premature infants. Am J Perinatol 12:34–38, 1995.
13. Juul SE, Haynes JW, McPherson RJ. Evaluation of neutropenia and neutrophilia in hospitalized preterm infants. J Perinatol 24:150–157, 2004.
14. Christensen RD, Calhoun DA, Rimsza LM. A practical approach to evaluating and treating neutropenia in the neonatal intensive care unit. Clin Perinatol 27:577–601, 2000.
15. Funke A, Berner R, Traichel B, et al. Frequency, natural course, and outcome of neonatal neutropenia. Pediatrics 106:45–51, 2000.
16. Manroe BL, Weinberg AG, Rosenfeld CR, Browne R. The neonatal blood count in health and disease. I. Reference values for neutrophilic cells. J Pediatr 95:89–98, 1979.
17. Mouzinho A, Rosenfeld CR, Sanchez PJ, Risser R. Effect of maternal hypertension on neonatal neutropenia and risk of nosocomial infection. Pediatrics 90:430–435, 1992.
18. Greer JP, Foerster J, Lukens JN, et al., eds. Wintrobe's Clinical Hematology, 11th edition. Lippincott Williams & Williams; 2003.
19. Nathan DG, Orkin SH, Look AT, Ginsburg D, eds. Nathan and Oski's Hematology of Infancy and Childhood, 6th edition. Elsevier; 2003.
20. Kostmann R. Infantile genetic agranulocytosis; agranulocytosis infantilis hereditaria. Acta Paediatr 45(Suppl 105):1–78, 1956.
21. Carlsson G, Fasth A. Infantile genetic agranulocytosis, morbus Kostmann: presentation of six cases from the original "Kostmann family" and a review. Acta Paediatr 90:757–764, 2001.
22. Aprikyan AA, Carlsson G, Stein S, Oganesian A, Fadeel B, Dale DC, Palmblad J, Henter JI. Neutrophil elastase mutations in severe congenital neutropenia patients of the original Kostmann family. Blood 103:389, 2004.
23. Zeidler C, Welte K. Kostmann syndrome and severe congenital neutropenia. Semin Hematol 39:82–88, 2002.
24. Ancliff PJ, Gale RE, Liesner R, et al. Mutations in the ELA2 gene encoding neutrophil elastase are present in most patients with sporadic severe congenital neutropenia but only in some patients with the familial form of the disease. Blood 98:2645–2650, 2001.
25. Bellanne-Chantelot C, Clauin S, Leblanc T, et al. Mutations in the ELA2 gene correlate with more severe expression of neutropenia: a study of 81 patients from the French Neutropenia Register. Blood 103:4119–4125, 2004.
26. Kollner I, Sodeik B, Schreek S, et al. Mutations in neutrophil elastase causing congenital neutropenia lead to cytoplasmic protein accumulation and induction of the unfolded protein response. Blood 108:493–500, 2006.
27. Zetterstrom R. Kostmann disease—infantile genetic agranulocytosis: historical views and new aspects. Acta Paediatr 91:1279–1281, 2002.
28. Carlsson G, Wahlin YB, Johansson A, et al. Periodontal disease in patients from the original Kostmann family with severe congenital neutropenia. J Periodontol 77:744–751, 2006.
29. Faber J, Lauener R, Wick F, et al. Shwachman-Diamond syndrome: early bone marrow transplantation in a high risk patient and new clues to pathogenesis. Eur J Pediatr 158:995–100, 1999.
30. Donadieu J, Michel G, Merlin E, et al. Hematopoietic stem cell transplantation for Shwachman-Diamond syndrome: experience of the French neutropenia registry. Bone Marrow Transplant 36:787–792, 2005.
31. Huhta JC, Pomerance HH, Barness EG. Clinicopathologic conference: Barth syndrome. Fetal Pediatr Pathol 24:239–254, 2005.
32. Barth PG, Van den Bogert C, Bolhuis PA, et al. X-linked cardioskeletal myopathy and neutropenia (Barth syndrome): respiratory-chain abnormalities in cultured fibroblasts. J Inherit Metabl Dis 19:157–160, 1996.
33. Barth PG, Valianpour F, Bowen VM, et al. X-linked cardioskeletal myopathy and neutropenia (Barth syndrome): an update. Am J Med Genet 126A:349–353, 2004.
34. Alter BP. Bone marrow failure syndromes. Clin Lab Med 19:113–133, 1999.
35. Dale DC, Bolyard AA, Aprikyan A. Cyclic neutropenia. Semin Hematol 39:89–94, 2002.
36. Sera Y, Kawaguchi H, Nakamura K, et al. A comparison of the defective granulopoiesis in childhood cyclic neutropenia and in severe congenital neutropenia. Haematologica 90:1032–1041, 2005.
37. Dale DC, Cottle TE, Fier CJ, et al. Severe chronic neutropenia: treatment and follow-up of patients in the Severe Chronic Neutropenia International Registry. Am J Hematol 72:82–93, 2003.
38. Chow JY. The molecular basis of type I glycogen storage diseases. Curr Mol Med 1:25–44, 2001.
39. Lalezari P, Khorshidi M, Petrosova M. Autoimmune neutropenia of infancy. J Pediatr 109:764–769, 1986.
40. Boxer LA. Leukocyte disorders: quantitative and qualitative disorders of the neutrophil, Part 1. Pediatr Rev 17:19–28, 1996.
41. Boxer LA. Immune neutropenias. Clinical and biological implications. Am J Pediatr Hematol Oncol 3:89–96, 1981.
42. Maheshwari A, Christensen RD, Calhoun DA. Immune-mediated neutropenia in the neonate. Acta Paediatr Suppl 91:98–103, 2002.
43. Makeshwari A, Christensen RD, Calhoun DA. Immune neutropenia in the neonate. Adv Pediatri 49:317–339, 2002.
44. Curtis BR, Reon C, Aster RH. Neonatal alloimmune neutropenia attributed to maternal immunoglobulin G antibodies against the neutrophil alloantigen HNA1c(SH): a report of five cases. Transfusion 45:1308–1313, 2005.

45. Davoren A, Saving K, McFarland JG, et al. Neonatal neutropenia and bacterial sepsis associated with placental transfer of maternal neutrophil-specific autoantibodies. Transfusion 44:1041–1046, 2004.
46. Calhoun DA, Rimsza LM, Burchfield DJ, et al. Congenital autoimmune neutropenia in two premature neonates. Pediatrics 108:181–184, 2001.
47. Bux J, Behrens G, Jaeger G, Welte K. Diagnosis and clinical course of autoimmune neutropenia in infancy; analysis of 240 cases. Blood 91:181–186, 1998.
48. Lekjowski M, Maheshwari A, Calhoun, et al. Persistent perianal abcess in early infancy as a presentation of autoimmune neutropenia. J Perinatol 23:428–430, 2003.
49. Conway LT, Clay ME, Kline WE, et al. Natural history of primary autoimmune neutropenia in infancy. Pediatrics 79:728–733, 1987.
50. Koenig JM, Christensen RD. Incidence, neutrophil kinetics, and natural history of neonatal neutropenia associated with maternal hypertension. N Engl J Med 321:557–562, 1989.
51. Koenig JM, Christensen RD. The mechanism responsible for diminished neutrophil production in neonates delivered of women with pregnancy-induced hypertension. Am J Obstet Gynecol 165:467–473, 1991.
52. Tsao PN, Teng RJ, Tang JR, Yau KI. Granulocyte colony-stimulating factor in the cord blood of premature neonates born to mothers with pregnancy-induced hypertension. J Pediatr 135:56–59, 1999.
53. Zuppa AA, Girlando P, Florio MG, et al. Influence of maternal preeclampsia on recombinant human granulocyte colony-stimulating factor effect in neutropenic neonates with suspected sepsis. Eur J Obstet Gynecol Reprod Biol 102:131–136, 2002.
54. Doron MW, Makhlouf RA, Katz VL, et al. Increased incidence of sepsis at birth in neutropenic infants of mothers with preeclampsia. J Pediatr 125:452–458, 1994.
55. Greco P, Manzionna M, Vimercati A, et al. Neutropenia in neonates delivered of women with preeclampsia. Acta Biomed Ateneo Parmense 68: Suppl 1:91–94, 1997.
56. Paul DA, Kepler J, Leef KH, et al. Effect of preeclampsia on mortality, intraventricular hemorrhage, and need for mechanical ventilation in very low-birth-weight infants. Am J Perinatol 15:381–386, 1998.
57. Kocherlakota P, La Gamma EF. Preliminary report: rhG-CSF may reduce the incidence of neonatal sepsis in prolonged preeclampsia-associated neutropenia. Pediatrics 102:1107–1111, 1998.
58. Christensen RD, Henry E, Wiedmeier SE, Stoddard RA, Lambert DK. Neutropenia among extremely low birth-weight neonates: data from a multihospital healthcare system. J Perinatol 26:682–687, 2006.
59. Koenig JM, Hunter DD, Christensen RD. Neutropenia in donor (anemic) twins involved in the twin-twin transfusion syndrome. J Perinatol 11:355–358, 1991.
60. Koenig JM, Christensen RD. Neutropenia and thrombocytopenia in infants with Rh hemolytic disease. J Pediatr 114:625–631, 1989.
61. Carr R, Modi N, Dore C. G-CSF and GM-CSF for treating or preventing neonatal infections. Cochrane Database Syst Rev (3):CD003066, 2003.
62. Ahmad A, Laborada G, Bussel J, Nesin M. Comparison of recombinant G-CSF, recombinant human GM-CSF and placebo for treatment of septic preterm infants. Pediatr Infect Dis J 21:1061–1065, 2002.
63. Bedford-Russell AR, Emmerson AJB, Wilkinson N, et al. A trial of recombinant human granulocyte colony stimulating factor for the treatment of very low birthweight infants with presumed sepsis and neutropenia. Arch Dis Child Fetal Neonatal Ed 84:F172–176, 2001.
64. Bilgin K, Yaramis A, Haspolat K, et al. A randomized trial of granulocyte-macrophage colony-stimulating factor in neonates with sepsis and neutropenia. Pediatrics 107:36–41, 2001.
65. Drossou-Agakidou V, Kanakoudi-Tsakalidou F, Taparkou A, et al. Administration of recombinant human granulocyte-colony stimulating factor to septic neonates induces neutrophilia and enhances the neutrophil respiratory burst and beta2 integrin expression. Results of a randomized controlled trial. Eur J Pediatr 157:583–588, 1998.
66. Miura E, Procianoy RS, Bittar C, et al. A randomized double-masked, placebo controlled trial of recombinant granulocyte colony-stimulating factor administration to preterm infants with the clinical diagnosis of early-onset sepsis. Pediatrics 107:30–35, 2001.
67. Schibler KR, Osborne KA, Leung LY, et al. A randomized placebo-controlled trial of granulocyte colony-stimulating factor administration to newborn infants with neutropenia and clinical signs of early-onset sepsis. Pediatrics 102:6–13, 1998.
68. Gillan ER, Christensen RD, Suen Y, et al. A randomized, placebo-controlled trial of recombinant human granulocyte colony-stimulating factor administration in newborn infants with presumed sepsis: significant induction of peripheral and bone marrow neutrophilia. Blood 84:1427–1433, 1994.
69. Cairo MS, Christensen RD, Sender LS, et al. Results of a phase I/II trial of recombinant human granulocyte-macrophage colony-stimulating factor in very low birthweight neonates: significant induction of circulatory neutrophils, monocytes, platelets, and bone marrow neutrophils. Blood 86:2509–2515, 1995.
70. Cairo MS, Agosti J, Ellis R, et al. A randomised double-blind placebo-controlled trial of prophylactic recombinant human GM-CSF to reduce nosocomial infection in very low birthweight neonates. J Pediatrics 134:64–70, 1999.
71. Carr R, Modi N, Doré CJ, et al. A randomised controlled trial of prophylactic GM-CSF in human newborns less than 32 weeks gestation. Pediatrics 103:796–802, 1999.

72. Rosenthal J, Healey T, Ellis R, et al. A two year follow-up of neonates with presumed sepsis treated with recombinant human G-CSF during the first week of life. J. Pediatr 128:135–137, 1996.
73. Bernstein HM, Pollock BH, Calhoun DA, Christensen RD. Administration of recombinant G-CSF to neonates with septicemia: a meta-analysis. Pediatrics 138:917–920, 2001.
74. Carr R, Modi N. Haemopoietic colony stimulating factors for preterm neonates. Arch Dis Child 76:F128–F133, 1997.
75. Carr R. Neutrophil production and function in newborn infants. Br J Haematol 110:18–28, 2000.
76. Carr R, Huizinga TWJ. Low sFcRIII demonstrates reduced neutrophil reserves in preterm neonates. Arch Dis Child Fetal Neonat Ed 83:F160, 2000.
77. Carr R, Modi N. Haemopoietic growth factors for neonates: assessing risks and benefits. Acta Paediatr Suppl 93:15–19, 2004.
78. Bracho F, Goldman S, Cairo MS. Potential use of granulocyte colony-stimulating factor and granulocyte-macrophage colony-stimulating factor in neonates. Curr Opin Hematol 5:215–220, 1998.
79. Parravicini E, van de Ven C, Anderson L, Cairo MS. Myeloid hematopoietic growth factors and their role in prevention and/or treatment of neonatal sepsis. Transfus Med Rev 16:11–24, 2002.
80. Modi N, Carr R. Promising stratagems for reducing the burden of neonatal sepsis. Arch Dis Child Fetal Neonat Ed 83:F150–F153, 2000.
81. Roberts RL, Szelc CM, Scates SM, et al. Neutropenia in an extremely premature infant treated with recombinant human granulocyte colony-stimulating factor. Am J Dis Child 145:808–812, 1991.
82. Lejeune M, Cantineux B, Harag S, et al. Defective functional activity and accelerated apoptosis in neutrophils from children with cancer are differentially corrected by granulocyte and granulocyte-macrophage colony stimulating factors in vitro. Br J Haematol 106:756–761, 1999.
83. Hutter JJ Jr, Hathaway WE, Wayne ER. Hematologic abnormalities in severe neonatal necrotizing enterocolitis. J Pediatr 88:1026–1031, 1976.
84. Kling PJ, Hutter JJ. Hematologic abnormalities in severe neonatal necrotizing enterocolitis: 25 years later. J Perinatol 23:523–530, 2003.
85. Juul SE, Calhoun DA, Christensen RD. "Idiopathic neutropenia" in very low birthweight infants. Acta Paediatr 87:963–968, 1998.
86. Juul SE, Christensen RD. Effect of recombinant granulocyte colony-stimulating factor on blood neutrophil concentrations among patients with "idiopathic neonatal neutropenia": a randomized, placebo-controlled trial. J Perinatol 23:493–497, 2003.
87. Chirico G, Motta M, Villani P, et al. Late-onset neutropenia in very low birthweight infants. Acta Paediatr Suppl 91:104–108, 2002.
88. Omar SA, Salhadar A, Wooliever DE, Alsgaard PK. Late-onset neutropenia in very low birth weight infants. Pediatrics 106:E55, 2000.
89. Calhoun DA, Christensen RD, Edstrom CS, et al. Consistent approaches to procedures and practices in neonatal hematology. Clin Perinatol 27:733–753, 2000.

Chapter 4

Why, When and How Should We Provide Red Cell Transfusions To Neonates?

Robin K. Ohls, MD

Oxygen Delivery and Consumption

Development of Transfusion Guidelines

Indications for Red Cell Transfusions

Selection of Red Cell Products

Guidelines to Decrease Transfusions in ELBW Infants and Suggested Transfusion Guidelines

Summary

Hospitalized neonates, especially preterm infants in the newborn intensive care unit (NICU), receive the greatest number of transfusions of any hospitalized patient group. During the first 2 weeks of life when blood draws are frequent, approximately 50% of infants weighing less than 1000 g at birth (extremely low birth weight, ELBW) will receive their first transfusion (1). By the end of hospitalization over 80% of ELBW infants will receive at least one transfusion (2–4). While the numbers of transfusions given to preterm infants remains significant, the numbers have decreased over the last 20 years, primarily due to the institution of restrictive transfusion guidelines (5, 6). This chapter will review the rationale of administering red cell transfusions, summarize studies evaluating the efficacy of restrictive transfusion guidelines, provide strategies to decrease red cell transfusions in neonates, and propose guidelines for administering red cell transfusions.

OXYGEN DELIVERY AND CONSUMPTION

The primary purpose of a red cell transfusion is to provide an immediate increase in oxygen delivery to the tissues. Oxygen delivery (DO_2) can be quantified as the product of cardiac output (CO) and arterial oxygen content (CaO_2):

$$CO \text{ (dL/min)} \times CaO_2 \text{ (mL/dL)} = DO_2 \text{ (mL/min)}$$

Arterial oxygen content is determined by the hemoglobin concentration, the arterial oxygen saturation (%), the oxygen-carrying capacity of hemoglobin (mL/g × g/dL Hgb), and the solubility of oxygen in plasma (in mL/dL):

$$CaO_2 = (SaO_2 \times 1.34 \times [Hgb]) + (0.0031 \times PaO_2)$$

Improving cardiac output, hemoglobin concentration, or arterial oxygen saturation increases oxygen supply to tissues. If cardiac output and oxygen saturation are both maximized, the only way to deliver more oxygen to tissues is to increase the hemoglobin concentrations by increasing red cell mass.

In young, healthy, conscious adults, the critical threshold below which oxygen delivery equals oxygen consumption occurs at less than 7.3 mL of oxygen per kg per min (7, 8). Any further decrease in oxygen delivery results in a decrease in oxygen consumption and tissue hypoxia. The ratio of oxygen consumption to oxygen delivery is known as the oxygen extraction ratio, and generally ranges from 0.15 to 0.33, meaning the body consumes 15–33% of the oxygen delivered. As the oxygen extraction ratio reaches or exceeds 0.4, organ and cellular function can begin to deteriorate (9). Neonates have the added burden of fetal hemoglobin, decreased concentrations of 2,3DPG, and the increased demands of accelerated growth. Despite these added burdens, neonates have an enhanced ability to compensate for a gradual decrease in hemoglobin. For example, neonates born with hemoglobin concentrations less than 4 gm/dL as a result of chronic severe fetomaternal hemorrhage can appear well compensated for this level of hemoglobin, and oxygen delivery appears adequate, in that the infant has a normal heart rate, normal perfusion and no acidosis (10).

Anemia occurs when the red cell mass is not adequate to meet the oxygen demands of the tissues, and the current treatment for anemia is an infusion of red cells. Until the administration of artificial oxygen carriers becomes available (11), the only way to acutely and significantly increase hemoglobin is by transfusing red cells. The difficulty comes in distinguishing a neonate who is anemic and requires immediate treatment with a red cell transfusion from a neonate with a low hematocrit. While the risk of transmission of known infectious agents such as HIV and hepatitis B and C is relatively low in the blood supplied to USA hospitals, the risk of infectious agents newly identified in transfused blood such as West Nile virus, *Trypanosoma cruzi*, *Plasmodium* spp., Parvovirus B19, and newly identified infectious agents such as avian flu, remains to be determined (12–14). The decision to transfuse should therefore be taken with deliberation, and caregivers should consistently (i) obtain consent and (ii) document benefit in the neonate following the transfusion.

DEVELOPMENT OF TRANSFUSION GUIDELINES

The evaluation and publication of increasingly conservative transfusion guidelines has occurred over the past two decades. The ability of critically ill adult patients to adapt to lower hemoglobin values has recently been evaluated, and studies in adults and neonates have sought to determine the safety and efficacy of transfusion guidelines.

Adult Transfusion Studies

Studies evaluating transfusion guidelines in critically ill adults have changed transfusion practices significantly over the last decade (15–19). The most significant of these was the TRICC (Transfusion Requirements in Critical Care) trial, a randomized, controlled clinical trial involving 838 critically ill adults (15). The investigators sought to determine whether a restrictive approach to transfusions was equivalent to a liberal approach. The 30 day mortality was similar between groups (18.7% restrictive versus 23.3% liberal); however, mortality rates were significantly lower in the restrictive group in those patients who were less acutely ill (8.7% versus 16.1%), and in patients less than 55 years of age. Mortality rates were similar between groups in patients with cardiovascular disease. The mortality rate during hospitalization was significantly lower in the restrictive group (22.2% versus 28.1%, $P = 0.05$). The authors concluded that a restrictive strategy of red cell transfusion is at least as effective as a liberal transfusion strategy, and possibly superior. Subsequent studies have all noted similar findings (16–19), and resulted in the development of more conservative transfusion guidelines for adult ICU patients.

Pediatric Transfusion Studies

Few studies have been performed in the pediatric population and none published to date was designed as a randomized trial. Pediatric ICUs have relied on adult ICU study results, and caregivers have been cautious about implementing more restrictive transfusion guidelines. In one retrospective cohort analysis, children admitted to pediatric intensive care units (PICUs) with Hgb =9 g/dL were evaluated (20). Of 240 children evaluated, 131 were transfused and 109 were not. Transfusions were associated with increased days of oxygen use, mechanical ventilation, vasopressor infusion, PICU stay, and hospital stay. The authors concluded that red cell transfusions were associated with increased use of resources in critically ill children.

A prospective study to determine incidence of red cell transfusions in critically ill children was performed in Canada (21). Of 985 children, at least one transfusion was given in 139 cases (14%). The most common reasons for transfusions in these patients were: hemoglobin <9.5 gm/dL, cardiac disease, increased illness severity, and multiple organ dysfunction

Optimal hemoglobin concentrations remain to be determined in pediatric intensive care patients, especially in those patients with cyanotic heart disease. A marked variability still exists among pediatric intensivists in terms of both hemoglobin thresholds for transfusions and the volume of transfusions ordered (22). A multicentered study performed in Canadian PICUs to evaluate the efficacy of restrictive versus liberal transfusion guidelines in critically ill pediatric patients will soon be published (known as the TRIPICU study).

Neonatal Transfusion Studies

Neonatal transfusion practices have changed significantly during the last three decades. In the 1970s and 1980s, standard transfusion practices in the NICU involved maintaining the infant's hematocrit at or above 40%. Care was taken to monitor the volume of blood removed through phlebotomy, and to replace that blood when losses reached 10 mL/kg. In most units in the USA, it was not until the mid 1990s that transfusion practices began to change, in large part following publication of a randomized erythropoietin (Epo) study performed in the USA by Kevin Shannon and colleagues (23). These investigators were able to create guidelines for the restrictive use of PRBC transfusions for VLBW infants. Infants randomized to Epo treatment received fewer transfusions. The additional significance of this study lay in its creation and publication of these guidelines (Table 4-1).

As a result of this and other studies, the number of transfusions given to neonates in the USA, especially ELBW infants, decreased from an average of 10 transfusions per hospitalization to four transfusions per hospitalization by the year 2000 (5). Decreases in transfusions administered to preterm infants also occurred in many countries throughout Europe to an even greater degree (6). The average number of transfusions given to similarly sized infants decreased to three per infant during an entire hospitalization. One reason for the lower number of transfusions was the volume of phlebotomy losses recorded. In numerous multicentered studies in which transfusion guidelines were employed and phlebotomy losses

Table 4-1   Red Cell Transfusion Guidelines from the USA Epo trial (23)

Do not transfuse for blood out alone

Do not transfuse for low hematocrit alone

Transfuse at Hct≤35% for infants who are:
- receiving >35% oxygen
- on CPAP or mechanical ventilation with mean airway pressure 6–8 cm H_2O

Transfuse at Hct≤30% for infants who are:
- receiving any supplemental oxygen
- on continuous positive airway pressure or mechanical ventilation with mean airway pressure < 6 cm H_2O
- having significant apnea and bradycardia (>9 episodes in 12 h or 2 episodes in 24 h requiring bagging while on therapeutic doses of methylxanthines)
- experiencing heart rates >180 beats/min or RR>80 breaths/min for 24 h
- experiencing weight gain <10 g/day over at least 4 days while receiving 100 kcal/kg/day
- undergoing surgery

Transfuse at Hct≤20% for infants who are:
- Asymptomatic with reticulocytes < 100 000/μL

determined, the phlebotomy volume in the USA averaged 80 mL/kg, while losses in European and South American multicentered studies averaged 40 mL/kg (2–4). Regardless of measures implemented to decrease transfusion needs, there will always be a correlation between blood removed for phlebotomy and blood transfused in critically ill ELBW infants (23). This relationship is graphically represented in Figure 4-1.

The Canadian Pediatric Society developed transfusion guidelines in 2002 that were more restrictive than the USA Epo study guidelines (24). This was due in part to a significant public health scandal in which thousands of patients became infected with HIV and hepatitis C following transfusions distributed by the Canadian Red Cross (25). The Canadian Paediatric Society guidelines are shown in Table 4-2.

Three randomized studies have been published evaluating the impact of restrictive transfusion guidelines in preterm infants. The first, performed by Ellen Bifano and colleagues and published in abstract form (26, 27), evaluated 50 infants with birth weights 650–1000 g. Infants were randomized from week 1 to 36 weeks post menstrual age (PMA) to a "high" hematocrit strategy (hematocrit maintained

Figure 4-1 Relationship between phlebotomy losses and volume of blood transfused. Despite advances in neonatal transfusion medicine, there will always be a direct relationship between the amount of blood drawn for phlebotomy, and the volume of blood returned in the form of a PRBC transfusion. The solid line (line 1) represents the general relationship without the institution of transfusion guidelines. The dashed line (line 2) represents the improvement in decreased blood transfused following instituting restrictive transfusion guidelines. The hatched line (line 3) represents further decrease in transfused blood volumes through the use of red cell growth factors.

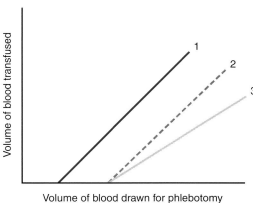

Table 4-2   Canadian Paediatric Society Recommendations for RBC transfusions (24)

RBC transfusions should be considered in newborn infants in the following specific clinical situations:

- Hypovolemic shock associated with acute blood loss
- Hematocrit between 30% and 35% or hemoglobin between 10 and 12 gm/dL in extreme illness conditions for which RBC transfusion may improve oxygen delivery to vital organs
- Hematocrit between 20% and 30% or hemoglobin between 6 and 10 gm/dL, and the infant is severely ill and/or on mechanical ventilation with compromised oxygen delivery
- Hematocrit falling below 20% or hemoglobin falling below 6 gm/dL with absolute reticulocyte count $100–150 \times 10^3/\mu L$ or less, suggesting low plasma concentration of erythropoietin, with the presence of the following clinical signs: poor weight gain, heart rate > 180 beats/min, respiratory distress and increased oxygen needs, and lethargy

greater than 32%) or a "low" hematocrit strategy (hematocrit maintained less than or equal to 30%). Hematocrits were maintained in the designated range with transfusions and erythropoietin in the high group, and with transfusions alone in the low group. Statistically significant differences in hematocrit were achieved by week 2 of the study and were maintained through 36 weeks PMA (Fig. 4-2).

There were no differences in baseline characteristics between the two groups, and the average birth weight of all infants enrolled in the study was 805 ± 86 g in the low and 837 ± 87 g in the high group (mean±SD; Table 4-3). At 36 weeks PMA, in comparing the 22 infants evaluated in the low hematocrit group with the 21 infants evaluated in the high hematocrit group, there was no difference in weight gain during hospitalization, the number of days spent on a ventilator, or the total number of hospital days (Table 4-3). At 1 year of age both weight gain and head growth were similar between groups (Table 4-3). In addition, there were no differences in neurodevelopmental impairments between the two groups, including a subgroup of infants with hematocrit =22% for greater than 3 weeks (Table 4-4). These investigators concluded that in ELBW infants, treatments aimed at

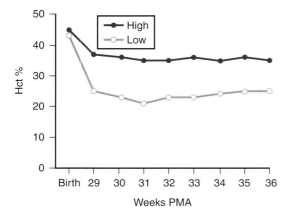

Figure 4-2 Differences in percent hematocrit (Hct) between infants randomized to the high hematocrit strategy (solid circles) and infants randomized to the low hematocrit strategy (open circles) were achieved by week 2 of the study, and maintained through 36 weeks postmenstrual age (PMA).

Table 4-3   Characteristics of Study Infants at the Start of Study, at 36 Corrected Weeks, and at 1 Year Corrected Age (26, 27)

	(n=22)	(n=21)
Study Entry:		
Birth weight (g)	805 ± 86	837 ± 8
Gestational age (weeks)	26 ± 2	26 ± 1
Male/female	14/8	16/5
Inborn (n,%)	16 (73%)	14 (67%)
Antenatal steroids (n,%)	18 (82%)	14 (67%)
36 Weeks:		
Weight gain (g/day)	22 ± 11	20 ± 4
Linear growth (cm/week)	1.1 ± 0.6	0.9 ± 0.4
Head growth (cm/week)	1.1 ± 0.5	0.8 ± 0.2
Mechanical ventilation (n,%)	32 ± 14	27 ± 13
Supplemental oxygen (n,%)	9 (41%)	9 (43%)
Postnatal steroids (n,%)	16 (73%)	16 (76%)
IVH (any) (n,%)	3 (14%)	4 (19%)
Grade III/IV (n,%)	0	1 (5%)
1-Year Follow-up:		
Bayley Scales of Infant Development		
Mental Developmental Index (MDI)	89 ± 16	86 ± 22
Psychomotor Developmental Index (PDI)	81 ± 19	84 ± 26
MDI or PDI < 68 (n,%)	6 (27%)	6 (29%)
Infant Neurological International Battery		
Normal (n,%)	16 (73%)	16 (76%)
Suspect (n,%)	2 (9%)	2 (10%)
Abnormal	4 (18%)	3 (14%)
Early Language Milestones:		
Pass (n,%)	19 (86%)	17 (81%)
Fail (n,%)	3 (14%)	4 (19%)

Values are mean ± SD.

maintaining hematocrit levels above 32% incurred additional cost without demonstrable benefit. Moreover, restrictive transfusion policies were not associated with adverse outcomes.

In July 2005, Bell and colleagues published their randomized study on liberal versus restrictive guidelines for red cell transfusion in preterm infants (28). In that study, 100 preterm infants 500–1300 g birth weight at the University of Iowa were randomized to a liberal or restrictive transfusion strategy. Infants received

Table 4-4   Outcome of Infants with Hct ≤ 22% for > 3 weeks (26, 27)

	Hematocrit ≤22% (n=11)	High hematocrit (n=21)
Growth		
Weight (percentile)	21 ± 23	23 ± 26
Length (percentile)	20 ± 19	20 ± 21
Head circumference (percentile)	50 ± 22	41 ± 26
Bayley Scales of Infant Development		
Mental Developmental Index	96 ± 12	86 ± 22
Psychomotor Developmental Index	81 ± 19	84 ± 26

Values are mean ± SD.

transfusions only when their hematocrit dropped below the assigned value, and transfusion thresholds decreased with improving clinical status. The primary outcome was a difference in the number of transfusions. In addition, morbidities associated with prematurity and hospital days were determined.

There were no differences in baseline characteristics between the two groups, and average birth weight for all infants enrolled was 956 g. Infants randomized to the restrictive strategy received fewer transfusions (an average of two fewer transfusions per patient), but had more episodes of apnea. In addition, infants in the restrictive strategy had a greater incidence of intraparenchymal brain hemorrhage or periventricular leukomalacia. Because of this finding, the authors concluded, "Although both transfusion programs were well tolerated, our findings of more frequent major adverse head ultrasound events in the restrictive RBC-transfusion group suggests that the practice of restrictive transfusions may be harmful to preterm infants." These findings were discussed in a series of letters to the editor following publication of the original study (29–31). All of the discussions centered on the conclusions reached by the investigators and the need for further study to confirm those conclusions.

Kirpalani and colleagues recently published the PINT study (Preterm Infant in Need of Transfusion) which sought to determine whether extremely low birth weight infants (ELBW) transfused at lower hemoglobin thresholds versus higher thresholds have different rates of survival or morbidity at discharge (32). This large, multicenter randomized clinical trial was designed to examine the impact of transfusion strategy on the incidence of a composite outcome – death, retinopathy of prematurity, bronchopulmonary dysplasia, or abnormal brain ultrasound – in ELBW infants. Four hundred and fifty-one ELBW infants were randomized to one of two transfusion strategies defined by the hemoglobin thresholds for RBC transfusion. The thresholds varied with age and with the level of respiratory support needed.

There were no baseline differences between the 223 infants randomized to the low transfusion threshold and the 228 infants randomized to the high transfusion threshold. The average birth weight of study participants was 770 g. Differences in hematocrit between groups were achieved by the first week of study. The composite primary outcome was similar for both groups: 74% in the low group, 70% in the high group ($P = 0.25$). In particular, the incidence of brain injury determined by ultrasound was 12.6% in the low group and 16% in the high group ($P = 0.53$). The authors concluded that in ELBW infants, maintaining a higher hemoglobin resulted in more infants receiving transfusions but conferred little evidence of benefit. The infants in the PINT study were smaller, sicker, with a greater risk of mortality and greater risk of brain injury than the infants enrolled in the Iowa study, yet there was no difference between the two groups in any morbidities. Because the Iowa study was published prior to the PINT study, controversy arose regarding the benefits and

Table 4-5	Summary of Neurologic Findings (26–28, 32)	
Study	Low-hematocrit strategy	High-hematocrit strategy
Bifano et al. ($n = 50$)	($n = 22$)	($n = 21$)
IVH (n)	0	1
Any NDI or growth deficiency (n,%)	12 (55%)	10 (48%)
Bell et al. ($n = 100$)	($n = 28$)	($n = 24$)
IVH (n,%)	5 (10%)	8 (16%)
PVL (n,%)	4 (14%)	0
PINT ($n = 451$)	($n = 175$)	($n = 188$)
"HUS brain injury" (n,%)	22 (12.6%)	30 (16%)

risks of restrictive transfusion guidelines. Table 4-5 summarizes the neurologic findings reported in the three randomized studies reviewed.

A difficulty in interpreting results of transfusion studies in neonates is that those studies measured what infants received, rather than what they actually needed. Neonatal (as well as adult and pediatric) transfusion practices would greatly benefit from studies that generate transfusion guidelines based on need, by identifying a useful transfusion marker. This work remains to be accomplished; however, a few investigators have attempted to define parameters, either through direct or indirect oxygen delivery (9), through resolution of signs of anemia (33–35), or through changes in cardiovascular parameters seen on echocardiography (36–38). These studies underscore the difficulty in determining which infants should receive PRBCs, and what signs, symptoms, and laboratory measurements should be used to determine that need.

The search for an ideal measure or marker for transfusion need continues. Work performed by Weiskopf and colleagues evaluated the effects of acute isovolemic hemodilution on neurocognititve functioning in healthy adults, and determined that the P300 latency period reflected changes in oxygen (39). Near infrared spectroscopy has also been evaluated as a tool to identify need for transfusions in preterm infants (40); however, lack of reproducibility in preterm infants still remains a significant factor preventing the use of this technique (41).

INDICATIONS FOR RED CELL TRANSFUSIONS

The indications for red cell transfusions in neonates differ primarily according to the rate of fall in hemoglobin, not according to any specific hemoglobin trigger. Neonates with significant acute blood loss require immediate volume resuscitation, but may or may not require a red cell transfusion. Term newborn infants may tolerate perinatal blood losses up to a third of their total blood volume. If acidosis persists in a neonate following volume resuscitation and adequate recirculation of the expanded blood volume, or if hemorrhage is ongoing, that neonate will probably benefit from a red cell transfusion. Infants with Hgb =10 gm/dL following volume expansion may have adequate oxygen delivery to tissues, and may simply require iron supplementation to replace iron stores lost due to the hemorrhage.

Determining the volume of PRBCs to transfuse in a neonate with known acute hemorrhage can be determined using the following formula (42): the volume of PRBCs to transfuse equals the desired rise in hematocrit times 1.6-times the infant's weight. Thus, a term, 3 kg infant with an acute drop in hematocrit at birth to 20% would need 120 mL PRBCs to achieve a desired hematocrit of 45%.

Caution should be taken in determining the transfusion needs of an infant born with a significantly low hematocrit, as it is vitally important to determine whether the infant experienced an acute fall in hematocrit, or a chronic fall in hematocrit. Infants with twin-to-twin transfusion syndrome or with chronic feto-maternal hemorrhage may be well compensated at birth, despite a hematocrit below 20%. An exchange transfusion should be considered in an infant with a low hematocrit in whom an immediate increase in oxygen delivery to tissues is necessary, as a significant increase in blood volume may result in the infant developing congestive heart failure.

Chronic Hemorrhage or a Chronic Drop in Hematocrit

All neonates undergo a natural adaptation to the extrauterine environment that allows them to compensate for a gradual drop in hematocrit. Immediately after birth increased oxygenation results in systemic oxygen delivery that far exceeds the tissues' demand for oxygen. Lacking the hypoxic stimulus, serum Epo concentrations fall and erythropoiesis rapidly declines. The hemoglobin concentration decreases over the first 2–3 months of life as the infant gains weight, remains stable over the next several weeks as erythropoiesis is reinitiated, then rises in the fourth to sixth month of life in response to a greater Epo stimulus (43). Term infants tolerate these changes in hemoglobin and hematocrit without consequence. Preterm infants experience a drop in hemoglobin lower than that seen in term infants, and the decrease appears proportional to the degree of prematurity. Hemoglobin concentrations between 7 and 8 gm/dL occur commonly in preterm infants who have not undergone significant phlebotomy losses. Epo concentrations in anemic preterm infants are still significantly lower than those found in adults, given the degree of their anemia (44, 45). This normocytic, normochromic anemia, termed the "anemia of prematurity", commonly affects infants ≤32 weeks gestation and is the most common anemia seen in the neonatal period. The anemia of prematurity is not specifically responsive to the addition of iron, folate, or vitamin E, although these substrates (as well as B-12) are administered to infants receiving erythropoietin to maximize erythropoiesis (4, 46). Some infants may be asymptomatic from their low hematocrit, while others demonstrate signs of anemia which are alleviated by transfusion. In preterm infants, determining when to transfuse can be problematic (47).

Transfusions affect erythropoiesis in newborns, and the decision to transfuse should not be based on hemoglobin concentration alone. For infants who undergo exchange transfusion or multiple transfusions, both erythropoietin concentrations and reticulocyte counts are lower at any given hemoglobin concentration. It is often assumed that oxygen delivery is decreased in newborns because of the presence of high-affinity fetal hemoglobin. In fact, a leftward shift in the hemoglobin–oxygen dissociation curve due to high levels of fetal hemoglobin might actually better maintain oxygen delivery during episodes of severe hypoxemia (44, 45).

When considering a transfusion in a preterm infant with a low hematocrit (not due to acute hemorrhage), the clinician should first determine whether the infant needs an immediate increase in oxygen to tissues (Fig. 4-3). If the answer is yes, then treatment consists of a transfusion of packed red cells. If there is no evidence that an immediate increase in oxygen delivery is necessary, then treatment with red cell growth factors and appropriate substrates might be considered. As the process of stimulating erythropoiesis requires at least a week to significantly impact the

TREATMENT OF AN INFANT WITH A LOW HEMATOCRIT

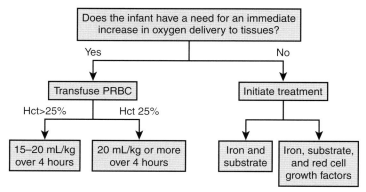

Figure 4-3 An approach to transfusions in neonates. When evaluating an infant with a low hematocrit (not due to an acute hemorrhage), the clinician should first determine whether the infant is in immediate need of increased oxygen delivery. If this is true, the treatment is a packed red blood cell (PRBC) transfusion. If the infant's hematocrit (Hct) is greater than 25% and further phlebotomy losses are estimated to be minimal, a volume of 15 mL/kg can be administered. All other infants receive 20 mL/kg. If it is determined that the infant does not need an immediate increase in oxygen delivery, treatment with red cell growth factors such as erythropoietin, and substrates such as iron, vitamin E, folate, and B-12 can be instituted.

reticulocyte count, and may not appreciably increase the hemoglobin concentration during that time, the infant should continue to be observed for signs of anemia.

SELECTION OF RED CELL PRODUCTS

Transfusions in neonates should be given as a means to rapidly increase oxygen delivery to tissues. Red cell transfusions may be given under acute settings, such as during resuscitation of an exsanguinated infant at delivery, or under more chronic settings, such as an infant in the NICU with a hemoglobin concentration that does not deliver adequate oxygen to tissues. In addition, red cell transfusions are used for severe hemolytic disease of the newborn, in the form of a double volume exchange transfusion, and are used to prime ECMO circuits. Finally, red cell transfusions are often used during neonatal surgery, especially cardiac surgery.

In the setting of severe acute hemorrhage when a red cell transfusion can be life-saving, O negative "trauma" PRBCs can be used. O negative whole blood should not be used. Type O negative whole blood will contain antibodies directed against A or B blood group, and will also contain leukocytes. It should only be used if the infant's blood type is known to be O negative. Matched whole blood has been used during major neonatal and pediatric cardiac surgery. In early studies whole blood was shown to be beneficial in decreasing post-surgical bleeding (48). Recent studies have reported no benefit of whole blood over reconstituted blood (49, 50). Infants receiving reconstituted blood spent less time in intensive care and had a smaller cumulative fluid balance (51).

Double Volume Exchange Transfusion

For infants requiring a double volume exchange transfusion to treat hemolytic disease of the newborn, whole blood should never be used. Blood type O Rh-negative washed PRBCs should be reconstituted with AB Rh-positive plasma to achieve a hematocrit of 45–50%. In this way the administration of antibodies directed against the infant's red cells (in the form of remaining plasma associated with O negative blood) is reduced to the greatest degree.

The volume of blood exchanged can be calculated based on a total blood volume of 85 mL/kg body weight. Thus, an infant weighing 2.6 kg would require a total volume of:

$$2.6 \text{ kg} \times 85 \text{ mL/kg} = 221 \text{ mL}$$

In many neonatal units, CMV-negative PRBCs are available for all infants. CMV-negative PRBCs should be used in specific populations, such as infants awaiting or undergoing transplant, immunocompromised infants, infants receiving in utero transfusions, and preterm infants born to CMV-negative mothers.

Leukoreduction, Stored Blood and Irradiation

Leukoreduced PRBCs should be used in neonates in order to decrease the spread of infection, and decrease the possibility of microchimerism, the addition of a small amount of foreign genetic material to the host's genetic material (52). The shelf life of PRBCs can be as great as 42 days, and there does not appear to be a significant difference in red cells transfused before 7–10 days compared with red cells transfused after 21 days (53, 54). Studies comparing potassium concentrations in blood stored for various periods show no significant increase in blood stored for greater than 21 days compared to blood stored for less than 7 days (54). Many blood banks will also irradiate PRBCs just prior to neonatal transfusion. Irradiation of RBCs is recommended for fetuses receiving in utero transfusions, for immunocompromised infants, and for infants receiving directed donor blood from a first- or second-degree relative. Irradiation may reduce the rare complication of graft versus host disease.

Cord Blood

Cord blood collection has been studied as a form of "autologous" donation, but most NICUs, labor and delivery services, and blood banks are not prepared for collection and storage of neonatal cord blood. An alternative to cord blood collection that reduces erythrocyte transfusions to ill neonates is delayed clamping of the umbilical cord. It is possible to promote placental transfer of blood to preterm infants by delaying the clamping of the umbilical cord for 30 s. In fact transfer of 10–15 mL/kg body weight can be expected using this method (55). In a randomized trial by Mercer and colleagues, this maneuver of delayed cord clamping among infants < 1500 g birth weight resulted in less intraventricular hemorrhage and less late-onset sepsis (56). Even a delay of 30 s results in improved iron status (57), fewer transfusions (58), and perhaps superior neurodevelopmental outcomes (56).

GUIDELINES TO DECREASE TRANSFUSIONS IN ELBW INFANTS AND SUGGESTED TRANSFUSION GUIDELINES

When a maternal patient has indicated that neonatal transfusions will be refused, and a premature birth is anticipated, an action plan can be created to optimize the preterm infant's chances of avoiding transfusion. A majority (85–90%) of ELBW infants receive transfusions. However, 10–15% of ELBW infants never receive a transfusion. This percentage can be increased through the use of such measures as delayed cord clamping, immediate red cell growth factor and iron therapy, judicious laboratory testing using micro-sampling, and a restrictive transfusion policy. Table 4-6 shows suggested guidelines to optimize the ELBW infant's chances of remaining transfusion-free. Most importantly, these measures can be identified and a plan created prenatally with the family. In addition, the neonatologists can

---

Table 4-6   Suggested Guidelines to Reduce Transfusions in ELBW Infants

- Discuss delayed cord clamping with the obstetrical team and document the plan in the mother's chart. The infant should be held below the placenta while the cord is intact for 30–45 s
- Initiate erythropoietin (Epo) treatment during the first day of life. This can be achieved by administering a subcutaneous injection of 400 units/kg Epo, or by adding 200 units/kg into a protein-containing intravenous solution (such as a 5% dextrose solution with 2% amino acids), to run over 4–24 h
- Administer parenteral iron, 3 mg/kg once a week or 0.5 mg/kg/day (added to TPN or administered IV over 4–6 h) until the infant is tolerating adequate volume feedings, then administer oral iron at 6 mg/kg/day
- Use in-line blood sampling such as the VIA system, or use micro-sampling devices such as the I-Stat to decrease the volume need for each lab
- Remove central lines as soon as possible
- Order labs judiciously (for example, no "blood gas q 6 hours" orders), and reconsider the need for "standard" or "routine" labs, such as weekly complete blood counts, daily blood gases or daily chemistry panels
- Monitor phlebotomy losses daily
- Communicate the lowest hemoglobin or hematocrit that will be tolerated for a variety of typical clinical scenarios and days of age, such as: (i) infant is on 100% oxygen, significant ventilator support, blood pressure support, and has a metabolic acidosis; (ii) infant is on minimal ventilator support or CPAP; (iii) infant is receiving enteral feeds and requiring oxygen; (iv) infant is on full feeds, growing well, no oxygen support. Consider these scenarios if the infant is less than 2 weeks of age, 2–4 weeks of age, or greater than 4 weeks of age

Table 4-7   Transfusion Guidelines

- A central hematocrit should be obtained on admission. No further hematocrits should be obtained unless specifically ordered
- Outside of rounds, transfusions should generally only be considered if acute blood loss of ≥10% associated with symptoms of decreased oxygen delivery occurs, or if significant hemorrhage of >20% total blood volume occurs
- In term and preterm infants, a transfusion should be considered if an immediate need for increased oxygen delivery to tissues is clinically suspected
- Infants should be transfused with 20 mL/kg PRBC unless the Hct is >29%. 20 mL/kg volume could also be used if significant phlebotomy losses are anticipated in smaller infants with Hct>29%
- For infants receiving Epo, considerations to the above guidelines should be made regarding the rate of decrease in hemoglobin or hematocrit, the infant's reticulocyte count, the postnatal day of age, the need for supplemental oxygen, and the overall stability of the infant
- Central measurements of hemoglobin or hematocrit are preferred; alternatively, heel stick measurements may be obtained after warming the heel adequately. An infant meeting the criteria below should not automatically be transfused. Transfusions can be considered for the following:

1) For infants **requiring moderate or significant mechanical ventilation**, defined as MAP >8 cmH$_2$O and FiO$_2$ > 0.40 on a conventional ventilator, or MAP>14 and FiO$_2$ > 0.40 on high-frequency ventilator, transfusions *can be considered* if the **hematocrit is ≤30% (hemoglobin ≤10 g/dL)**

2) For infants **requiring minimal mechanical ventilation**, defined as MAP ≤8 cmH$_2$O and/or FiO$_2$ ≤ 0.40, or MAP<14 and/or FiO$_2$ < 0.40 on high frequency, transfusions *can be considered* if the **hematocrit is ≤25% (hemoglobin ≤ 8 g/dL)**

3) For infants on supplemental oxygen who are **not requiring mechanical ventilation**, transfusions *can be considered* if the **hematocrit is ≤20% (hemoglobin ≤7 g/dL), and** one or more of the following is present:

   - ≥24 h of tachycardia (heart rate >180) or tachypnea (RR >60)
   - a doubling of the oxygen requirement from the previous 48 h
   - lactate ≥2.5 mEq/L or an acute metabolic acidosis (pH<7.20)
   - weight gain <10 g/kg/day over the previous 4 days while receiving ≥120 kcal/kg/day
   - the infant will undergo major surgery within 72 h

4) For infants **without any symptoms**, transfusions *can be considered* if the **hematocrit is ≤18% (hemoglobin ≤6 g/dL)** associated with an absolute reticulocyte count <100 000 cells/μL (<2%)

establish a relationship with the family and discuss their NICU transfusion thresholds. This is much better done proactively, so that the need for last-minute court orders to transfuse can be minimized.

Transfusion guidelines currently used by several NICUs (all located at or above 5000 feet elevation) are provided (Table 4-7). These guidelines have been implemented in our unit for 30 months. During that time no differences from previous years in ELBW outcomes have been recorded.

SUMMARY

Previously, limitations in the knowledge of the pathophysiology of anemia contributed to unfounded and liberal transfusion practices in preterm infants and to uncertain risk-benefit ratios (1). Over the last two decades, researchers have explored an array of strategies to minimize transfusions in the most critically ill. Currently, the ideal test for transfusion need does not exist. Studies on the efficacy and outcomes of restrictive transfusion guidelines in adults, children and neonates should and will continue.

Acknowledgment

I wish to thank Anne Debuyserie for her assistance in completing the manuscript.

REFERENCES

1. Bifano EM, Curran TR. Minimizing donor blood exposure in the neonatal intensive care unit. Current trends and future prospects. Clin Perinatol 22:657, 1995.
2. Maier RF, Obladen M, Muller-Hansen I, et al. Early treatment with erythropoietin beta ameliorates anemia and reduces transfusion requirements in infants with birth weights below 1000 g. J Pediatr 141:8, 2002.
3. Donato H, Vain N, Rendo P, et al. Effect of early versus late administration of human recombinant erythropoietin on transfusion requirements in premature infants: results of a randomized, placebo-controlled, multicenter trial. Pediatrics 105:1066, 2000.
4. Ohls RK, Ehrenkranz RA, Das A, et al. National Institute of Child Health and Human Development Neonatal Research Network. Neurodevelopmental outcome and growth at 18 to 22 months' corrected age in extremely low birth weight infants treated with early erythropoietin and iron. Pediatrics 114:1287, 2004.
5. Widness JA, Seward VJ, Kromer IJ, et al. Changing patterns of red blood cell transfusion in very low birth weight infants. J. Pediatr 129:680, 1996.
6. Maier RF, Sonntag J, Walka MM, et al. Changing practices of red blood cell transfusions in infants with birth weights less than 1000 g. J Pediatr 136:220, 2000.
7. Lieberman JA, Weiskopf RB, Kelley SD, et al. Critical oxygen delivery in conscious humans is less than 7.3 mL O2 kg(-1) min(-1). Anesthesiology 92:407, 2000.
8. Madjdpour C, Spahn DR, Weiskopf RB. Anemia and perioperative red blood cell transfusion: A matter of tolerance. Crit Care Med 34:S102, 2006.
9. Alverson DC. The physiologic impact of anemia in the neonate. Clin Perinatol 22:609, 1995.
10. Willis C, Forman CS Jr. Chronic massive fetomaternal hemorrhage: a case report. Obstet Gynecol 71:459, 1988.
11. Inayat MS, Bernard AC, Gallicchio VS, et al. Oxygen carriers: a selected review. Transfus Apher Sci 34:25, 2006.
12. Pealer LN, Marfin AA, Petersen LR, et al. Transmission of West Nile virus through blood transfusion in the United States in 2002. N Engl J Med 349:1236, 2003.
13. Dodd RY. Emerging infections, transfusion safety, and epidemiology. N Engl J Med 349:1205, 2003.
14. Alter HJ, Stamer SL, Dodd RY. Emerging infectious diseases that threaten the blood supply. Semin Hematol 44:32, 2007.
15. Hebert PC, Wells G, Blajchman MA, et al. A multicenter, randomized, controlled clinical trial of transfusion requirements in critical care. Transfusion Requirements in Critical Care Investigators, Canadian Critical Care Trials Group. N Engl J Med 340:409, 1999.
16. Napolitano LM, Corwin HL. Efficacy of red blood cell transfusion in the critically ill. Crit Care Clin 20:255, 2004.
17. Chant C, Wilson G, Friedrich JO. Anemia, transfusion, and phlebotomy practices in critically ill patients with prolonged ICU length of stay: a cohort study. Crit Care 10:R140, 2006.
18. Croce MA, Tolley EA, Claridge JA, Fabian TC. Transfusions result in pulmonary morbidity and death after a moderate degree of injury. J Trauma 59:19, 2005.
19. Malone DL, Dunne J, Tracy JK, et al. Blood transfusion, independent of shock severity, is associated with worse outcome in trauma. J Trauma 54:898, 2003.
20. Goodman AM, Pollack MM, Patel KM, Luban NLC. Pediatric red blood cell transfusions increase resource use. J Pediatr 142:123, 2003.
21. Armano R, Gauvin F, Ducruet T, et al. Determinants of red blood cell transfusions in a pediatric critical care unit: a prospective, descriptive epidemiological study. Crit Care Med 33:2637, 2005.
22. Nahum E, Ben-Ari J, Schonfeld T. Blood transfusion policy among European pediatric intensive care physicians. J Intensive Care Med 19:38, 2004.
23. Shannon KM, Keith JF 3rd, Mentzer WC, et al. Recombinant human erythropoietin stimulates erythropoiesis and reduces erythrocyte transfusions in very low birth weight preterm infants. Pediatrics 95:1, 1995.
24. Red blood cell transfusions in newborn infants: Revised guidelines. Paediatr Child Health 7:553, 2002.
25. Kondro W. Canadian Red Cross found negligent. Lancet 350:1154, 1997.
26. Bifano EM. The effect of hematocrit (HCT) level on clinical outcomes in Extremely Low Birthweight (ELBW) infants. Pediatr Res 49:311A, 2001.
27. Bifano EM, Bode MM, D'Eugenio DB. Prospective randomized trial of high vs. low hematocrit in Extremely Low Birth Weight (ELBW) infants: one year growth and neurodevelopmental outcome. Pediatri Res 51:325A, 2002.
28. Bell EF, Strauss RG, Widness JA. Randomized trial of liberal versus restrictive guidelines for red blood cell transfusion in preterm infants. Pediatrics 115:1685, 2005.
29. Boedy RF, Mathew OP. Letter to editor: Randomized trial of liberal versus restrictive guidelines for red blood cell transfusion in preterm infants. Pediatrics 116:1048, 2005.
30. Murray N, Roberts I, Stanworth S. Letter to editor: Red blood cell transfusion in neonates. Pediatrics 116:1609, 2005.
31. Swamy RS, Embleton ND. Letter to editor: Red blood cell transfusions in preterm infants: is there a difference between restrictive and liberal criteria? Pediatrics 115:257, 2005.
32. Kirpalani H, Whyte RK, Andersen C. The Premature Infants in Need of Transfusion (PINT) study: a randomized, controlled trial of a restrictive (low) versus liberal (high) transfusion threshold for extremely low birth weight infants. J Pediatr 149:301, 2006.

33. Wardle SP, Garr R, Yoxall CW, Weindling AM. A pilot randomised controlled trial of peripheral fractional oxygen extraction to guide blood transfusions in preterm infants. Arch Dis Child Fetal Neonatal Ed 86:F22, 2002.
34. Bifano EM, Smith F, Borer J. Relationship between determinants of oxygen delivery and respiratory abnormalities in preterm infants with anemia. J Pediatr 120:292, 1992.
35. Izraeli S, Ben-Sira L, Harell D, et al. Lactic acid as a predictor for erythrocyte transfusion in healthy preterm infants with anemia of prematurity. J Pediatr 122:629, 1993.
36. Bard H, Fouron JC, Chessex P, Widness JA. Myocardial, erythropoietic, and metabolic adaptations to anemia of prematurity in infants with bronchopulmonary dysplasia. J Pediatr 132:630, 1998.
37. Bohler T, Janecke A, Linderkamp O. Blood transfusion in late anemia of prematurity: effect on oxygen consumption, heart rate, and weight gain in otherwise healthy infants. Infusionsther Transfusionsmed 21:376, 1994.
38. Alkalay AL, Galvis S, Ferry DA, et al. Hemodynamic changes in anemic premature infants: Are we allowing the hematocrits to fall too low? Pediatrics 112:838, 2003.
39. Weiskopf RB, Toy P, Hopf HW, et al. Acute isovolemic anemia impairs central processing as determined by P300 latency. Clin Neurophysiol 116:1028, 2005.
40. Soul JS, Taylor GA, Wypij D, Duplessis AJ, et al. Noninvasive detection of changes in cerebral blood flow by near-infrared spectroscopy in a piglet model of hydrocephalus. Pediatr Res 48:445, 2000.
41. Menke J, Voss U, Moller G, Jorch G. Reproducibility of cerebral near infrared spectroscopy in neonates. Biol Neonate 83:6, 2003.
42. Morris KP, Naqvi N, Davies P, et al. A new formula for blood transfusion volume in the critically ill. Arch Dis Child 90:724, 2005.
43. Kling PJ, Schmidt RL, Roberts RA, et al. Serum erythropoietin levels during infancy: associations with erythropoiesis. J Pediatr 128:791, 1996.
44. Brown MS, Garcia JF, Phibbs RH, et al. Decreased response of plasma immunoreactive erythropoietin to "available oxygen" in anemia of prematurity. J Pediatr 105:793, 1984.
45. Stockman JA, Graeber JE, Clark DA, et al. Anemia of prematurity: Determinants of the erythropoietin response. J Pediatr 105:786, 1984.
46. Haiden N, Schwindt J, Cardona F, et al. Effects of a combined therapy of erythropoietin, iron, folate, and vitamin B12 on the transfusion requirements of extremely low birth weight infants. Pediatrics 118:2004, 2006.
47. Keyes WG, Donohue PK, Spivak JL, et al. Assessing the need for transfusion of premature infants and the role of hematocrit, clinical signs, and erythropoietin level. Pediatrics 84:412, 1989.
48. Manno CS, Hedberg KW, Kim HC, et al. Comparison of the hemostatic effects of fresh whole blood, stored whole blood, and components after open heart surgery in children. Blood 77:930, 1991.
49. Williams GD, Bratton SL, Ramamoorthy C. Factors associated with blood loss and blood product transfusions: a multivariate analysis in children after open-heart surgery. Anesth Analg 89:57, 1999.
50. Kwiatkowski JL, Manno CS. Blood transfusion support in pediatric cardiovascular surgery. Transfus Sci 21:63, 1999.
51. Mou SS, Giroir BP, Molitor-Kirsch EA, Leonard SR, et al. Fresh whole blood versus reconstituted blood for pump priming in heart surgery in infants. N Engl J Med 351:1635, 2004.
52. Lee TH, Reed W, Mangawang-Montalvo L, et al. Donor WBCs can persist and transiently mediate immunologic function in a murine transfusion model: effects of irradiation, storage, and histocompatibility. Transfusion 41:637, 2001.
53. Strauss RG, Burmeister LF, Johnson K, et al. Feasibility and safety of AS-3 red blood cells for neonatal transfusions. J Pediatr 136:215, 2000.
54. Fernandes da Cunha DH, Nunes Dos Santos AM, Kopelman BI, et al. Transfusions of CPDA-1 red blood cells stored for up to 28 days decrease donor exposures in very low-birth-weight premature infants. Transfus Med 15:467, 2005.
55. Aladangady N, McHugh S, Aitchison TC, et al. Infant's blood volume in a controlled trial of placental transfusion at preterm delivery. Pediatrics 117:93, 2006.
56. Mercer JS, Vohr BR, McGrath MM, et al. Delayed cord clamping in very preterm infants reduces the incidence of intraventricular hemorrhage and late-onset sepsis: a randomized, controlled trial. Pediatrics 117:1235, 2006.
57. Chaparro CM, Neufeld LM, T Alavez G. Effect of timing of umbilical cord clamping on iron status in Mexican infants: a randomized controlled trial. Lancet 367:1997, 2006.
58. Philip A. Delayed cord clamping in preterm infants. Pediatrics 117:1434, 2006.

Chapter 5

Controversies in Neonatal Thrombotic Disorders

Marilyn J. Manco-Johnson, MD

Hemostatic System

Genetic and Acquired Thrombophilias

Catheter-Related Thrombosis

Neonatal Stroke

Antithrombitic Therapies

Summary

While this chapter will deal with current controversies surrounding neonatal thrombosis, it may be useful to summarize what is generally agreed upon regarding thrombosis in newborn infants. Although rare in comparison to adult case rates, the incidence of thromboembolism in the pediatric population is increased during the perinatal period as well as in adolescents (1, 2). Cooperative studies in Germany and The Netherlands have reported the rates of neonatal thromboembolism at 5.1 and 0.7 per 100 000 births, respectively, while the Canadian registry reported a rate of neonatal thrombosis of 24 per 10 000 admissions to neonatal intensive care units (3–5). The German cooperative group reported the thrombosis-related neonatal mortality at 12% for renal vein thrombosis and 4% for other venous thromboembolic events (3). The recurrence rate of thromboembolism following symptomatic neonatal thrombotic events has been reported at 3.3 and 7% in two studies (4, 6).

Neonatal thrombotic disorders range in severity from asymptomatic thrombi to fatal events. Mortality rates of 9–18 % have been reported (3–5). The majority of neonatal thromboses are related to catheters, and many of these are determined in asymptomatic infants (4, 5). Causes of increased thromboses during the perinatal period are believed to be related to developmental characteristics of the hemostatic system, thrombophilic traits, medical conditions affecting the fetus and neonate, and complications of intensive supportive care. Optimal treatment has not been determined. Many controversies remain regarding neonatal thrombosis, as discussed below.

HEMOSTATIC SYSTEM

1. *Does the unique balance of the fetal and neonatal hemostatic system predispose to thrombosis during and shortly following the process of birth? Does the unique fetal hemostatic system require any different approach to interpretation of diagnostic coagulation tests?*

Ontogeny of the Hemostatic System

The hemostatic balance between bleeding and clotting is unique in the fetus and newborn infant. Perhaps the most striking feature of developmental hemostasis is the paradoxical gain of function in assays of whole blood clotting contrasted with deficiencies in individual components of the coagulation system.

The development of hemostasis in the fetus and neonate has been recently summarized and is displayed in Table 5-1 (7). Certain coagulation proteins develop early in gestation. Platelet number and mean concentrations of certain procoagulant proteins such as factor VIII, factor V, the von Willebrand factor (VWF), fibrinogen, thrombomodulin and tissue factor are within or above the normal adult range even in extremely preterm infants (8). Other proteins, notably the vitamin-K-dependent coagulation proteins, factors II, VII, IX, X, protein C and protein S, as well as the physiologic inhibitors, tissue factor pathway inhibitor (TFPI) and antithrombin (AT), are low at term birth and the various proteins do not achieve normal adult levels until later in infancy through adolescence (8–10). The differential rates of protein expression may be predicted to favor coagulation activation and thrombus formation. However, the concentration of $\alpha2$-macroglobulin is also increased in neonatal plasma partially offsetting the relative deficiency of other coagulation inhibitory proteins.

A few neonatal proteins have shown true qualitative differences in comparison to the adult molecular forms. In the adult, VWF is secreted from the endothelial cell in ultra-large multimers that are cleaved following their release into plasma by the ADAMTS13 metalloproteinase (11). VWF in cord blood demonstrates increased-molecular-weight multimers resembling intracellular VWF and that found in the plasma of patients with thrombotic thrombocytopenic purpura (TTP), a condition caused by deficiency of or auto-antibodies directed against ADAMTS 13 (12). Adult-sized VWF multimers are achieved by 3 weeks of postnatal age. It was hypothesized that physiologically decreased levels of the ADAMTS13 proteinase at birth may cause the ultra-large neonatal VWF multimers in the neonate, but experimental data have been conflicting and it is unlikely that low levels of ADAMTS 13 are solely responsible for fetal VWF (13, 14). Neonatal platelets display decreased aggregation to agonists ADP and thrombin as compared to older children and adults, due to maturational deficiencies in intracellular signaling (15, 16). Despite diminished intrinsic platelet function, the ultra-large multimers of VWF in neonatal plasma mediate accelerated platelet adhesion to collagen in the newborn infant that is manifest, paradoxically, in

Table 5-1	**Neonatal Hemostatic Balance**		
Elevated plasma concentrations and early development	**Deficient plasma concentration and delayed development**	**Fetal molecular forms with gain of function**	**Fetal molecular forms with loss of function**
Procoagulant factors VIII, V, XIII, fibrinogen, tissue factor	Vitamin-K-dependent factors II, VII, IX, X, protein C, protein S	VWF	Fibrinogen Plasminogen/ plasmin
VWF, platelet count	AT, TFPI		
Tissue factor Thrombomodulin	TAFI		

VWF, von Willebrand factor; AT, antithrombin; TFPI, tissue factor pathway inhibitor; TAFI, thrombin activatable fibrinolytic inhibitor.

shorter bleeding times and platelet function analyzer (PFA)-100 closure times in the neonate relative to healthy children and adults (17, 18).

The effective concentration of some fetal proteins is enhanced by decreased concentrations of their regulatory cofactors. For example, plasma concentrations of total protein S are low in the newborn infant (mean 20 U/dL), However, free or functional protein S, which functions as a cofactor to protein C, averages 40 U/dL owing to the very low concentrations of C4b-binding protein that, in the older child and adult, binds approximately half of protein S (19). Bound protein S does not function in hemostasis. Likewise, the functional fibrinolytic capacity of plasminogen is maximized in neonatal plasma by very low levels of the plasminogen-binding protein, histidine-rich glycoprotein (20).

Fetal fibrinogen has been shown to contain increased sialic acid and phosphorus, shorter and thinner fibrils, and decreased N-terminal alanine in the Aα chain in comparison to adult fibrinogen (21). The thrombin time is prolonged in cord blood plasma and reaches adult values at approximately 3 weeks. Like fetal fibrinogen, fetal plasminogen contains increased sialic acid. Activation of fetal plasminogen to plasmin is reduced in comparison to the adult molecule; however, fetal plasminogen also demonstrates decreased rates of inactivation in comparison to the adult molecule (22).

Global whole blood assays of coagulation such as the thromboelastogram show increased coagulability as manifest by a shortened lag time and increased maximal amplitude of clot formation in neonatal whole blood, while tests of plasma clot formation and thrombin generation are decreased in neonatal plasma from which red cells, white cells and platelets have been removed (23–26). Increased coagulability of fetal and neonatal blood has been related to increased levels of circulating tissue factor along with relatively decreased levels of the inhibitors tissue factor pathway inhibitor and antithrombin (24, 25). In addition, the increased red cell mass of blood in term infants supports more rapid fibrin formation. In spite of low plasma concentration and decreased activation of fetal plasminogen, the newborn manifests brisk fibrinolysis both on whole blood thromboelastogram as well as by euglobulin clot lysis time and other global measures of fibrinolysis (26, 27). Postnatal loss of fibrinolytic activity in preterm infants with respiratory distress syndrome has been shown to correlate with disease severity (28).

Interpretation of coagulation tests in the newborn infant requires knowledge of normal values for developmental age as well as alterations associated with acquired neonatal disorders.

2. Does the unique fetal hemostatic system predispose newborn infants to thrombosis? If so, should neonatal replacement therapies be given to achieve normal adult levels of coagulation proteins either to reduce the risk of or to treat established thromboses?

Are newborn infants more prone to bleed or clot? On balance, the hemostatic system of the newborn infant is intact, and excessive bleeding and clotting rarely occur in well term infants. Sick infants frequently manifest dysregulated thrombin generation, consumptive coagulopathy and an increased rate of thrombus formation (29). Sepsis and catheters are the most common correlates of thrombosis in the neonatal intensive care nursery (1, 2, 4). Infection promotes clotting activation and catheters provide a nidus for thrombus propagation. Several other medical conditions in sick newborn infants increase the prothrombotic tendency of the neonate. Hypoxia and acidosis in preterm infants with respiratory distress syndrome activate coagulation and are a risk factor for disseminated intravascular coagulation (DIC). Clotting activation is also associated with hemolytic anemia, most commonly caused by Rh or ABO incompatibility, hyperviscosity syndrome and maternal diabetes mellitus. Rarely extreme elevations in white blood cell or platelet counts may cause ischemia, usually in the central nervous system, in newborn infants.

Bleeding in sick preterm infants is commonly related to consumptive coagu-lopathy (30). Extreme acquired deficiencies of regulatory proteins, especially pro-tein C, are not infrequent in sick newborn infants (31, 32). Most small clinical trials performed to date to replace coagulation inhibitors using fresh frozen plasma or antithrombin concentrate have not shown clear benefit (33). In addition, some interventive trials employing antithrombin concentrate or recombinant activated protein C have yielded unexpected rates of intracranial hemorrhage in neonates and very young infants, raising safety concerns regarding inhibitor replacement (34, 35). Although young infants on these trials were critically ill with numerous confound-ing risk factors for hemorrhage, the serious adverse events raise safety concerns regarding inhibitor replacement (34, 35). However, one observational study of an-tithrombin repletion in neonatal cardiac surgery showed benefit in reduction of symptomatic venous thrombosis without excess bleeding (36). Ongoing investiga-tions into the ontogeny and regulation of thrombin generation in the newborn infant will guide future efforts to determine whether supplementation of physio-logic coagulation components in certain high-risk infants may prevent thrombus formation or help treat established thrombi with reduced toxicity.

GENETIC AND ACQUIRED THROMBOPHILIAS

3. *Do thrombophilic genes of the mother or fetus or acquired thrombophilic conditions predispose the fetus to thrombosi in utero and during labor and delivery?*

Spontaneous venous and arterial thrombosis detected at or shortly following birth is rare and primarily involves the renal veins, inferior vena cava, aorta and middle cerebral arteries. Renal vein thrombosis usually follows some evidence of fetal distress and is more frequent in infants of diabetic mothers (37, 38). Placentas of mothers with antiphospholipid antibody syndrome (APAS) are often small with histological evidence of thrombosis and infarction (39). However many perinatal thromboembolic events appear to be idiopathic. Vascular obstruction and resultant hypoperfusion are suspected but cannot be confirmed. This has led pediatric hema-tologists and perinatologists to search for constitutional factors that may predispose to thrombosis.

Genetic Thrombophilias

Thrombophilic gene mutations are common in the Caucasian population (40). Increased plasma factor VIII activity is found in 10% of the population, although the mechanism has not been delineated (41). Five to ten percent of Europeans carry the factor V Leiden mutation, which decreases the rate of inactivation of activated factor V by its physiologic regulator, activated protein C (42). One to two percent of Caucasians are heterozygous for the prothrombin 20210 mutation, which augments thrombin generation potential by increasing circulating concentrations of pro-thrombin by 15–30% (43).

A homozygous mutation in the methylene tetrahydrofolate reductase gene resulting in a thermolabile molecular variant (MTHFR 677TT) is present in about 9% of the USA population. However, due to universal folic acid enrichment of flour in the USA, blood levels of homocysteine are rarely increased even in persons homozygous for the MTHFR 677TT variant. Most epidemiologic studies have associated an increased thrombotic risk with elevated homocysteine levels and not with the genetic mutation per se (44). However, the effect of the MTHFR gene mutation on pediatric thrombosis and other adverse pregnancy outcomes remains controversial and a positive association has been found in some studies (45, 46). Elevations in plasma concentrations of procoagulant proteins, including factors IX and XI, have also been implicated in thrombophilia (47, 48). Mutations that result in quantitative or qualitative deficiencies of the physiologic anticoagulants anti-thrombin, protein C and protein S are rare but contribute a greater thrombotic potential to affected individuals than the more common mutations (49).

Newborn infants may present with signs of in utero and perinatal DIC and thrombosis related to genetic thrombophilia, most importantly homozygous deficiencies of protein C, protein S or antithrombin, or combined multiple-trait thrombophilia (50, 51). Some, but not all, investigations of neonates with throm-boembolic events report an increased risk for genetic thrombophilia (3, 4, 52–54). While odds ratios for thrombotic disorders are increased in series of infants with single thrombophilic traits, conversely, a very small minority of all babies carrying these traits develop thrombosis. Although not precisely known, the recurrence risk of perinatal thrombotic events for future pregnancies clinically appears to be low. It is likely that thrombophilic mutations, when inherited as a single thrombophilic trait, decrease the threshold for thrombosis in fetuses and babies in the context of other triggers, rather than being a sufficient etiology for spontaneous thrombosis. Optimal management of pregnancy and the perinatal period for infants of parents who carry thrombophilic mutations has not been determined. Women carrying thrombophilic traits manifest an increased risk for fetal loss, but evidence does not support routine use of anticoagulation during pregnancy in asymptomatic mothers to prevent fetal loss (55).

Active research is currently ongoing regarding potential relationships between maternal and/or fetal thrombophilia and diverse pregnancy outcomes including fetal demise, intrauterine growth restriction, placental abruption, severe pre-eclampsia and fetal thrombosis (56–58). The results of these investigations will contribute important information regarding the pathophysiology of fetal and neo-natal thrombosis. The high prevalence of thrombophilic mutations in the popula-tion and the relatively low incidence of thrombotic perinatal disease in affected fetuses and neonates raises an ethical dilemma in routine thrombophilia screening and genetic counseling specifically related to pregnancy and childbirth.

Acquired Thrombophilias

Maternal antiphospholipid antibodies (APAs), including the lupus anticoagulant, anticardiolipin antibody and anti-β2-glycoprotein-I antibodies have been associat-ed with pregnancy-associated complications, including maternal thrombosis, recur-rent miscarriage, and fetal demise (59, 60). Maternal APAs are transported across the placenta along with other IgG immunoglobulins and may be a cause of peri-natal thrombosis. Most infants respond to standard antithrombotic therapies. The evaluation of perinatal thrombosis should include an assessment of maternal APAs. The incidence of thrombosis in live-born infants of mothers with APAs is unknown but appears to be low, and the role of interventions to prevent thrombosis in affected infants is completely unknown.

CATHETER-RELATED THROMBOSIS

4. What causes catheter-related thrombosis and can catheter-related thrombosis in the newborn infant be prevented?

The use of indwelling arterial and venous catheters is almost universal in intensively supported ill newborn infants. A large proportion of thrombi in new-born infants are catheter-related (61). Tyson and colleagues reported pathologic evidence of thromboatheromatous changes of the aorta in 33 of 56 neonates (59%) who had an umbilical artery catheter (UAC) in place prior to death (62). In addi-tion, it is generally suspected that neonatal sepsis is promoted by fibrin strands at the catheter tip or lining catheter sheaths, which may serve as a nidus for infection.

The use of UACs, umbilical venous catheters (UVCs), and central venous catheters (CVCs) in neonates has been associated with thromboembolism, infarction, sepsis, cardiac perforation, catheter malfunction and death. UVCs carry a particular risk of portal vein thrombosis. Estimates of the frequency and causes vary greatly but most studies concur that the risk is increased with catheter malposition, and morbidity can be substantial (63–66). Symptomatic thrombosis, confirmed with objective imaging, was reported in 10 (23%) of 44 newborn and older infants with CVCs (67). Other series have reported mechanical complications in peripherally inserted CVCs of 15–48% (68). Neonates undergoing cardiac surgery in a Finnish study were at increased risk of CVC thrombosis, and a relationship to the factor V Leiden mutation was suggested (69). The results of one prospective German study of pediatric patients with cardiac disease, including many neonates, suggested that catheter-related thrombosis following cardiac catheterization or surgery was more common in infants and children carrying thrombophilic traits (70). Many factors contribute to neonatal catheter-related thrombosis, including the small caliber of the vessel, endothelial damage, abnormal blood flow, catheter composition, design, and site, duration of catheterization and composition of infusate. There is no controversy regarding the magnitude of the problem of catheter-related thrombosis in newborn infants. However, there is debate regarding the most important factors contributing to catheter-related thrombosis in neonates that may be impacted by clinical practice. Several recent Cochrane Systematic Reviews have addressed these issues. Table 5-2 displays data regarding factors predisposing to catheter thrombi. Currently, there is no strong evidence on which to base decisions regarding catheter composition, design, or placement although practice is shifting toward high UAC placement. Many attempts have been made to decrease the risk of catheter thrombosis and infection by minimally inhibiting coagulation with heparin by continuous infusion through the catheter or directly bonded to the polyurethane catheter. Table 5-3 displays a summary of data regarding strategies to decrease the rate of catheter-related thrombosis. It is clear that use of heparin by infusion and/or catheter bonding prolongs the duration of catheter patency. Rates of infection and thrombosis, however, continue to cause clinical concern and warrant attempts at improvement.

An interesting new polyurethane catheter incorporates bonding with a heparin-antithrombin complex. This complex has been found to extend the durability of antithrombotic effect and is showing promising early results in a rabbit model of catheter thrombosis (81). Another newer approach is the instillation of thrombolytic agents into the void volume of catheters to clear fibrin sheaths that form on the surface of catheters and fibrin strands that occlude catheter openings. Recombinant TPA has been used in two open-label studies to clear occluded CVCs in infants and children, including newborn infants (82, 83). Efficacy in restoration of catheter patency was 80–90% and toxicity was minimal. There were no bleeding complications. While published reports deal with local instillation of thrombolytic agents to restore patency of occluded catheters, the same approach can be used periodically in functioning catheters to prevent occlusion.

Currently, catheter use should be limited to explicit need and they should be removed as soon as feasible. Inclusion of unfractionated heparin in very low concentrations (approximately 1 U/mL) to the catheter infusate does not alter the rate of catheter-related thrombi, but prolongs catheter patency. The optimal agent, route and dose intensity of prophylaxis for catheter-related thrombosis in the neonate has not been determined. Risks of major bleeding complications, especially intracranial bleeding, limit clinical studies of thrombus prophylaxis in the population of preterm infants at highest risk for thrombosis. Future studies are needed to determine whether the safest and most effective prevention of catheter-related thrombosis will be found in a better catheter design or in better prophylactic antithrombotic therapies administered to the infant.

Table 5-2   Data Regarding Contribution of Catheter Characteristics to Thrombosis

Catheter Factor	Type of study	N	Conclusions
Catheter material	Cochrane review (71)		This meta-analysis found no basis for choosing PVC vs. heparin-bonded PU
	1 RCT	125	No difference
PVC vs. Silastic	1 Comparison study	20	Silastic had fewer thromboses
Silicone elastomer	Single-arm open label (72)	83	Infections 1.2 per 1000 catheter days; 1 (1.2%) thrombosis; 8 (9.6%) occlusion
UAC catheter position	Cochrane review (73) 5 trials reviewed	790	Fewer clinical vascular complications with high UAC position
Central venous catheter position	Retrospective review (74)	587	Complications in 28% of catheters with 2 deaths
			Caval thrombosis in 1%; sepsis in 4%; higher rate of complications with proximal placement and infant weight < 2500 g; no difference in silicone vs. PU, or surgical vs. percutaneous placement
Broviac catheterization	Case series (75)	52	Rate of infection or thrombosis 2.08 per 100 catheter days
Catheter hole position	Cochrane review (76) 1 randomized clinical trial	71	Relative risk of thrombosis with end-hole was 0.27 (95% CI 0.11, 0.67)
Multiple vs. single lumen	Cochrane review (77) 3 RCT	99	Multiple lumen catheter use was associated with fewer peripheral IVs but more catheter malfunction; there was no difference in rates of sepsis or thrombosis but studies were not powered to detect differences or did not report this outcome

PVC, polyvinyl chloride; PU, polyurethane; RCT, randomized clinical trial; UAC, umbilical artery catheter.

Table 5-3   Data Considering the Efficacy of Various Strategies to Prevent Neonatal Catheter-Related Thrombosis

Intervention	Type of study	N	Conclusions
Heparin infusion, 1 U/mL in UAC	Cochrane review (78) 4 RCT	252	Low-dose heparin infusates clearly reduce catheter occlusion, RR 0.20 (95% CI 0.11, 0.35) and hypertension; non-significant trend toward decreased aortic thrombosis
Heparin infusion, 1 U/mL in peripherally inserted CVC	Cochrane review (68) 1 RCT	66	No difference in catheter occlusion, thrombosis, duration of catheter patency or sepsis
Heparin-bonded PU vs. PVC UAC catheters	RCT (79)	125	No difference in mechanical complications, thrombosis
Heparin-bonded PU peripherally inserted CVC	Double-blinded RCT (80)	200	20% of subjects were neonatal, 80% pediatric Significantly reduced rate of infection and thrombosis

CVC, central venous catheter.

5. What causes neonatal stroke and are there any treatments that improve outcomes?

Perinatal and prenatal arterial ischemic strokes (AIS) are potentially devastating disorders affecting 0.25–1 infants per thousand live births (84–86). Approximately 60% of cases are perinatal and present with symptoms in the first few days of life, chiefly seizures and apnea, while presumed prenatal stroke presents with pathologic hand preference, hemiplegia or seizures several months postnatally (87). Perinatal cerebral sinovenous thrombosis (CSVT), principally affecting the lateral and superficial venous sinuses, has been reported at 0.4 cases per thousand live births (88). The mortality rate from neonatal AIS or cerebral sinovenous thromboembolism is < 10% (84, 86). The recurrence rate of thromboembolism following neonatal symptomatic AIS in one report was 3.3%, primarily consisting of venous thrombosis (89), while recurrence following cerebral sinovenous thrombosis in another study was 13% (88). Both entities are more common in male neonates (90).

Although many newborn infants with symptomatic AIS appear clinically normal after recovery from the acute event, on follow-up approximately one-third exhibit hemiparesis and another third have cognitive abnormalities, primarily affecting speech and language (84, 91). Infants with presumed pre- or perinatal AIS are evaluated based upon persistent abnormalities of neurologic examination detected later in infancy and, understandably, suffer a worse outcome than infants with neonatal symptoms, many of which resolve. Essentially all infants with presumed pre- or perinatal AIS manifest motor deficits, half exhibit speech, cognitive or behavioral deficits, and approximately one-quarter have seizures (87).

The cause of neonatal stroke has been elusive. Both arterial and venous perinatal cerebral thromboembolisms share common clinical characteristics. In both disorders, perinatal complications are increased and include fetal distress, abnormal fetal heart tracings, coagulopathy, maternal diabetes, complications of pregnancy and delivery, and, especially, infection (84–88). Both genetic and acquired thrombophilias are risk factors for perinatal stroke (84, 87, 88, 92, 93).

Thrombin generation in utero may be a common denominator in the diverse pathophysiologic pathways to neonatal stroke. Clotting activation originating from either the maternal or fetal side of the placenta could release thrombin or small fibrin clots into the fetal circulation via the umbilical vein. Physiologically, the patent foramen ovale (PFO) of the fetal heart forms a conduit from the systemic fetal venous circulation directly to the brain prior to spontaneous closure in the infant. Because small fibrin thrombi formed in the placenta or venous circulation of the fetus could lodge in the cerebral arterial circulation, fetal AIS in a pregnancy complicated by maternal or fetal thrombophilia could be the equivalent of venous thromboembolism that characterizes thrombophilia in later life. Fetal circulation passes from the placenta through the umbilical vein and ductus venosus to the right heart, where 27% of blood crosses the PFO and enters the ascending aorta. Entry to the left carotid is least angled. Two-thirds of neonatal strokes involve the left hemisphere. Embolization from the portal vein to the brain in a neonate has been described, confirming this theoretic model of fetal stroke in vivo (94).

Most commonly, the diagnosis of perinatal stroke traditionally has been made using computerized tomography (CT), which reveals ischemia early (low-density lesion) progressing to organized infarction (lower-density cystic lesion). CT with contrast offers potential delineation of intravascular thrombus or congenital cerebral arterial hypoplasia or stenosis (computerized tomography angiography, CTA). MRI is an attractive alternative to CT owing to its lack of radiation exposure. Advanced magnetic resonance imaging (MRI) techniques using diffusion weighted imaging (DWI) and diffusion tensor imaging (DTI) allow greater delineation of brain architectural detail, including integrative neuronal pathways such as the internal capsule and optic radiation. The principles of DWI and DTI and their application to neonatal stroke have been recently reviewed (95, 96). As the internal capsule is myelinated around the time of term gestation, the movement of water across axons is increasingly restricted and water will move more freely along the length of axons. The diffusion of water can be measured with an apparent diffusion coefficient (ADC). Abnormalities of perinatal stroke are best seen on DWI 1–4 days following birth, when conventional MRI may still be normal. DTI, a development of DWI, makes use of the directional movement of water to provide information on white matter tract integrity that is expressed as mean diffusivity, a directionally averaged measure of water diffusion and fractional anisotrophy which measures the directionality of diffusion. Fractional anisotrophy is reduced in acute stroke and may help time the onset of ischemia. Using DWI and DTI, a study of 40 infants with neonatal stroke determined that lesions involving the combination of the cerebral hemisphere, basal ganglia and posterior limb of the internal capsule result in hemiplegia while infarctions involving any one or two of these anatomic structures do not (95). These results contrast with childhood stroke where involvement of one or two of these anatomic structures may result in hemiplegia (97). Powerful imaging techniques such as DWI and DTI will be important to elucidate the pathophysiology of stroke in neonates, indicate prognosis, and guide future interventional trials.

Anticoagulation is standard therapy for venous thrombosis. A review of two small trials of anticoagulation for cerebral sinovenous thrombosis, one using unfractionated heparin and the other low-molecular-weight heparin, found a non-statistical trend favoring treatment (98). While the efficacy of anticoagulant therapy for cerebral sinovenous thrombosis has not been established, bleeding complications in this population of neonates is low (88). The Seventh American College of Chest Physicians (ACCP) Conference on Antithrombotic and Thrombolytic Therapy recommends initial therapy with unfractionated or low-molecular-weight heparin followed by low-molecular-weight heparin for a total of 3 months, based upon Grade 2C evidence (99). In contrast, there are no trials addressing the safety or efficacy of anticoagulant therapy for AIS in newborn infants. The ACCP recommendations for neonatal AIS call for withholding anticoagulation and aspirin in general, also based on Grade 2C evidence. However, 3 months of anticoagulation are recommended for neonates with defined cardioembolic AIS. In adults with AIS, TPA has shown efficacy in restoring cerebral blood flow and reversing clinical signs of stroke when delivered within 3 h of onset of symptoms (100). TPA is not an attractive therapeutic for neonatal stroke due to the increased risk of intracranial hemorrhage in the newborn infant and general lack of recognizable symptoms at the time of initial vascular occlusion.

The traditional rationale of antithrombotic therapy is to limit thrombus progression and embolization. The mortality and recurrence rates of neonatal AIS are both relatively low. A more appropriate goal for neonates with acute AIS may be to limit the cellular damage incurred by ischemia, applying a broader perspective to pathophysiology and potential intervention. Infarction following vascular ischemia in stroke is mediated by cellular inflammation, disruption of metabolic processes and endothelial cell barrier function, and apoptosis. Interventional strategies targeted to prevent neuronal apoptosis and to decrease cellular dysfunction could provide neuroprotective strategies with no effect on plasma coagulation.

Activated protein C (APC) is a vitamin-K-dependent coagulation regulatory protein that dampens thrombin generation in the clotting cascade by inactivating cofactors FVa and FVIIIa, which are responsible for the 1000-fold augmentation in thrombin generation. Protein C is activated by a complex of thrombin with thrombomodulin on the endothelial cell surface. The anticoagulant effect of activated protein C is mediated by its binding to the endothelial protein C receptor (EPCR). Activated protein C also binds to the cellular receptor protease-activatable receptor 1 (PAR-1), resulting in the generation of pleiotrophic cytoprotective effects that have been recently reviewed, including alteration of gene expression profiles, anti-inflammatory activities, anti-apoptotic activity and protection of endothelial cell barrier function (101). The prospective epidemiologic Atherosclerosis Risk in Communities study (ARIC) suggested that higher levels of plasma protein C may be protective against AIS [OR 0.65 (0.4–1.0)] (102). Neuroprotective effects of APC when given 6 h after the onset of brain ischemia (103) have been confirmed in murine and rat models of AIS.

Nitric oxide (NO) produced by endothelial cells also demonstrates a neuro-protective effect. NO also has a wide range of effects that include vasodilatation, increased cerebral blood flow, platelet inhibition, and anti-inflammation. The rationale for increasing NO in acute stroke has been recently summarized (104). NO is increased by statins, steroids, nutrients and exercise. Rat models have demonstrated a neuroprotective effect of statins when administered following arterial vascular occlusion in adult animals (105). Unfortunately, a neuroprotective effect in neonatal animals was achieved only by administration of the agent prior to the vascular insult.

Erythropoietin is a growth factor that induces red cell precursor differentiation and proliferation in the bone marrow. Erythropoietin and its receptor are also expressed in brain tissue, where it exerts angiogenic, neurogenic and anti-apoptotic activities through activation of intracellular anti-apoptotic signaling pathways (106–109). Recombinant erythropoietin is being evaluated as a potential neuroprotective therapeutic agent for stroke. In neonatal rats subjected to focal cortical infarct by occlusion of the middle cerebral artery, treatment with erythropoietin decreased both infarction volume and neuronal apoptosis (109). Erythropoietin is widely used in extremely preterm infants to limit blood transfusion requirements. While it is unclear whether doses used to prevent anemia of prematurity may be adequate for neuroprotection, this usage has an established safety profile (110, 111).

Kallikrein, a serine protease in the contact system of coagulation, bridges activation pathways of blood clotting and inflammation. Kallikrein, acting on the kinin B2 receptor, has also demonstrated neuroprotective effects in AIS through decreases in apoptosis and inflammation (112).

Currently unknown is whether perinatal AIS occurs in a substantial proportion of cases as a result of genetic or acquired coagulopathy that can be suspected and treated using standard antithrombotic approaches to prevent or limit brain damage. Also unknown is what neuroprotective benefits other potential therapeutic strategies discussed above will confer to newborn infants affected with AIS.

ANTITHROMBITIC THERAPIES

6. What are the risks and benefits of antithrombotic therapies in the neonate compared with treatment of the child and adult? What antithrombotic agents should be administered to neonates, in what intensity and for what duration?

Historically, standard antithrombotic therapy has been withheld in many neonates with thrombosis, particularly venous thrombosis, for fear of morbidity and mortality caused by bleeding. As data have emerged regarding the appropriate use and monitoring of anticoagulant and thrombolytic agents in newborn infants, the perceived and real toxicity of antithrombotic therapies has decreased (2–5, 113, 114). The German registry of neonatal thrombosis reported rates of major hemorrhage of 2% for heparin anticoagulation and 15% thrombolysis (3).

Initial dosing recommendations for unfractionated heparin (UH), enoxaparin low-molecular-weight heparin (LMWH) and tissue plasminogen activator (TPA)

Table 5-4   IV Dosing for Antithrombotic Therapies in Newborn Infants

	Unfractionated heparin: continuous IV	Enoxaparin: q12 h subcutaneous	Tissue plasminogen activator: continuous IV
Loading dose	Newborn < 37 weeks: 50 U/kg Newborn > 37 weeks: 100 U/kg Infant/child > 1 month: 50 U/kg	None	None
Initial maintenance dose	Newborn < 28 weeks: 15 U/kg/hr Newborn 28–36 weeks: 20 U/kg/h (may require up to 30 U/kg/h to achieve therapeutic anti-Xa level) Newborn > 37 weeks: 28 U/kg/h (may need up to 50 U/kg/h to achieve therapeutic anti-Xa level)	Newborn to < 12 months: 1.5 mg/kg (may require 1.25 to 2.0 mg/kg/dose to achieve therapeutic anti-Xa level)	Infants to < 3 months: 0.06 mg/kg/h (may double if not effect in 12–24 h)
Monitoring	Anti-Xa activity 0.3–0.7 U/mL	Anti-Xa activity 0.5–1.0 U/mL	Clot decrease in extent or lysis by imaging increase in D-dimer or FSP

IV, intravenous.

are listed in Table 5-4 as previously described (113). Table 5-5 includes important contraindications to the use of each of these agents. While anticoagulant therapy is aimed at achieving the adult therapeutic range, it is important to recognize that these data were derived in adults and were empiric. There are no trials comparing varying intensities of anticoagulation in newborn infants with thrombosis.

UH is effective in newborn infants when used appropriately. However, infants are often resistant to the anticoagulant effects of heparin due to physiologically decreased levels of antithrombin, an increased volume of distribution, rapid heparin clearance, and nonspecific protein binding in plasma (115, 116). Term infants with thrombosis manifest requirements for extraordinarily high rates of UH, up to

Table 5-5   Contraindications to Specific Antithrombotic Therapies in Infants

Unfractionated heparin	Low-molecular-weight heparin	Systemic TPA
Known allergy History of HIT	Known allergy History of HIT; invasive procedure < 24 h	Known allergy Active bleeding CNS ischemia/surgery < 10 days (includes birth asphyxia); surgery < 7 days; invasive procedure < 3 days; seizures < 48 h
*Fibrinogen < 100 mg/dL; platelet count < 50 000/μL	*Fibrinogen < 100 mg/dL; platelet count < 50 000/μL	*Fibrinogen < 100 mg/dL; platelet count < 50 000/μL; INR > 2

HIT, heparin-induced thrombocytopenia and/or thrombosis.
CNS, central nervous system.
*With transfusion support, if necessary.

50 U/kg/h, to maintain the target therapeutic range. Dose requirements in heparin-resistant neonates have been decreased by repletion of antithrombin although there is no evidence in the literature to support this indication. UH can be particularly attractive in the initiation of anticoagulation, especially in critically ill children, because it has a very short half-life and can be rapidly adjusted or discontinued in the event that the child begins to hemorrhage or requires surgery or an invasive procedure. The activated partial thromboplastin time (PTT) is not used by some pediatric hematologists to monitor UH in the newborn infant because the baseline PTT is prolonged at birth by low levels of the contact factors of coagulation and the PTT prolongation is not linear with heparin anticoagulant effect. Anti-Xa activity levels effectively monitor UH in newborn infants. Other pediatric hematologists continue to use the PTT to monitor UH and reserve the anti-Xa activity assay for LMWH.

Most infants with thrombosis can be treated adequately with LMWH (114). Enoxaparin anticoagulant effect is also dependent upon antithrombin and must be determined by monitoring. LMWH can be given twice daily by subcutaneous injection and monitored using anti-Xa activity levels. Similar to UH, the dose of LMWH needed to achieve the therapeutic range in newborn infants is both higher than that in older infants and more variable. We have determined a dosing range for enoxaparin from 1.25 to more than 2.0 mg/kg/dose in newborn infants, with most infants requiring 1.5–1.625 mg/kg/dose. Because the kinetics of intravenous and subcutaneous enoxaparin are similar, infants lacking subcutaneous fat have been treated using intravenous dosing (117). There are minimal published data on this route of administration. Peak and trough levels should be assayed to determine a safe and effective intravenous dosing schedule.

Although bleeding risks are a grave concern in ill preterm infants, babies with acute thrombosis at risk for loss of life or limb may be considered for thrombolysis. Thrombolysis has been especially helpful for occlusive clots of the aorta, peripheral arteries and acute atrial clots when careful attention is paid to the contraindications and risks (118–122).

Outcome of Neonatal Thrombosis

Pediatric thrombosis centers have been recently organized to study thrombosis in infants and children. Reports regarding outcome are beginning to emerge (113, 123). Complete resolution rates of non-renal vein venous thromboembolism in neonates have been reported at about one-third and similar in infants treated with anticoagulation or thrombolysis (123). Neonatal renal vein thrombosis, a particularly difficult clinical entity, was reported to cause renal infarction in most affected newborn infants in a large series of German infants (124). Treatment with anticoagulation, antithrombin replacement or thrombolysis has not been associated with improved outcomes (124, 125). Renal enlargement at birth is a poor prognostic sign for renal outcome (126). It appears that many, if not most, episodes of renal vein thrombosis begin prior to delivery and clot may be organized, and for this reason resistant to antithrombotic therapy, at the time of treatment initiation.

The recurrence risk of neonatal thrombosis has not been adequately assessed to date. The prevalence of post-thrombotic syndrome, a clinical entity characterized by chronic limb pain and swelling following an episode of venous thrombosis, has not been determined following perinatal thrombosis. Inferior vena cava thrombosis secondary to placement of central venous catheters has been associated with serious long-term post-thrombotic complications in affected newborn and older infants in another German series (127). In two reports, adolescents with a history of inferior vena cava or renal venous thrombosis in the perinatal period presented with lower-extremity deep venous thrombosis and/or post-thrombotic syndrome during adolescence (124, 128). Post-thrombotic syndrome also appears to be common and often is severe, following occlusive superior vena cava thrombosis related to cardiac surgery or catheterizations. It is evident that neonatal thrombotic disorders cause significant morbidity and mortality and have long-term consequences in affected infants. Optimal prediction, prevention and treatment have not been determined. The intrauterine origin of many neonatal thrombotic events, particularly AIS and renal vein thrombosis, adds increased complexity to the challenges of early detection and intervention.

SUMMARY

The newborn infant, especially the ill preterm infant, is at increased risk for thrombosis from a variety of causes, including physiologic immaturity of the hemostatic system, genetic and acquired thrombophilias, pregnancy complications, underlying medical conditions and use of indwelling catheters. Due to bleeding risks and the relatively low rate of thrombotic complications, anticoagulant prophylaxis is not attractive in at-risk infants. However, infants with vascular thrombosis can be safely treated with UH and LMWH anticoagulation as well as TPA thrombolysis, provided appropriate considerations are given to dosing, monitoring and contraindications. The greatest challenge to future understanding of neonatal thrombotic disorders is the lack of evidence from well-organized clinical trials in this vulnerable population. Pediatric hematologists have recently organized national and international professional organizations to conduct and analyze clinical trials on thrombotic disorders in infants, with a high regard for the safety issues of such studies. Support for prospective investigations of neonatal thrombotic disorders is necessary for continued progress in this field.

Acknowledgment

This work was supported by a Grant from the Centers for Disease Control and Prevention #UR6/CCU820552.

REFERENCES

1. Manco-Johnson MJ. Etiopathogenesis of pediatric thrombosis. Hematology 10 (suppl 1):167, 2005.
2. Journeycake JM, Manco-Johnson MJ. Thrombosis during infancy and childhood: what we know and what we do not know. Hematol Clinics North Am 18:1315, 2004.
3. Nowak-Gottl U, von Kries R, Gobel U. Neonatal symptomatic thromboembolism in Germany: two year survey. Arch Dis Child 76:F163, 1997.
4. Van Ommen CH, Heijboer H, Buller H, et al. Venous thromboembolism in childhood: a prospective two-year registry in The Netherlands. J Pediatrics 139:676–681, 2001.
5. Schmidt B, Andrew M. Neonatal thrombosis: report of a prospective Canadian and international registry. Pediatrics 96:939–943, 1995.
6. Kurnik K, Kosch A, Strater R, et al. for the Childhood Stroke Study Group. Recurrent thromboembolism in infants and children suffering from symptomatic neonatal arterial stroke. A prospective follow-up study. Stroke 34:2887, 2003.
7. Manco-Johnson MJ. Development of hemostasis in the fetus. Thromb Res 115 (Suppl 1):P55, 2005.
8. Reverdiau-Moalic P, Delahousse B, Body G, et al. Evolution of blood coagulation activators and inhibitors in the healthy human fetus. Blood 88(3):900–906, 1996.
9. Andrew M, Paes B, Milner R, et al. Development of the human coagulation system in the full-term infant. Blood 70(1):165–172, 1987.
10. Andrew M, Vegh P, Johnston M, et al. Maturation of the hemostatic system during childhood. Blood 80(8):1998–2005, 1992.
11. Bowen DJ, Collins PW. Insights into von Willebrand factor proteolysis: clinical implications. Br J Haematol 133(5):457–467, 2006.
12. Weinstein MJ, Blanchard R, Moake JL, et al. Fetal and neonatal von Willebrand factor (vWF) is unusually large and similar to the vWF in patients with thrombotic thrombocytopenic purpura. Br J Haematol 72(1):68–72, 1989.
13. Kavakli K, Canciani MT, Mannucci PM. Plasma levels of the von Willebrand factor-cleaving protease in physiological and pathological conditions in children. Pediatr Hematol Oncol 19:467–473, 2002.

14. Tsai HM, Sarode R, Downes KA. Ultralarge von Willebrand factor multimers and normal ADAMTS activity in the umbilical cord blood. Thromb Res 108:121–125, 2002.
15. Israels SJ, Rand ML, Michelson AD. Neonatal platelet function. Semin Thromb Hemost 29:363–372, 2003.
16. Saxonhouse MA, Sola MC. Platelet function in term and preterm neonates. Clin Perinatol 31:15–28, 2004.
17. Del Vecchio A, Sola, MC. Performing and interpreting the bleeding time in the neonatal intensive care unit. Clin Perinatol 27:643–654, 2000.
18. Rand ML, Carcao MD, Blanchette VS. Use of the PFA-100 in the assessment of primary, platelet-related hemostasis in a pediatric setting. Semin Thromb Hemost 24:523–529, 1998.
19. Sthoeger D, Nardi M, Karpatkin M. Protein S in the first year of life. Br J Haematol 72:424–428, 1989.
20. Corrigan JJ Jr, Jeter MA. Histadine-rich glycoprotein and plasminogen plasma levels in term and preterm newborns. Am J Dis Child 144:825–828, 1990.
21. Hathaway WE, Bonnar J. Hemostatic disorders of the pregnant woman and newborn infant. New York, NY: Elsevier; 1987: 60–61.
22. Ries M. Molecular and functional properties of fetal plasminogen and its possible influence on clot lysis in the neonatal period. Semin Thromb Hemost 23:247–252, 1997.
23. Markarian M, Githens JH, Rosenblut E, et al. Hypercoagulability in premature infants with special reference to the respiratory distress syndrome and hemorrhage. I. Coagulation studies. Biol Neonate 17:84–97, 1971.
24. Streif W, Paes B, Berry L, et al. Influence of exogenous factor VIIa on thrombin generation in cord plasma of full-term and pre-term newborns. Blood Coagul Fibrinolysis 11(4):349–357, 2000.
25. Cvirn G, Gallistl S, Leschnik B, et al. Low tissue factor pathway inhibitor (TFPI) together with low antithrombin allows sufficient thrombin generation in neonates. J Thromb Haemost 1(2):263–268, 2003.
26. Goldenberg NA, Hathaway WE, Jacobson L, et al. A new global assay of coagulation and fibrinolysis. Thromb Res 116:345–356, 2005.
27. Smith AA, Jacobson LJ, Miller BI, et al. A new euglobulin clot lysis assay for global fibrinolysis. Thromb Res 112:329–337, 2003.
28. Markarian M, Githens JH, Jackson JJ, et al. Fibrinolytic activity in premature infants. Relationship of the enzyme system to the respiratory distress syndrome. Am J Dis Child 113(3):312–321, 1967.
29. Manco-Johnson MJ. Disseminated intravascular coagulation and other hypercoagulable syndromes. Int J Pediatr Hematol Oncol 1:1–23, 1994.
30. McDonald MM, Johnson ML, Rumack CM, et al. Role of coagulopathy in newborn intracranial hemorrhage. Pediatrics 74(1):26–31, 1984.
31. Manco-Johnson MJ, Marlar RA, Jacobson LJ, et al. Severe protein C deficiency in newborn infants. J Pediatr 113:359–363, 1988.
32. Manco-Johnson MJ, Abshire TC, Jacobson LJ, et al. Severe neonatal protein C deficiency: prevalence and thrombotic risk. J Pediatr 119:793–798, 1991.
33. Goldenberg NA, Manco-Johnson MJ. Pediatric hemostasis and use of plasma components. Best Prac Res Clin Haematol 19:143–155, 2006.
34. Schmidt B, Gillie P, Mitchell L, et al. A placebo-controlled randomized trial of antithrombin therapy in neonatal respiratory distress syndrome. Am J Respir Crit Care Med 158:470–476, 1998.
35. Goldstein B, Nadel S, Peters M, et al. ENHANCE: results of a global open-label trial of drotrecogin alfa (activated) in children with severe sepsis. Pediatr Crit Care Med 7:277–278, 2006.
36. Petaja J, Peltola K, Rautiainen P. Disappearance of symptomatic venous thrombosis after neonatal cardiac operations during antithrombin II substitution. J Thorac Cardiovasc Surg 118:955–956, 1999.
37. Oppenheimer EH, Esterly JR. Thrombosis in the newborn: comparison between infants of diabetic and nondiabetic mothers. J Pediatr 67:549–556, 1965.
38. Winyard PJD, Bharucha T, De Bruyn R, et al. Perinatal renal venous thrombosis: presenting renal length predicts outcome. Arch Dis Child Fetal Neonatal Ed 91:273–278, 2006.
39. Van Horn JT, Craven C, Ward K, et al. Histologic features of placentas and abortion specimens from women with antiphospholipid and antiphospholipid-like syndromes. Placenta 25(7):642–648, 2004.
40. Rosendaal FR. Venous thrombosis: the role of genes, environment and behavior. Hematology Am soc Hematol State of the Art 1–12, 2005.
41. Kraaijenhagen RA, In't Anker PS, Koopman MM, et al. High plasma concentration of factor VIIIc is a major risk factor for venous thromboembolism. Thromb Haemost 83:5–9, 2000.
42. Zoller B, Hillarp A, Berntorp E, et al. Activated protein C resistance due to a common factor V gene mutation is a major risk factor for venous thrombosis. Annu Rev Med 48:45–58, 1997.
43. Poort SR, Rosendaal FR, Reitsma PH, et al. A common genetic variation in the 3′-untranslated region of the prothrombin gene is associated with elevated plasma prothrombin levels and an increase in venous thrombosis. Blood 88:3698–3703, 1996.
44. Den Heijer M, Koster T, Blom HJ, et al. Hyperhomocysteinemia as a risk factor for deep-vein thrombosis. N Engl J Med 334(12):759–762, 1996.
45. Rook JL, Nugent DJ, Young G. Pediatric stroke and methylenetetrahydrofolate reductase polymorphisms: an examination of C677T and A1298C mutations. J Pediatr Hematol Oncol 27(11):590–593, 2005.
46. Brenner G. Thrombophilia and adverse pregnancy outcome. Obstet Gynecol Clin North Am 33(3):443–456, ix, 2006.

47. Meijers JC, Tekelenburg WL, Bouma BN, et al. High levels of coagulation factor XI as a risk factor for venous thrombosis. N Engl J Med 342:696–701, 2000.

48. Van Hylckama Vlieg A, van der Linden IK, Bertina RM, et al. High levels of factor IX increase the risk of venous thrombosis. Blood 95(12):3678–3682, 2000.

49. Bucciarelli P, Rosendaal FR, Tripodi A, et al. Risk of venous thromboembolism and clinical manifestations in carriers of antithrombin, protein C, protein S deficiency, or activated protein C resistance: a multicenter collaborative family study. Arterioscler Thromb Vasc Biol 19(4):1026–1033, 1999.

50. Petaja J, Manco-Johnson MJ. Protein C pathway in infants and children. Semin Thromb Hemost 29:349–361, 2003.

51. Manco-Johnson MJ, Nuss R. Thrombophilia in the infant and child. Adv Pediatr 48:363–384, 2001.

52. Kosch A, Kuwertz-Bröking E, Heller C, et al. Renal venous thrombosis in neonates: prothrombotic risk factors and long-term follow-up. Blood 104:1356–1360, 2004.

53. Van Ommen CH, Peters M. Venous thromboembolic disease in childhood. Semin Thromb Hemost 29:391–403, 2003.

54. Hagstrom JN, Walter J, Bluebond-Langner R, et al. Prevalence of the factor V Leiden mutation in children and neonates with thromboembolic disease. J Pediatr 133:777–781, 1998.

55. Vossen CY, Preston FE, Conard J, et al. Hereditary thrombophilia and fetal loss: a prospective follow-up study. J Thromb Haemost 2:592–596, 2004.

56. Brenner B, Grabowski EF, Hellgren M, et al. Thrombophilia and pregnancy complications. Thromb Haemost 92:678–681, 2004.

57. Rosendaal FR. Venous thrombosis: a multicausal disease. The Lancet 353:1167–1173, 1999.

58. Robertson L, Wu O, Langhorne P, et al. Thrombophilia in pregnancy: a systematic review. Br J Haematol 132:171–196, 2006.

59. Kutteh WH. Antiphospholipid antibodies and reproduction. J Reprod Immunol 35:151–171, 1997.

60. deKlerk OL, deVries TW, Sinnige LG. An unusual case of neonatal seizures in a newborn infant. Pediatrics 100:E8, 1997.

61. Hermansen MC, Hermansen MG. Intravascular catheter complications in the neonatal intensive care unit. Clin Perinatol 32:141–156,vii, 2005.

62. Tyson JE, deSa DJ, Moore S. Thromboatheromatous complications of umbilical arterial catheterization in the newborn period. Clinicopathological study. Arch Dis Child 51:744–754, 1976.

63. Schwartz DS, Gettner PA, Konstantino MM, et al. Umbilical venous catheterization and the risk of portal vein thrombosis. J Pediatr 131:760–762, 1997.

64. Kim JH, Lee YS, Kim SH, et al. Does umbilical vein catheterization lead to portal venous thrombosis? Prospective US evaluation in 100 neonates. Radiology 219:645–650, 2001.

65. Morag I, Epelman M, Daneman A, et al. Portal vein thrombosis in the neonate: risk factors, course and outcome. J Pediatr 148:745–749, 2006.

66. Butler-O'Hara M, Buzzard CJ, Reubens L, et al. A randomized trial comparing long-term and short-term use of umbilical venous catheters in premature infants with birth weights of less than 1251 grams. Pediatrics 118:e25–e35, 2006.

67. Salonvaara M, Riikonen P, Kekomaki R, et al. Clinically symptomatic central venous catheter-related deep venous thrombosis in newborns. Acta Paediatr 88:642–646, 1999.

68. Shah P, Shah V. Continuous heparin infusion to prevent thrombosis and catheter occlusion in neonates with peripherally placed percutaneous central venous catheters. Cochrane Database Sys Rev 3, 2005.

69. Petäjä J, Lundström U, Sairanen H, et al. Central venous thrombosis after cardiac operations in children. J Thorac Cariovasc Surg 112:883–889, 1996.

70. Nowak-Göttl U, Dübbers A, Kececioglu D, et al. Factor V Leiden, protein C and lipoprotein (a) in catheter-related thrombosis in childhood: a prospective study. J Pediatr 131:608–612, 1997.

71. Barrington KJ. Umbilical artery catheters in the newborn: effects of catheter materials. Cochrane Database Sys Rev 1, 1999. Art. No.: CD000949. DOI: 10.1002/14651858.CD000949.

72. Gilhooly J, Lindenberg J, Reynolds JW. Central venous silicone elastomer catheter placement by basilic vein cutdown in neonates. Pediatrics 78:636–639, 1986.

73. Barrington KJ. Umbilical artery catheters in the newborn: effects of position of the catheter tip. Cochrane Database Sys Rev 1, 1999. Art. No.: CD000505. DOI: 10.1002/14651858.CD000505.

74. Goutail-Flaud MF, Sfez M, Berg A, et al. Central venous catheter-related complications in newborns and infants: a 587-case survey. J Pediatr Surg 26:645–650, 1991.

75. Sadiq HF, Devaskar S, Keenan WJ, Weber TR. Broviac catheterization in low birth weight infants: incidence and treatment of associated complications. Crit Care Med 15:47–50, 1987.

76. Barrington KJ. Umbilical artery catheters in the newborn: effects of catheter design (end vs side hole). Cochrane Database Sys Rev 1, 1999. Art. No.: CD000508. DOI: 10.1002/14651858.CD000508.

77. Kabra NS, Kumar M, Shah SS. Multiple versus single lumen umbilical venous catheters for newborn infants. Cochrane Database Sys Rev 3, 2005. Art. No.: CD004498. DOI: 10.1002/14651858.CD004498.

78. Barrington KJ. Umbilical artery catheters in the newborn: effects of heparin. Cochrane Database Sys Rev 1, 1999. Art. No.: CD000507. DOI: 10.1002/14651858.CD000507.

79. Jackson JC, Truog WE, Watchko JF, et al. Efficacy of thromboresistant umbilical artery catheters in reducing aortic thrombosis and related complications. J Pediatr 110:102–105, 1987.

80. Pierce CM, Wade A, Mok Q. Heparin-bonded central venous lines reduce thrombotic and infective complications in critically ill children. Intens Care Med 26:967–972, 2000.

81. Klement P, Du YJ, Berry LR, et al. Chronic performance of polyurethane catheters covalently coated with ATH complex: a rabbit jugular vein model. Biomaterials 27:5107–5117, 2006.

82. Blaney M, Shen V, Kerner JA, et al. for the CAPS investigators. Alteplase for the treatment of central venous catheter occlusion in children: results of a prospective, open-label, single-arm study (the Cathflo Activate Pediatric Study). J Vasc Interv Radiol 17:1745–1751, 2006.

83. Jacobs BR, Haygood M, Hingl J. Recombinant tissue plasminogen activator in the treatment of central venous catheter occlusion in children. J Pediatr 139:593–596, 2001.

84. Chalmers EA. Perinatal stroke – risk factors and management. Brit J Haematol 130:333–343, 2005.

85. Lee J, Croen LA, Backstrand KH, et al. Maternal and infant characteristics associated with perinatal arterial stroke in the infant. JAMA 292:723–729, 2005.

86. deVeber G. Canadian paediatric ischaemic stroke registry: analysis of children with arterial ischaemic stroke. The Canadian Pediatric Stroke Study Group. Ann Neurol 48:526, abstr., 2000.

87. Golomb MR, MacGregor DL, Domi T, et al. Presumed pre- or perinatal arterial ischemic stroke: risk factors and outcomes. Ann Neurol 50:163–168, 2001.

88. deVeber G, Andrew M. Cerebral sinovenous thrombosis in children. New Engl J Med 345:417–423, 2001.

89. Kurnik K, Kosch A, Sträter R, et al. for the Childhood Stroke Study Group. Recurrent thromboembolism in infants and children suffering from symptomatic neonatal arterial stroke. a prospective follow-up study. Stroke 34:2887–2893, 2003.

90. Golomb MR, Dick PT, MacGregor DL, et al. Neonatal arterial ischemic stroke and cerebral sinovenous thrombosis are more commonly diagnosed in boys. J Child Neurol 19:493–497, 2004.

91. Mecuri E, Barnett A, Rutherford M, et al. Neonatal cerebral infarction and neuromotor outcome at school age. Pediatrics 113:95–100, 2004.

92. Günther G, Junker R, Sträter R, et al. for the Childhood Stroke Study Group. Symptomatic ischemic stroke in full-term neonates: role of acquired and genetic prothrombotic risk factors. Stroke 31:2437–2441, 2000.

93. deVeber G, Monagle P, Chan A, et al. Prothrombotic disorders in infants and children with cerebral thromboembolism. Arch Neurol 55:1539–1543, 1998.

94. Parker MJ, Joubert GI, Levin SD. Portal vein thrombosis causing neonatal cerebral infarction. Arch Dis Child Fetal Neonatal Ed 87:125–127, 2002.

95. Rutherford MA, Ward P, Malamatentiou C. Advanced MR techniques in the term-born neonate with perinatal brain injury. Semin Fetal Neonatal Med 10:445–460, 2005.

96. Cowan FM, deVries LS. The internal capsule in neonatal imaging. Semin Fetal Neonatal Med 10:461–474, 2005.

97. Boardman JP, Ganesan V, Rutherford MA, et al. Magnetic resonance imaging correlates of hemiparesis after perinatal and childhood middle cerebral artery stroke. Pediatrics 115:321–326, 2005.

98. Stam J, deBruijn S, deVeber G. Anticoagulation for cerebral sinus thrombosis. Stroke 34:1054–1055, 2003.

99. Monagle P, Chan A, Massicotte P, et al. Antithrombotic therapy in children. The seventh ACCP conference on antithrombotic and thrombolytic therapy. Chest 126:645S–687S, 2004.

100. Saver JL, Yafeh B. Confirmation of tPA treatment effect by baseline severity-adjusted end point reanalysis of the NINDS-tPA stroke trials. Stroke 38:414–416, 2007.

101. Mosnier LO, Zlokovic BV, Griffin JH. The cytoprotective protein C pathway. Blood 2007, in print: prepublished online November 16, 2006; DOI 10.1182/blood-2006–09–003004.

102. Folsom AR, Rosamond WD, Shahar E, et al. Prospective study of markers of hemostatic function with risk of ischemic stroke. The Atherosclerosis Risk in Communities (ARIC) Study Investigators. Circulation 199:736–742, 1999.

103. Zlokovic BV, Zhang C, Liu D, et al. Functional recovery after embolic stroke in rodents by activated protein C. Ann Neurol 58:474–477, 2005.

104. Endres M, Laufs U, Liao J, et al. Targeting eNOS for stroke protection. Trends Neurosci 27:283–289, 2004.

105. Cimino M, Balduini W, Carloni S, et al. Neuroprotective effect of Simvastatin in stroke: a comparison between adult and neonatal rat models of cerebral ischemia. Neuro Toxicology 26:929–933, 2005.

106. Siren A-L, Fratelli M, Brines M, et al. Erythropoietin prevents neuronal apoptosis after cerebral ischemia and metabolic stress. Proc Natl Acad Sci USA 98:4044–4049, 2001.

107. Wen TC, Sadamoto Y, Tanaka J, et al. Erythropoietin protects neurons against chemical hypoxia and cerebral ischemic injury by upregulating Bcl-xL expression. J Neurosci Res 67:795–803, 2002.

108. Carmichael ST. Cellular and molecular mechanisms of neural repair after stroke: Making waves. Ann Neurol 59:735–742, 2006.

109. Sola A, Rogido M, Lee BH, et al. Erythropoietin after focal cerebral ischemia activates the Janus kinase-signal transducer and activator of transcription signaling pathway and improves brain injury in postnatal day 7 rats. Pediatr Res 57:481–487, 2005.

110. Ohls R, Ehrenkranz RA, Das A, et al. for the National Institute of Child Health and Human Development Neonatal Research Network. Neurodevelopmental outcome and growth at 18 to 22 months' corrected age in extremely low birth weight infants treated with early erythropoietin and iron. Pediatrics 114:1287–1291, 2004.

111. Bierer R, Peceny MC, Hartenberger CH, et al. Erythropoietin and neurodevelopmental outcome in preterm infants. Pediatrics 118:e635–e640, 2006.

112. Chao J, Chao L. Kallikrein-kinin in stroke, cardiovascular and renal disease. Exp Physiol 90(3):291–298, 2004.
113. Manco-Johnson MJ. How I treat venous thrombosis in children. Blood 107:21–29, 2006.
114. Revel-Vilk S, Sharanthkumar A, Massicotte P, et al. Natural history of arterial and venous thrombosis in children treated with low molecular weight heparin: a longitudinal study by ultrasound. J Thromb Haemost 2:42–46, 2004.
115. McDonald MM, Jacobson LJ, Hay WW JR, et al. Heparin clearance in the newborn. Pediatr Res 15:1015–1018, 1981.
116. McDonald MM, Hathaway WE. Anticoagulant therapy by continuous heparininzation in newborn and older infants. J Pediatr 101:451–457, 1982.
117. Dunaway KK, Gal P, Ransom JL. Use of enoxaparin in a preterm infant. Ann Pharmacother 34(12):1410–1413, 2000.
118. Albisetti M. Thrombolytic therapy in children. Thromb Res 118:95–105, 2006.
119. Wang M, Hays T, Balasa V, et al. for the Pediatric Coagulation Consortium. Experience using low-dose tissue plasminogen activator thrombolysis in children. J Pediatr Hematol Oncol 25:379–386, 2003.
120. Harmann, Becker, Hussein, et al. Treatment of neonatal thrombus formation with recombinant tissue plasminogen activator: six years experience and review of the literature. Arch Dis Child Neonatal Ed 85:F18–F22, 2001.
121. Gupta AA, Leaker M, Andrew M, et al. Safety and outcomes of thrombolysis with tissue plasminogen activator for the treatment of intravascular thrombosis in children. J Pediatr 139:682–688, 2001.
122. Ferari F, Vagnarelli F, Gargano G, et al. Early intracardiac thrombosis in preterm infants and thrombolysis with recombinant tissue type plasminogen activator. Arch Dis Child Fetal Neonatal Ed 85:F66–F72, 2001.
123. Goldenberg NA. Long-term outcomes of venous thrombosis in children. Curr Opin Hematol 12:370–376, 2005.
124. Kosch A, Kuwertz-Bröking, Heller C, et al., for the Childhood Thrombophilia Study Group. Renal venous thrombosis in neonates: prothrombotic risk factors and long-term follow-up. Blood 104:1356–1360, 2004.
125. Nuss R, Hays T, Manco-Johnson M. Efficacy and safety of heparin anticoagulation for neonatal renal vein thrombosis. Am J Pediatr Hematol Oncol 16(2):127–131, 1994.
126. Winyard PJD, Bharucha T, De Bruyn R, et al. Perinatal renal venous thrombosis: presenting renal length predicts outcome. Arch Dis Child Fetal Neonatal Ed 91:273–278, 2006.
127. Hausler M, Hubner D, Delhaas T, et al. Long term complications of inferior vena cava thrombosis. Arch Dis Child 85:228–233, 2001.
128. Ramanaathan R, Hughes TMD, Richardson AJ. Perinatal inferior vena cava thrombosis and absence of the infrarenal inferior vena cava. J Vasc Surg 33:1097–1099, 2001.

Chapter 6

Practical Approaches to the Neutropenic Neonate

Akhil Maheshwari, MD

Definition of Neutropenia in Neonates

Clinical Evaluation of Neutropenia in Neonates

Clinical Management of a Neonate with Neutropenia

Neutropenia is a commonly detected problem among ill neonates, affecting up to 8% of all patients in neonatal intensive care units (NICUs) (1–4). Since nearly 400 000 neonates are admitted annually to NICUs in the USA, as many as 32 000 infants may be recognized as neutropenic. The incidence is higher among preterm infants than among term infants, with estimates ranging between 6 and 58% depending on the definition of neutropenia (5). In many neonates the neutropenia is transient and does not appear to convey a survival disadvantage. However, in others it is prolonged and severe and constitutes a serious deficiency in antimicrobial defense.

DEFINITION OF NEUTROPENIA IN NEONATES

The diagnosis of neutropenia is based on a low blood neutrophil concentration. An absolute neutrophil count (ANC) can be calculated from a routine complete blood count as follows:

absolute neutrophil count = white cell count (/µL) × neutrophil percentage

where the neutrophil percentage is calculated as the sum of the percentage figures for segmented neutrophils, band neutrophils, metamyelocytes, and any other neutrophil precursors that may be seen on the differential count.

The interpretation of an ANC value in a neonate usually involves comparison with available reference ranges. In a statistical sense, neutropenia is defined as an ANC two standard deviations below the mean value for the age (6) or, alternatively, as an ANC below the lower limit of normal on an age-defined population (7, 8). The reference ranges used most commonly were provided by Manroe and colleagues from the Southwestern Medical Center at Dallas, and these figures are based on the latter definition (9). This data set was derived from a cohort of 434 neonates born at 38.9 ± 2.4 weeks gestation obtained during the first 28 days following birth. Peak neutrophil counts occurred between 12 and 24 h postnatally, with 95% confidence limits of 7800–14500 cells/µL (Fig. 6-1). The neutrophil count then decreased, achieving a stable lower value of 1750 by 72 h of life. The stable upper limit of the next 28 days was not achieved until 6.6 days of age.

The reference ranges reported by Manroe and coworkers are widely accepted for term and near-term infants, but are less appropriate for very-low-birth-weight (VLBW) infants (10–13). Mouzinho and colleagues (8) revised the reference ranges

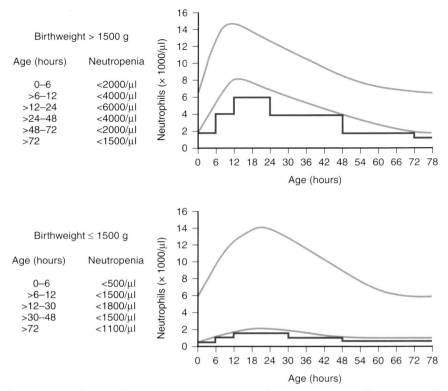

Birthweight > 1500 g

Age (hours)	Neutropenia
0–6	<2000/µl
>6–12	<4000/µl
>12–24	<6000/µl
>24–48	<4000/µl
>48–72	<2000/µl
>72	<1500/µl

Birthweight ≤ 1500 g

Age (hours)	Neutropenia
0–6	<500/µl
>6–12	<1500/µl
>12–30	<1800/µl
>30–48	<1500/µl
>72	<1100/µl

Figure 6-1 Definition of neutropenia. The upper panel gives the normal reference range for neutrophils (in between tinted lines) as established by Manroe et al. (9). Values below the solid line were considered neutropenic for neonates with a birth weight > 1500 g. The lower panel gives the normal reference range for neutrophils (in between tinted lines) as established by Mouzinho et al. (8) for neonates with a birth weight of 1500 g. Values below the solid line were considered neutropenic. (Reproduced with permission from Funke A, et al. Frequency, natural course, and outcome of neonatal neutropenia. Pediatrics 106:45–51, 2000.)

for blood neutrophil concentrations in VLBW infants (Fig. 6-1). Serial counts ($N =$ 1788) were obtained prospectively between birth and 28 days of age from 63 normal infants of 29.9 ± 2.3 weeks gestation. No difference in the upper limit of normal (neutrophilia) was observed between those VLBW infants and their more mature counterparts reported in 1979. However, there was greater variation at the lower end of the ranges and neutropenia was defined as a concentration less than 2000/µL at 12 h of life and less than 1000/µl after 48 h. In a recent study (14) comparing the reference ranges in septic VLBW infants, the figures from Manroe and colleagues were observed to provide greater sensitivity, but the ranges reported by Mouzinho and coworkers were more specific when neonates with early-onset group B streptococcal infection were compared with a matched control group.

The reference ranges are useful for accurate interpretation and follow-up of neutrophil counts. The definition of neutropenia, the lower limit of normal for blood neutrophil concentrations, has been variously reported as 1500/µL (15), 1800/µL (9), and 1100/µL (8). These 'cut-off' values are aimed to provide the clinician with a critical threshold to initiate investigation and, if possible, treatment. However, the relationship between blood neutrophil concentration and risk of developing an infection is not well established in neonates. Extrapolating from the chronic severe neutropenia registry and chemotherapy studies in children, neonates with neutrophil counts above 1000/µL are not likely to be at an increased risk. Neonates with blood neutrophil concentrations less than 500/µL probably are at increased risk, particularly if the severe neutropenia persists many days or

Table 6-1   Causes of Neutropenia in Neonates

DECREASED NEUTROPHIL PRODUCTION

Infants of hypertensive women (exact etiology unknown; possible causes include presence of a placenta-derived inhibitor of neutrophil production, decreased responsiveness of precursors to G-CSF)

Donors of twin-twin transfusions

Neonates with Rh hemolytic disease (progenitor "steal" where precursors may be diverted towards erythroid differentiation)

Congenital neutropenias/Bone marrow failure syndromes

Kostmann syndrome (maturation arrest and increased apoptosis of precursors; neutrophil elastase mutations which lead to exclusive membrane localization of the enzyme)

Reticular dysgenesis (inherited immunodeficiency with impairment of both myeloid and lymphoid series)

Barth syndrome (organic aciduria, dilated cardiomyopathy, and neutropenia; neutropenia presumably due to a neutrophil membrane defect)

Shwachman-Diamond syndrome (exocrine pancreatic insufficiency and neutropenia; defect in SBDS protein which may be involved in ribosomal biogenesis)

Cartilage-hair hypoplasia (short-limbed dwarfism; impairment of proliferation in neutrophil precursors)

Cyclic neutropenia (cyclic hematopoiesis with nadirs at 3-week intervals; neutrophil elastase mutations which prevent membrane localization of the enzyme)

Inherited errors of metabolism

Organic acidemias (metabolic intermediates inhibit proliferation of neutrophil precursors)

Glycogen storage disease type 1b (increased neutrophil apoptosis)

Viral infections (infection of neutrophil progenitors, hypersplenism)

Rubella

Cytomegalovirus

Copper deficiency

Alloimmune neutropenia associated with anti-NB1 antibodies (NB1 antigen is present on neutrophil precursors)

INCREASED NEUTROPHIL DESTRUCTION

Bacterial or fungal sepsis (increased tissue migration; low marrow production in overwhelming sepsis)

Necrotizing enterocolitis (circulating neutrophil pool depleted due to increased migration into the intestines and peritoneum, increased emargination)

Alloimmune neonatal neutropenia (analogous to Rh-hemolytic disease of erythrocytes, where mother produces antibody against an antigen present on fetal neutrophils which has been inherited from the father)

Neonatal autoimmune neutropenia (passively acquired anti-neutrophil antibodies from mother, who has autoimmune neutropenia)

Autoimmune neutropenia of infancy (infant becomes sensitized to self-antigens present on neutrophils and produces antibody against own neutrophils)

OTHER CAUSES

Idiopathic neutropenia of prematurity (a diagnosis of exclusion; readily reversible with G-CSF therapy)

Drug-induced neutropenia (can occur with a large number of drugs; those commonly incriminated in the NICU include β-lactam antibiotics, thiazide diuretics, ranitidine, acyclovir)

Pseudoneutropenia (a benign condition where circulating neutrophil pool is smaller than the vascular emarginated pool)

Artefactual neutropenia (a benign condition where neutrophils agglutinate upon exposure to the EDTA, which is used as anticoagulant in blood samples in vitro)

weeks (16–20). Neonates with blood neutrophil counts between 500 and 1000/μL are at some intermediate risk.

CLINICAL EVALUATION OF NEUTROPENIA IN NEONATES

Neutropenia can be secondary to decreased production of neutrophils, increased neutrophil destruction, or a combination of these mechanisms (Table 6-1). The most commonly encountered causes of neonatal neutropenia are those related to maternal hypertension, sepsis, twin-twin transfusion, alloimmunization, and hemolytic disease (21).

Evaluation for Etiology

(1) Perinatal information: maternal history of hypertension with fetal growth retardation, multiple gestation with disparity between twins, or an infectious illness during pregnancy can be diagnostic. Similarly, presence of high-risk factors for early onset sepsis such as prolonged rupture of membranes or chorioamnionitis can provide useful clues. The presence of neutropenia or autoimmune disease in the mother can suggest the presence of transplacental transfer of anti-neutrophil autoantibodies.

(2) Concurrent illness such as necrotizing enterocolitis, bacterial or fungal sepsis, immunodeficiency, cardiomyopathy (Barth syndrome), intractable metabolic acidosis or other derangements or the presence of anemia and/or thrombocytopenia can provide useful information.

(3) Physical examination: characteristic dysmorphic features such as skeletal dysplasia, radial or thumb hypoplasia (congenital bone marrow failure syndromes), hepatosplenomegaly (TORCH, storage disorders), or skin/hair pigmentary abnormalities (Chédiak-Higashi syndrome) can be helpful.

(4) Chronological age: several disorders are associated with specific periods. Neutropenia associated with maternal hypertension is usually observed in the first week, and persistence beyond 5 days should trigger further work-up. Congenital bone marrow failure syndromes also can present early. Inborn errors of metabolism usually present late in the first week and beyond. Copper deficiency may be rarely seen in growing premature infants dependent on parenteral nutrition. Idiopathic neutropenia of prematurity also occurs late in the hospital course of growing VLBW infants, and resolves spontaneously.

Evaluation of Neutrophil Kinetics

In the bone marrow, the neutrophil population is composed of a neutrophil proliferative pool (consisting of myeloblasts, promyelocytes, and myelocytes) and a postmitotic neutrophil storage pool (consisting of metamyelocytes, band neutrophils and segmented neutrophils). The release of mature segmented neutrophils is tightly regulated in a differentiation-dependent process (22). Thus, the appearance of bands and other immature neutrophil precursors in the circulation indicates that the bone marrow pool of mature neutrophils has already been depleted (Fig. 6-2). In neutropenia, an approximate kinetic evaluation can be performed by calculating the "immature to total neutrophil ratio (I/T)" from the differential white blood cell count:

$$(bands + metamyelocytes + myelocytes)$$

$$(segmented\ neutrophils + bands + metamyelocytes + myelocytes)$$

Schelonka and colleagues reported that normal I/T ratios in term neonates have a mean value of 0.16 (SD 0.10), with a 10–90th percentile range extending from 0.05 to 0.27 (23). An elevated I/T ratio (= 0.3) in the presence of neutropenia suggests depletion of the bone marrow neutrophil storage pool due to increased peripheral destruction/tissue recruitment of neutrophils, and also, in most

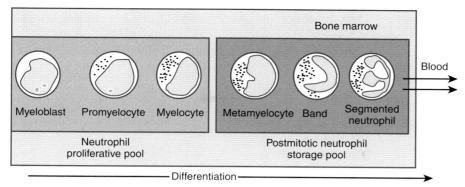

Figure 6-2 Mature segmented neutrophils are released from the bone marrow into the bloodstream in a series of differentiation-dependent events. Appearance of earlier, less mature forms (such as bands) suggests that the post-mitotic storage pool of mature neutrophils has been depleted. Such depletion can be assessed by calculating the "immature to total neutrophil (I/T) ratio".

instances, an increase in the marrow production of neutrophils. A normal or low I/T ratio in the presence of severe neutropenia suggests that the neutropenia is from decreased production, just as would be inferred for erythrocytes in an anemic patient with a low reticulocyte count.

The I/T neutrophil ratio is best known for its value in screening tests for sepsis in neonates, even though elevated ratios can be seen in many other conditions. Unlike the absolute neutrophil count, which shows a wider spread, the I/T ratio retains its discriminatory value for sepsis even in VLBW infants and can be successfully employed in conjunction with other screening tests such as C-reactive protein concentrations.(8, 9, 13, 24–26)

A bone marrow biopsy can be useful in cases with prolonged (> 2 weeks), unusual, or refractory neutropenia. The procedure is usually performed in the tibial marrow using an Osgood needle (27). The marrow is evaluated for proliferative and postmitotic storage pools of neutrophils. Reduction in both cellular populations suggests decreased marrow activity, while increased numbers of proliferative precursors with a depleted storage pool is consistent with increased peripheral destruction of neutrophils. A combination of an expanded proliferative pool with a normal storage pool is generally seen during marrow recovery, and is relatively non-specific (28, 29). However, it needs to be considered that although marrow findings can provide vital kinetic information, the observations are rarely of diagnostic value. For instance, marrow findings can be very similar in hyporegenerative states as disparate as Kostmann syndrome and in an infant born to a hypertensive mother, even when the clinical conditions might be completely dissimilar in etiology and outcome.

Evaluation of Clinical Severity

The risk of infection and mortality in neutropenic neonates correlates with:
   (a) severity of neutropenia (risk related inversely to the ANC) (30);
   (b) overall severity of sickness/concurrent illnesses, as it would increase the probability of invasive monitoring and lower tissue resistance (31); in VLBW infants, the risk of infection secondary to neutropenia and the mortality attributable to infection and neutropenia are significantly higher than in term newborns (30);
   (c) duration of neutropenia: the risk of infection increases with duration, and persistent neutropenia should trigger evaluation and/or treatment even if of a moderate severity (20).

CLINICAL MANAGEMENT OF A NEONATE WITH NEUTROPENIA

The clinical approach to the neonate with neutropenia should depend on the severity, duration, and etiology of the disorder. In an ill neutropenic neonate sepsis should always be considered as a possibility, and antibiotic therapy should be started pending culture maturation. If the neutropenia is severe and prolonged, reverse isolation procedures may be considered.

The role of prophylactic antibiotics in neonatal neutropenia is unclear. In children with chronic idiopathic or chemotherapy-associated neutropenia, antibiotics are often recommended until neutrophil counts rise to above 1000/μL (32–34). Since most causes of neutropenia in neonates are transient conditions, and in view of the fear of emergence of multidrug-resistant bacterial strains, routine antibiotic prophylaxis is not recommended in newborn infants at this time.

Hematopoietic Growth Factors

Granulocyte colony-stimulating factor (G-CSF) and granulocyte-macrophage colony-stimulating factor (GM-CSF) are naturally occurring cytokines that are in routine clinical use in adults and children to accelerate neutrophil recovery following anti-cancer therapy. G-CSF increases the number of circulating neutrophils by stimulating the release of neutrophils from bone marrow, inducing myeloid proliferation, and reducing neutrophil apoptosis (35). GM-CSF was initially defined by its ability to generate both granulocyte and macrophage colonies from precursor cells as a result of proliferation and differentiation (36). Under physiologic conditions, G-CSF is the primary systemic regulator of the circulating concentrations of neutrophils (35). GM-CSF, in contrast, does not play a major role in steady-state conditions but is upregulated at tissue sites of inflammation to enhance neutrophil and macrophage maturation (37).

Recombinant G-CSF and GM-CSF have been evaluated in neonates with neutropenia. Both agents hold promise in correction of circulating neutrophil concentrations, although the efficacy varies with the etiology. The effect of these growth factors on clinical outcome remains unresolved.

Role in Neonatal Sepsis

Recombinant G-CSF has been evaluated in neonatal sepsis and neutropenia in several trials. Gillan and colleagues reported a dose-dependent biologic effect of G-CSF (38). They studied 42 neonates with presumed bacterial infection during their first 3 days of life. These infants were randomized to receive a placebo or 1, 5, 10, or 20 μg/kg/day of G-CSF for three consecutive days. A dose-dependent increase in blood neutrophil concentrations was observed. Since then the efficacy of G-CSF in neonatal sepsis has been examined by Schibler et al., Bedford-Russell et al., Miura et al., Barak et al., and Kocherlakota and La Gamma (39–43). In a meta-analysis based on these studies, Bernstein and colleagues reported that 73 G-CSF recipients had a lower mortality than 82 infants in the control arms. However, when the non-randomized studies were excluded, the analysis did not remain statistically adequate (44).

Recombinant GM-CSF therapy has also been tried in neonatal sepsis. Cairo and associates observed dose-dependent increases in circulating neutrophil and monocyte concentrations within 48 h of GM-CSF administration (5 or 10 μg/kg/day). Tibial marrow aspirates revealed an increase in neutrophil reserves, and neutrophil C3bi receptor expression was increased within 24 h of beginning treatment (45). Bilgin and coworkers, in a prospective, randomized study, administered GM-CSF to 30 patients for 7 consecutive days. Twenty-five patients from the GM-CSF group and

24 from the conventionally treated group had early-onset sepsis, and the remaining 11 patients had late-onset sepsis. The GM-CSF-treated group showed significantly higher absolute neutrophil counts and a lower mortality rate (46).

There has been considerable interest in the use of GM-CSF therapy as prophylaxis against nosocomial infections in VLBW infants. Both neutrophils and mononuclear phagocytes are known to be functionally immature in neonates, and hence prophylactic use of GM-CSF was well supported by pathophysiological considerations. Carr and colleagues initiated a 5-day course of prophylactic GM-CSF therapy (10 μg/kg) in 75 non-infected VLBW neonates within the first 72 h. GM-CSF therapy abolished neutropenia in treated infants, including those with and without sepsis, during a 4-week period following study entry. Although the GM-CSF recipients had fewer symptomatic, blood culture-positive septic episodes than controls, the difference did not reach statistical significance (47). In another large, randomized, placebo-controlled trial in 264 ELBW neonates, prophylactic GM-CSF administration at 8 μg/kg for the first 7 days and then every other day for 21 days led to higher ANCs, but did not change the incidence of confirmed nosocomial infections (48).

It appears that G-CSF may be more efficacious in raising neutrophil counts than GM-CSF. When cord blood neutrophils are treated with these agents in vitro, only G-CSF delays apoptosis (49). In a small study, Ahmad and coworkers (50) compared the relative efficacy of G-CSF and GM-CSF in correcting sepsis-induced neutropenia. Twenty-eight patients were randomized: 10 received G-CSF (10 μg/kg/day); 10 received GM-CSF (8 μg/kg/day) and 8 received placebo for a maximum of 7 days or until an absolute neutrophil count (ANC) of 10 000 cells/mm was reached. The neutrophil count in the G-CSF-treated group increased more rapidly than in the GM-CSF group.

Carr and colleagues have reviewed existing evidence for the use of G-CSF/GM-CSF in neonatal sepsis (51). In preterm infants with suspected systemic infection, G-CSF or GM-CSF did not provide additional survival advantage beyond antibiotic therapy [typical relative risk of death 0.71 (95% CI 0.38, 1.33)]. However, in a subgroup analysis of 97 infants who, in addition to systemic infection, had clinically significant neutropenia at trial entry ($< 1.7 \times 10^9$/L), the investigators did find a significant reduction in mortality by day 14 [relative risk 0.34 (95% CI 0.12, 0.92); risk difference −0.18 (95% CI −0.33, −0.03); number needed to treat 6 (95% CI 3–33)]. In prophylactic studies, recombinant GM-CSF did not reduce mortality [relative risk 0.59 (95% CI 0.24, 1.44); risk difference −0.03 (95% CI −0.08, 0.02)].

Role in Neonatal Immune-mediated Neutropenias

Recombinant G-CSF has been successfully used in correcting immune-mediated neutropenia in infants. Besides its effects on neutrophil production and delaying apoptosis, G-CSF has additional beneficial effects in immune-mediated neutropenias by downregulating antigen expression, thus rendering the neutrophils less vulnerable to circulating antibodies (52). This effect may be most pronounced with the antigens located on the FcRγIIIb, such as HNA-1a and HNA-1b. G-CSF might also increase additional antibody mopping sites by increasing the levels of soluble FcRγIII (53). G-CSF activates neutrophils, and might also correct some of the functional impairments in neutrophils induced by anti-neutrophil antibodies (54). It is also notable that in patients with immune-mediated neutropenias, serum G-CSF levels may not rise appropriately unless they have an infection, providing further justification for recombinant therapy (55). A review of these disorders may be found elsewhere (56).

G-CSF may need to be used with caution in patients with immune-mediated neutropenias secondary to antibodies against the neutrophil antigen HNA-2a (NB1). Stroncek and coworkers demonstrated that, unlike the downregulating effect on HNA-1a and -1b, G-CSF increased the expression of HNA-2a in healthy adult volunteers (57). We reported a neonate with alloimmune neutropenia secondary to anti-HNA-2a antibodies where the response was delayed, and was achieved only with an unusually high dose (58).

Role in Congenital Neutropenias

G-CSF is highly effective in patients with congenital neutropenias (59). This group of disorders broadly includes various inherited forms of neutropenia, including Kostmann syndrome (severe congenital neutropenia), cyclic neutropenia, Shwachman-Diamond syndrome, and inborn errors of metabolism such as glycogen storage disease 1b and organic acidemias. These conditions are associated with absolute neutrophil counts below 500/µL and an increased susceptibility to bacterial infections (59, 60).

Kostmann syndrome is marked by several neutropenias presenting in early infancy with absolute neutrophil counts of less than 200/µL and recurrent bacterial infections. These patients have mutations in the neutrophil elastase gene *ELA2* (61). G-CSF therapy is highly effective in patients with Kostmann syndrome. Data on more than 400 patients collected by the Severe Chronic Neutropenia International Registry (SCNIR) since 1994 have shown that recombinant G-CSF therapy was effective in more than 90% of patients in maintaining the neutrophil counts at approximately 1000/µL (60, 62). All responding patients required significantly fewer antibiotics and days of hospitalization (63). Over the last two decades, recombinant G-CSF therapy has significantly improved the survival of these patients (64).

Human cyclic neutropenia is a rare hematological disorder characterized by regular fluctuation in the serial count of blood neutrophils (65). The oscillations occur at subnormal levels at 3-week intervals, when neutrophil counts often fall to <250/µL. Bone marrow examination reveals a variable morphology, appearing normal during periods of higher neutrophil counts and with "maturation arrest" of neutrophilic series during or just before onset of severe neutropenia. Other blood cells, such as platelets or reticulocytes, often also vary in a cyclical pattern. G-CSF is considered in these infants if infections occur during periods of severe neutropenia. Continuous G-CSF therapy can elevate blood neutrophil counts to safe levels with lower risk of infections. Although the characteristic cycles are not eliminated by G-CSF, the period of the oscillations is shortened to 12–14 days (66). In contrast to G-CSF, these patients respond very poorly to GM-CSF (67). Shwachman-Diamond syndrome (SDS) is characterized by exocrine pancreatic insufficiency, neutropenia and growth retardation. Neutropenia might be seen in the neonatal period, and is the most common hematological abnormality, occurring in 88–100% of patients (68). The neutropenia is usually intermittent, fluctuating from severely low to normal levels. G-CSF therapy is effective in inducing a clinically beneficial neutrophil response. GM-CSF has also been used, but has inconsistent benefit (69). Glycogen-storage disease type 1b is a rare metabolic disorder which affects the transport system of glucose-6-phosphatase metabolism. These patients present with hepatomegaly, failure to thrive, renal dysfunction and recurrent infections. Chronic neutropenia in these patients is accompanied by functional defects in chemotaxis and phagocytosis. G-CSF therapy corrects neutropenia in these patients and also restores some of the functional activity of these cells (70).

Role in Neutropenia Related to Maternal Pregnancy-induced Hypertension

G-CSF has been used successfully in the neutropenia of PIH. Makhlouf and colleagues treated nine neutropenic infants born to mothers with preeclampsia with G-CSF (10 µg/kg/day) starting within 24 h of birth and for a maximum of three doses if neutropenia persisted. The absolute neutrophil count increased significantly in eight of the nine infants within 6 h, and neutrophilia was sustained for at least 72 h after administration of a single dose of G-CSF (71). Similar results were reported by La Gamma and coworkers, who treated four infants with G-CSF for up to 3 days. Absolute neutrophil counts increased nearly 4-fold within 48 h; maximal values were recorded on the 9th day after initiation of therapy. Total leukocyte counts subsequently decreased but remained in the normal range (72).

There are conflicting reports on whether neonates with neutropenia related to maternal PIH are at a higher risk of infection (73, 74). It is possible that G-CSF therapy may reduce the incidence of infection in these infants (75). However, infants born to preeclamptic mothers may have a slower neutrophilic response with G-CSF when compared to their counterparts born to normotensive mothers (76). It remains unclear which neonates with the neutropenia of PIH would be well served by G-CSF treatment.

Role in "Idiopathic" Neutropenia

Juul and Christensen reported a severe, prolonged, idiopathic, but self-resolving, variety of neutropenia among preterm neonates (77). These infants were neutropenic at or shortly following delivery, and remained neutropenic (generally < 500/μL) for 1–9 weeks. Blood and bone marrow studies indicated that the neutropenia was: (i) the kinetic result of diminished neutrophil production; (ii) not alloimmune; (iii) not cyclic; and (iv) not associated with recognized inborn errors, bacterial or viral infections, or medications. Treatment with G-CSF in these patients led to an immediate, marked increase in blood neutrophil concentration. This effect persisted to day 5, but counts were not different from those of the five placebo recipients on days 12 and 15. These patients apparently have a substantial G-CSF-mobilizable marrow neutrophil reserve, and on this basis the authors speculated that idiopathic neonatal neutropenia may not constitute a significant deficiency in antibacterial defense (78). The decision to treat these well infants may have to be individualized, depending on the duration and severity of neutropenia.

Dosage and Treatment Protocol for G-CSF Therapy

The usual dose of G-CSF is 5–10 μg/kg/day, administered by intravenous or subcutaneous injection. In most situations, the response is evident within 24–48 h. In well neutropenic infants, treatment may be considered only if neutropenia persists for more than 2–3 days, as many of these babies will recover spontaneously, and the overall risk of sepsis in otherwise healthy neonates has been reported to be about 8.5%. G-CSF therapy is not used routinely in sepsis-induced neutropenia as it is often a transient phenomenon, endogenous G-CSF levels are often high in these patients, and there is lack of definite evidence for benefit in these patients. In patients with neutropenia related to maternal hypertension, treatment is considered if ANCs are < 500/μL and persist at this level for many days. Neonates with immune-mediated neutropenia usually respond promptly to G-CSF, and often need continued treatment for a total of 2–3 weeks. The diagnosis of idiopathic neutropenia remains one of exclusion, and is often considered in retrospect following a dramatic resolution of neutropenia with G-CSF therapy.

In an occasional patient, G-CSF therapy will not raise blood neutrophil counts. In these apparently refractory cases, a bone marrow examination should be considered. G-CSF doses may be increased in increments of 10 μg/kg at 7–14-day intervals if the ANC remains below 1000/μL (58, 63). Doses can be reduced or withheld once ANCs reach 5000/μL or above, and attempts should be made to use the lowest dose necessary for maintaining a "safe" neutrophil count high enough to overcome infections. Non-responders to G-CSF are defined as those patients who fail to respond to doses exceeding 120 μg/kg/day.

The adverse effects of short-term G-CSF administration to neutropenic neonates are minimal, although Gilmore and coworkers noted that one of their infants with alloimmune neutropenia was irritable after the first two doses (79). These authors considered the possibility of bone pain, as is often seen with older children receiving G-CSF for other indications. This, however, did not necessitate cessation of therapy, and quickly resolved after the completion of the treatment. With longer-term G-CSF therapy as in congenital neutropenias, mild splenomegaly, moderate thrombocytopenia, osteoporosis, malignant transformation into myelodysplastic syndrome/leukemia, and anti-GCSF antibodies have been described (60, 80, 81).

Intravenous Immunoglobulins

Intravenous immunoglobulins (IVIG) have been used with success in alloimmune and autoimmune neutropenia, with a response rate of about 50% (17, 82–85). The elevation in neutrophil counts is often transient, lasting for about a week, although long-term remissions have been reported (85, 86). Mascarin and Ventura used anti-Rh (D) immunoglobulin in a 7-month-old infant with autoimmune neutropenia and achieved an improvement in the neutrophil counts, but the effect again lasted for only about 10 days and multiple doses were required (87). In view of logistic difficulties in outpatient administration of IVIG, lack of a titrable dose-reponse effect, and the fact that IVIG can rarely induce neutropenia by itself, it has been used less often than G-CSF in patients with immune neutropenia (88).

Intravenous immunoglobulin has been used with moderate success in neonatal sepsis, and efforts are on to evaluate microorganism-specific antibody preparations (89). Administration of IVIG can successfully mobilize neutrophils from the marrow storage pool into the circulation and thereby help, at least transiently, ameliorate neutropenia (90).

Corticosteroids

Steroids have been tried in the management of immune-mediated neutropenias and in congenital bone marrow failure syndromes. In alloimmune neutropenia, steroids are not very effective. Of the five infants reported independently by Lalezari and Buckwold and Emson, only one showed a partial response (91, 92). The response has been slightly better in autoimmune neutropenia of infancy, but is still inconsistent. Bux and coworkers treated seven patients and documented a sustained rise in neutrophil counts in four during the treatment period (85).

Steroids have been used in conjunction with G-CSF in a patient with Kostmann syndrome who was refractory to treatment with G-CSF alone (93). Activation of the glucocorticoid receptor can synergize with G-CSF signals to promote proliferation of myeloid cells.

Other Modalities

Exchange transfusions have not been successful in treating immune-mediated neutropenia (94). Granulocyte transfusions with cells negative for the implicated antigen can be helpful to tide over acute crises, but the effect often lasts for only a few hours. Current evidence does not show a clear beneficial role for granulocyte transfusions. (95) Nevertheless, the ability to stimulate neutrophilia rapidly in granulocyte donors using G-CSF has renewed interest in neutrophil transfusions for septic, neutropenic patients and may be useful in selected patients with short-term needs.

REFERENCES

1. Aladjidi N, Casanova JL, Canioni D, et al. Severe aplastic anemia of neonatal onset: a single-center retrospective study of six children. J Pediatr 132:600–605, 1998.
2. Christensen RD, Rothstein G. Exhaustion of mature marrow neutrophils in neonates with sepsis. J Pediatr 96:316–318, 1980.
3. Baley JE, Stork EK, Warkentin PI, Shurin SB. Neonatal neutropenia. Clinical manifestations, cause, and outcome. Am J Dis Child 142:1161–1166, 1988.
4. Gessler P, Luders R, Konig S, et al. Neonatal neutropenia in low birthweight premature infants. Am J Perinatol 12:34–38, 1995.
5. al-Mulla ZS, Christensen RD. Neutropenia in the neonate. Clin Perinatol 22:711–739, 1995.
6. Athens JW. Disorders of neutrophil proliferation and circulations: a pathophysiological view. Clin Haematol 4:553–566, 1975.
7. Manroe BL, Rosenfeld CR, Weinberg AG, Browne R. The differential leukocyte count in the assessment and outcome of early-onset neonatal group B streptococcal disease. J Pediatr 91:632–637, 1977.
8. Mouzinho A, Rosenfeld CR, Sanchez PJ, Risser R. Revised reference ranges for circulating neutrophils in very-low-birth-weight neonates. Pediatrics 94:76–82, 1994.
9. Manroe BL, Weinberg AG, Rosenfeld CR, Browne R. The neonatal blood count in health and disease. I. Reference values for neutrophilic cells. J Pediatr 95:89–98, 1979.
10. Coulombel L, Dehan M, Tchernia G, et al. The number of polymorphonuclear leukocytes in relation to gestational age in the newborn. Acta Paediatr Scand 68:709–711, 1979.
11. Lloyd BW, Oto A. Normal values for mature and immature neutrophils in very preterm babies. Arch Dis Child 57:233–235, 1982.
12. Faix RG, Hric JJ, Naglie RA. Neutropenia and intraventricular hemorrhage among very low birth weight (less than 1500 grams) premature infants. J Pediatr 114:1035–1038, 1989.
13. Prober CG, Stevenson DK, Neu J, Johnson JD. The white cell ratio in the very low birth weight infant. Clin Pediatr (Phila) 18:481–486, 1979.
14. Engle WD, Rosenfeld CR, Mouzinho A, et al. Circulating neutrophils in septic preterm neonates: comparison of two reference ranges. Pediatrics 99:E10, 1997.
15. Xanthou M. Leucocyte blood picture in healthy full-term and premature babies during neonatal period. Arch Dis Child 45:242–249, 1970.
16. Boxer LA, Yokoyama M, Lalezari P. Isoimmune neonatal neutropenia. J Pediatr 80:783–787, 1972.
17. Cartron J, Tchernia G, Celton JL, et al. Alloimmune neonatal neutropenia. Am J Pediatr Hematol Oncol 13:21–25, 1991.
18. Dale DC. Immune and idiopathic neutropenia. Curr Opin Hematol 5:33–36, 1998.
19. Engle WD, Rosenfeld CR. Neutropenia in high-risk neonates. J Pediatr 105:982–986, 1984.
20. Gray PH, Rodwell RL. Neonatal neutropenia associated with maternal hypertension poses a risk for nosocomial infection. Eur J Pediatr 158:71–73, 1999.
21. Christensen RD, Calhoun DA, Rimsza LM. A practical approach to evaluating and treating neutropenia in the neonatal intensive care unit. Clin Perinatol 27:577–601, 2000.
22. van Eeden SF, Miyagashima R, Haley L, Hogg JC. A possible role for L-selectin in the release of polymorphonuclear leukocytes from bone marrow. Am J Physiol 272:H1717–1724, 1997.
23. Schelonka RL, Yoder BA, desJardins SE, et al. Peripheral leukocyte count and leukocyte indexes in healthy newborn term infants. J Pediatr 125:603–606, 1994.
24. Christensen RD, Bradley PP, Rothstein G. The leukocyte left shift in clinical and experimental neonatal sepsis. J Pediatr 98:101–105, 1981.
25. Spector SA, Ticknor W, Grossman M. Study of the usefulness of clinical and hematologic findings in the diagnosis of neonatal bacterial infections. Clin Pediatr (Phila) 20:385–392, 1981.
26. Rodwell RL, Leslie AL, Tudehope DI. Early diagnosis of neonatal sepsis using a hematologic scoring system. J Pediatr 112:761–767, 1988.
27. Sola MC, Rimsza LM, Christensen RD. A bone marrow biopsy technique suitable for use in neonates. Br J Haematol 107:458–460, 1999.
28. Christensen RD. Neutrophil kinetics in the fetus and neonate. Am J Pediatr Hematol Oncol 11:215–223, 1989.
29. Christensen RD. Granulocytopoiesis in the fetus and neonate. Transfus Med Rev 4:8–13, 1990.
30. Funke A, Berner R, Traichel B, et al. Frequency, natural course, and outcome of neonatal neutropenia. Pediatrics 106:45–51, 2000.
31. Auriti C, Maccallini A, Di Liso G, et al. Risk factors for nosocomial infections in a neonatal intensive-care unit. J Hosp Infect 53:25–30, 2003.
32. Trifilio S, Verma A, Mehta J. Antimicrobial prophylaxis in hematopoietic stem cell transplant recipients: heterogeneity of current clinical practice. Bone Marrow Transplant 33:735–739, 2004.
33. Bernini JC, Wooley R, Buchanan GR. Low-dose recombinant human granulocyte colony-stimulating factor therapy in children with symptomatic chronic idiopathic neutropenia. J Pediatr 129:551–558, 1996.
34. Calhoun DA, Christensen RD, Edstrom CS, et al. Consistent approaches to procedures and practices in neonatal hematology. Clin Perinatol 27:733–753, 2000.
35. Calhoun DA, Christensen RD. Human developmental biology of granulocyte colony-stimulating factor. Clin Perinatol 27:559–576, vi, 2000.
36. Burgess AW, Metcalf D. The nature and action of granulocyte-macrophage colony stimulating factors. Blood 56:947–958, 1980.

37. Hamilton JA, Anderson GP. GM-CSF Biology. Growth Factors 22:225–231, 2004.

38. Gillan ER, Christensen RD, Suen Y, et al. A randomized, placebo-controlled trial of recombinant human granulocyte colony-stimulating factor administration in newborn infants with presumed sepsis: significant induction of peripheral and bone marrow neutrophilia. Blood 84:1427–1433, 1994.

39. Schibler KR, Osborne KA, Leung LY, et al. A randomized, placebo-controlled trial of granulocyte colony-stimulating factor administration to newborn infants with neutropenia and clinical signs of early-onset sepsis. Pediatrics 102:6–13, 1998.

40. Bedford Russell AR, Emmerson AJ, Wilkinson N, et al. A trial of recombinant human granulocyte colony stimulating factor for the treatment of very low birthweight infants with presumed sepsis and neutropenia. Arch Dis Child Fetal Neonatal Ed 84:F172–F176, 2001.

41. Miura E, Procianoy RS, Bittar C, et al. A randomized, double-masked, placebo-controlled trial of recombinant granulocyte colony-stimulating factor administration to preterm infants with the clinical diagnosis of early-onset sepsis. Pediatrics 107:30–35, 2001.

42. Barak Y, Leibovitz E, Mogilner B, et al. The in vivo effect of recombinant human granulocyte-colony stimulating factor in neutropenic neonates with sepsis. Eur J Pediatr 156:643–646, 1997.

43. Kocherlakota P, La Gamma EF. Human granulocyte colony-stimulating factor may improve outcome attributable to neonatal sepsis complicated by neutropenia. Pediatrics 100:E6, 1997.

44. Bernstein HM, Pollock BH, Calhoun DA, Christensen RD. Administration of recombinant granulocyte colony-stimulating factor to neonates with septicemia: A meta-analysis. J Pediatr 138:917–920, 2001.

45. Cairo MS, Christensen R, Sender LS, et al. Results of a phase I/II trial of recombinant human granulocyte-macrophage colony-stimulating factor in very low birthweight neonates: significant induction of circulatory neutrophils, monocytes, platelets, and bone marrow neutrophils. Blood 86:2509–2515, 1995.

46. Bilgin K, Yaramis A, Haspolat K, et al. A randomized trial of granulocyte-macrophage colony-stimulating factor in neonates with sepsis and neutropenia. Pediatrics 107:36–41, 2001.

47. Carr R, Modi N, Dore CJ, et al. A randomized, controlled trial of prophylactic granulocyte-macrophage colony-stimulating factor in human newborns less than 32 weeks gestation. Pediatrics 103:796–802, 1999.

48. Cairo MS, Agosti J, Ellis R, et al. A randomized, double-blind, placebo-controlled trial of prophylactic recombinant human granulocyte-macrophage colony-stimulating factor to reduce nosocomial infections in very low birth weight neonates. J Pediatr 134:64–70, 1999.

49. Molloy EJ, O'Neill AJ, Grantham JJ, et al. Granulocyte colony-stimulating factor and granulocyte-macrophage colony-stimulating factor have differential effects on neonatal and adult neutrophil survival and function. Pediatr Res 57:806–812, 2005.

50. Ahmad A, Laborada G, Bussel J, Nesin M. Comparison of recombinant granulocyte colony-stimulating factor, recombinant human granulocyte-macrophage colony-stimulating factor and placebo for treatment of septic preterm infants. Pediatr Infect Dis J 21:1061–1065, 2002.

51. Carr R, Modi N, Dore C. G-CSF and GM-CSF for treating or preventing neonatal infections. Cochrane Database Syst Rev CD003066, 2003.

52. Rodwell RL, Gray PH, Taylor KM, Minchinton R. Granulocyte colony stimulating factor treatment for alloimmune neonatal neutropenia. Arch Dis Child Fetal Neonatal Ed 75:F57–58, 1996.

53. Kerst JM, de Haas M, van der Schoot CE, et al. Recombinant granulocyte colony-stimulating factor administration to healthy volunteers: induction of immunophenotypically and functionally altered neutrophils via an effect on myeloid progenitor cells. Blood 82:3265–3272, 1993.

54. de Haas M, Kerst JM, van der Schoot CE, et al. Granulocyte colony-stimulating factor administration to healthy volunteers: analysis of the immediate activating effects on circulating neutrophils. Blood 84:3885–3894, 1994.

55. Bux J, Hofmann C, Welte K. Serum G-CSF levels are not increased in patients with antibody-induced neutropenia unless they are suffering from infectious diseases. Br J Haematol 105:616–617, 1999.

56. Maheshwari A, Christensen RD, Calhoun DA. Immune neutropenia in the neonate. Adv Pediatr 49:317–339, 2002.

57. Stroncek DF, Jaszcz W, Herr GP, Clay ME, McCullough J. Expression of neutrophil antigens after 10 days of granulocyte-colony stimulating factor. Transfusion 38:663–668, 1998.

58. Maheshwari A, Christensen RD, Calhoun DA. Resistance to recombinant human granulocyte colony-stimulating factor in neonatal alloimmune neutropenia associated with anti-human neutrophil antigen-2a (NB1) antibodies. Pediatrics 109:E64, 2002.

59. Christensen RD, Calhoun DA. Congenital neutropenia. Clin Perinatol 31:29–38, 2004.

60. Zeidler C. Congenital neutropenias. Hematology 10 (Supp 1):306–311, 2005.

61. Dale DC, Person RE, Bolyard AA, et al. Mutations in the gene encoding neutrophil elastase in congenital and cyclic neutropenia. Blood 96:2317–2322, 2000.

62. Dale DC, Cottle TE, Fier CJ, et al. Severe chronic neutropenia: treatment and follow-up of patients in the Severe Chronic Neutropenia International Registry. Am J Hematol 72:82–93, 2003.

63. Zeidler C, Boxer L, Dale DC, et al. Management of Kostmann syndrome in the G-CSF era. Br J Haematol 109:490–495, 2000.

64. Freedman MH. Safety of long-term administration of granulocyte colony-stimulating factor for severe chronic neutropenia. Curr Opin Hematol 4:217–224, 1997.

65. Dale DC, Hammond WPt. Cyclic neutropenia: a clinical review. Blood Rev 2:178–185, 1988.

66. Schmitz S, Franke H, Wichmann HE, Diehl V. The effect of continuous G-CSF application in human cyclic neutropenia: a model analysis. Br J Haematol 90:41–47, 1995.

67. Schmitz S, Franke H, Loeffler M, et al. Model analysis of the contrasting effects of GM-CSF and G-CSF treatment on peripheral blood neutrophils observed in three patients with childhood-onset cyclic neutropenia. Br J Haematol 95:616–625, 1996.

68. Dror Y. Shwachman-Diamond syndrome. Pediatr Blood Cancer 45:892–901, 2005.

69. van der Sande FM, Hillen HF. Correction of neutropenia following treatment with granulocyte colony-stimulating factor results in a decreased frequency of infections in Shwachman's syndrome. Neth J Med 48:92–95, 1996.

70. Lesma E, Riva E, Giovannini M, et al. Amelioration of neutrophil membrane function underlies granulocyte-colony stimulating factor action in glycogen storage disease 1b. Int J Immunopathol Pharmacol 18:297–307, 2005.

71. Makhlouf RA, Doron MW, Bose CL, et al. Administration of granulocyte colony-stimulating factor to neutropenic low birth weight infants of mothers with preeclampsia. J Pediatr 126:454–456, 1995.

72. La Gamma EF, Alpan O, Kocherlakota P. Effect of granulocyte colony-stimulating factor on pre-eclampsia-associated neonatal neutropenia. J Pediatr 126:457–459, 1995.

73. Paul DA, Leef KH, Sciscione A, Tuttle DJ, Stefano JL. Preeclampsia does not increase the risk for culture proven sepsis in very low birth weight infants. Am J Perinatol 16:365–372, 1999.

74. Doron MW, Makhlouf RA, Katz VL, et al. Increased incidence of sepsis at birth in neutropenic infants of mothers with preeclampsia. J Pediatr 125:452–458, 1994.

75. Kocherlakota P, La Gamma EF. Preliminary report: rhG-CSF may reduce the incidence of neonatal sepsis in prolonged preeclampsia-associated neutropenia. Pediatrics 102:1107–1111, 1998.

76. Zuppa AA, Girlando P, Florio MG, et al. Influence of maternal preeclampsia on recombinant human granulocyte colony-stimulating factor effect in neutropenic neonates with suspected sepsis. Eur J Obstet Gynecol Reprod Biol 102:131–136, 2002.

77. Juul SE, Calhoun DA, Christensen RD. "Idiopathic neutropenia" in very low birthweight infants. Acta Paediatr 87:963–968, 1998.

78. Juul SE, Christensen RD. Effect of recombinant granulocyte colony-stimulating factor on blood neutrophil concentrations among patients with "idiopathic neonatal neutropenia": a randomized, placebo-controlled trial. J Perinatol 23:493–497, 2003.

79. Gilmore MM, Stroncek DF, Korones DN. Treatment of alloimmune neonatal neutropenia with granulocyte colony-stimulating factor. J Pediatr 125:948–951, 1994.

80. Taniguchi S, Shibuya T, Harada M, Niho Y. Decreased levels of myeloid progenitor cells associated with long-term administration of recombinant human granulocyte colony-stimulating factor in patients with autoimmune neutropenia. Br J Haematol 83:384–387, 1993.

81. Yakisan E, Schirg E, Zeidler C, et al. High incidence of significant bone loss in patients with severe congenital neutropenia (Kostmann's syndrome). J Pediatr 131:592–597, 1997.

82. Huizinga TW, Kuijpers RW, Kleijer M, et al. Maternal genomic neutrophil FcRIII deficiency leading to neonatal isoimmune neutropenia. Blood 76:1927–1932, 1990.

83. Kemp AS, Lubitz L. Delayed umbilical cord separation in alloimmune neutropenia. Arch Dis Child 68:52–53, 1993.

84. Yoshida N, Shikata T, Sudo S, et al. Alloimmune neonatal neutropenia in monozygous twins. High-dose intravenous gammaglobulin therapy. Acta Paediatr Scand 80:62–65, 1991.

85. Bux J, Behrens G, Jaeger G, Welte K. Diagnosis and clinical course of autoimmune neutropenia in infancy: analysis of 240 cases. Blood 91:181–186, 1998.

86. Bussel J, Lalezari P, Fikrig S. Intravenous treatment with gamma-globulin of autoimmune neutropenia of infancy. J Pediatr 112:298–301, 1988.

87. Mascarin M, Ventura A. Anti-Rh(D) immunoglobulin for autoimmune neutropenia of infancy. Acta Paediatr 82:142–144, 1993.

88. Lassiter HA, Bibb KW, Bertolone SJ, et al. Neonatal immune neutropenia following the administration of intravenous immune globulin. Am J Pediatr Hematol Oncol 15:120–123, 1993.

89. Lamari F, Anastassiou ED, Stamokosta E, et al. Determination of slime-producing S. epidermidis specific antibodies in human immunoglobulin preparations and blood sera by an enzyme immunoassay: correlation of antibody titers with opsonic activity and application to preterm neonates. J Pharm Biomed Anal 23:363–374, 2000.

90. Christensen RD, Brown MS, Hall DC, et al. Effect on neutrophil kinetics and serum opsonic capacity of intravenous administration of immune globulin to neonates with clinical signs of early-onset sepsis. J Pediatr 118:606–614, 1991.

91. Lalezari P. Alloimmune neonatal neutropenia and neutrophil-specific antigens. Vox Sang 46:415–417, 1984.

92. Buckwold AE, Emson HE. Acute neonatal neutropenia in siblings. Can Med Assoc J 80:116–119, 1959.

93. Dror Y, Ward AC, Touw IP, Freedman MH. Combined corticosteroid/granulocyte colony-stimulating factor (G-CSF) therapy in the treatment of severe congenital neutropenia unresponsive to G-CSF: Activated glucocorticoid receptors synergize with G-CSF signals. Exp Hematol 28:1381–1389, 2000.

94. Hinkel GK, Schneider I, Gebhardt B, Leverenz S. Alloimmune neonatal neutropenia: clinical observations and therapeutic consequences. Acta Paediatr Hung 27:31–41, 1986.

95. Mohan P, Brocklehurst P. Granulocyte transfusions for neonates with confirmed or suspected sepsis and neutropaenia. Cochrane Database Syst Rev CD003956, 2003.

Chapter 7

What Evidence Supports Dietary Interventions to Prevent Infant Food Hypersensitivity and Allergy?

David A. Osborn, MBBS, MMed (Clin Epi), FRACP, PhD •
John Sinn, MBBS (Syd), DCH, Dip Paed, MMed (Clin Epi), FRACP

Nomenclature

Allergy and Food Hypersensitivity

Prevention

Future Directions

Conclusions

Food hypersensitivity and allergy are prevalent and a substantial health problem that may be increasing in developed countries (1, 2). A major focus is now on the mechanisms for development of immune tolerance and allergen sensitization in the fetus and newborn, and on primary prevention strategies. This chapter focuses on the evidence for use of dietary interventions in pregnant and breast-feeding women, and feed-related interventions in infants for the prevention of food hypersensitivity and allergy. The mechanisms for the in utero development of immune tolerance and allergy, consensus nomenclature for food hypersensitivity and allergy, and the mechanisms, epidemiology and risk factors for development of food hypersensitivity and allergy are addressed.

NOMENCLATURE

The terminology used to describe allergy and allergy-like reactions is confusing. As a result, the World Allergy Organization in 2003 reported an update of standardized nomenclature of allergy (3). Briefly, the term hypersensitivity has been advocated to describe "objectively reproducible symptoms or signs initiated by exposure to a defined stimulus at a dose tolerated by a normal person." Allergy is a "hypersensitivity reaction initiated by immunological mechanisms." Atopy is a "personal and/or familial tendency to become sensitized and produce IgE antibodies in response to ordinary exposures to allergens, usually proteins. As a consequence, these infants can develop typical symptoms of asthma, rhinoconjunctivitis, or eczema." Therefore, eczema may be atopic, which is IgE-mediated, or non-atopic, which more commonly presents as chronic eczema associated with a lymphocytic infiltrate on skin biopsy. The presence of allergen-specific IgE is established either by allergen skin-prick tests or by in vitro allergen-specific IgE measurements (e.g., radioallergosorbent test – RAST). In infants with food hypersensitivity, food-specific IgG antibodies are not clinically important but indicate previous exposure to the food. If IgE is involved, the term IgE-mediated food allergy is used.

ALLERGY AND FOOD HYPERSENSITIVITY

Several population-based studies using identical methods of ascertainment at intervals of 10–15 years have shown significant increases in the prevalence of allergic disease in children in the last 30 years in developed countries (2, 4, 5). The manifestations of allergic disease are age-dependent. Infants commonly present with symptoms and signs of atopic eczema, gastrointestinal symptoms and recurrent wheezing. Asthma and rhinoconjunctivitis become prevalent in later childhood. Sensitization to allergens tends to follow a characteristic pattern, with sensitization to food allergens in the first 2–3 years of life, then indoor allergens (e.g., house dust mite and pets) and subsequently outdoor allergens (e.g., rye and Timothy grass). The cumulative prevalence of allergic disease in childhood is high, with up to 7–8% developing a food allergy, 15–20% atopic eczema, and 31–34% developing asthma or recurrent wheezing. Of these, 7–10% will continue to have asthma symptoms beyond 5 years of age (2).

Food hypersensitivities affect around 6% of infants < 3 years of age, with prevalence decreasing over the first decade (6, 7). Despite the vast array of food allergens that we are exposed to, relatively few account for the majority of food reactions. Cow's milk, soy, egg and peanut account for the majority of food hypersensitivities in children, whereas peanut, tree nuts, fish and shellfish are the most common food allergies in adults. The majority of infants who develop cow's milk reactions do so in the first year. Between 40 and 60% of these infants will have IgE-mediated reactions to proteins, including casein, ß-lactoglobulin, bovine serum albumin, IgG heavy chains and lactoferrin (8). Many children outgrow their food hypersensitivity, although around 25% retain sensitivities in the second decade and around 35% develop sensitizations to other foods. Clinical tolerance develops for most food allergens over time, with the exceptions of peanuts, nuts and seafood (2, 6, 7, 9). However, prospective studies have reported that early sensitization to cow's milk, egg and house dust mite are highly predictive of subsequent clinical allergic disease, including persistent atopic eczema and asthma, particularly in high-risk infants.

The Fetus: Immune Tolerance versus Sensitization

The fetus is capable of mounting sophisticated immune responses (10). Circulating B lymphocytes can be detected with IgM surface immunoglobulin from as early as 19–20 weeks, implying that the full sensitization process, from antigen presentation to T cell proliferation to B cell stimulation and antibody production, has occurred. There is almost universal priming to environmental antigens in utero, with most infants subsequently being tolerant to exposures to the same antigens. However, the balance is altered towards sensitization in infants destined to have allergic disease. A minority of all infants will already have raised cord blood total IgE and specific IgE. IgE is reasonably specific but not very sensitive for predicting later allergic disease.

Studies to date suggest infants who develop allergies have a disturbance in the balance between cytokines that suppress an allergic response as characterized by T helper-1 (Th-1) phenotypic responses, and allergy-promoting Th-2 responses. This balance appears to be affected by factors such as maternal atopy (risk), maternal IgG responses (protective), and potentially maternal and fetal nutritional factors. Two potential routes of fetal antigen exposure are from ingested antigens in the amniotic fluid and transplacentally. Although antigen-presenting cells are present in the fetal gut, they are not in the skin or airways. It is thought sensitization is more likely to occur in the gut, where mature active immune cells are found (11). The second major route is via the placenta. Antigen is mostly complexed with maternal IgG and occurs maximally in the third trimester of pregnancy. However, transplacental passage of dietary antigens, including cow's milk ß-lacto-globulin and egg ovalbumin, occurs as early as 26 weeks gestation. The passage of antigens is enhanced across the preterm placenta, increased by dose of exposure and decreasing molecular weight (12). However, for immunological priming to occur the antigen must have access to sites where it can be taken up by dendritic cells for processing and presentation to naïve T cells. The specifics of these interactions, and how they are affected by genetic and environmental factors, are likely to be important in the understanding of fetal sensitization to allergens.

The Infant: Food Tolerance versus Sensitization

Food allergy is a manifestation of an abnormal mucosal immune response to ingested dietary antigens (6). The gastrointestinal barrier is a complex physio-chemical barrier and cellular barrier. Innate (natural killer cells, neutrophils, macrophages, epithelial cells) and adaptive (intraepithelial and lamina propria lymphocytes, Peyer's patches, secretory IgA and cytokines) immune responses provide an active barrier to antigens. Even so, around 2% of ingested food antigens are absorbed. The efficiency of this gut barrier is reduced in the newborn period. Perinatal risk factors reported for asthma and/or allergy have included prematurity (13–15) and fetal growth restriction (13), both of which are associated with an immature and potentially injured gut mucosal barrier. Maternal smoking may explain some of these effects (14).

Mechanisms and Risk Factors for Development of Childhood Allergy and Food Hypersensitivity

A substantial proportion of children with clinical allergic disease are non-atopic, although this differs with the phenotypic expression of the disease (2). In the Isle of Wight study (16), of infants with a diagnosed allergic phenotype, only 32% were found to be atopic (identified by skin-prick test and serum-specific IgE). Of these, 14% had early transient sensitization at 4 years, 52% had persistent sensitization at 4 and 10 years and 35% had delayed sensitization at 10 years. These atopic phenotypes had different risk factors, with sibling food allergy being the only heredity risk factor in regression analysis for delayed childhood atopy. Chronically atopic children were much more likely to have diagnosed asthma, eczema, and rhinoconjunctivitis. Their symptoms were more likely to be persistent and be diagnosable as clinical allergy. The development of atopic disease is likely to be dependent on a complex interaction between genetic and environmental factors. Genetic factors are estimated to account for over 50% of asthma and allergy (2, 17), but are unlikely to explain the increasing prevalence in the last 30 years (2). Dietary and environmental exposures to allergens, as well as modifying factors such as immaturity at birth (13, 15), high head to weight ratios (13), infections (18, 19), intestinal miroflora, tobacco smoke (14, 18, 20–22), dietary factors (23) and pollution (24), may well contribute to the development of asthma and allergy. Peat and Li (24) have developed a useful classification of risk factors for childhood asthma which assist in the identification of high-risk children and serve as a guide to primary prevention.

Identifying Infants at High Risk of Food Sensitization or Allergy

Less than half of those who develop childhood allergic disease have a first-degree family history of allergy. However, the risk of development of allergic diseases increases substantially with family heredity. Around 10% of children without a first-degree allergic relative develop allergic disease, compared to 20–30% with single allergic heredity (parent or sibling) and 40–50% with double allergic heredity (18, 25–27). Maternal and sibling allergy is a stronger predictor of childhood allergic disorders than paternal allergy (23), although paternal allergy was a stronger predictor of atopic sensitization (21).

The use of cord blood IgE levels results in improved predictive ability for subsequent allergy. Although the combination of atopic family heredity and cord blood IgE levels has frequently been used in dietary preventive studies in infants, they are still not seen as sufficiently predictive for routine clinical use (2). Defining a high-risk group as either double parental allergic predisposition or severe single parent allergy combined with an infant cord blood IgE = 0.3 kU/L results in the high-risk group comprising 8–10% of the total birth cohort, compared with 16–20% if cord blood IgE is not used and 30–40% if all those with at least single atopic predisposition are included (26). Studies of dietary interventions for prevention of food hypersensitivity and allergy have variably defined high risk as a single first-degree relative with allergy, dual first-degree heredity, or a combination of first-degree heredity and cord blood IgE = 0.3 kU/L or 0.5 kU/L. Clearly, there is a balance between achieving a high positive predictive value and having adequate sensitivity for allergy. To date, there is no highly accurate method for predicting food hypersensitivity and allergy in children. Current recommendations generally define high-risk infants in terms of atopic heredity (29, 30).

PREVENTION

By consensus (30), prevention of allergy is divided into primary prevention: the prevention of immunological sensitization (development of IgE antibodies); secondary prevention: preventing the onset of allergic disease following sensitization such as the progression from eczema and rhinoconjunctivitis to more severe disease such as asthma; and tertiary prevention: the treatment of allergic disease so as to prevent complications. The focus on the newborn is with primary prevention. The basis for primary prevention measures requires meeting the following criteria (30):

1. have the potential to benefit a major proportion of the population;
2. be of no known harm to anyone; and
3. not involve unreasonable costs.

Factors facilitating primary prevention include the finding that infants with a family history of allergy have an increased risk of IgE sensitization, and the risk of developing IgE-mediated disease is related to family history for a specific allergic phenotype. Genetic factors are thought to contribute in excess of 50% of the development of IgE sensitization and IgE-mediated allergic disease. However, specific genes allowing identification of high-risk infants are yet to be adequately described. In addition, although sensitization to foods and other allergens precedes the development of allergy, the exposure to dietary and environmental allergens is ubiquitous and usually a harmless phenomenon associated with tolerance (31). In many infants, early sensitization to dietary allergens, although predictive of allergic disease, is frequently followed by loss of sensitization. Therefore, the aim of primary prevention is to prevent not just sensitization, but also allergic disease. Primary prevention measures include those aimed at reducing or changing exposures to antigens, and modifying adjuvant risk factors and exposures. This review focuses on the evidence for dietary and adjuvant treatments that have the potential to be used for the primary prevention of clinical allergic disease, not just sensitization.

Table 7-1   Randomized Trials of Maternal Dietary Allergen Avoidance During Pregnancy for Prevention of Allergy in Infants

Trial	N	Participants	Maternal allergen avoidance	Control
Falth-Magnusson et al. 1987 (91–93)	212	Pregnant women with history of allergy in self, husband or previous children	Cow's milk and egg avoidance diet from 28 weeks gestation	Normal diet
Lilja et al. 1988 (94, 95)	171	Pregnant women with history of respiratory allergy to pollen and/or dander	Low milk and low egg diet during third trimester	High milk and high egg diet during third trimester
Lovegrove et al. 1994 (35)	44	Pregnant women with atopic histories in self or partner	Milk-free diet from 36 weeks gestation and during lactation	Normal diet

Maternal Dietary Allergen Avoidance in Pregnancy

A systematic review (32) found three randomized trials enrolling 334 pregnant women that examined the effect of maternal dietary allergen avoidance in pregnancy for prevention of infant allergy. All studies enrolled pregnant women with a first-degree family history of allergy (Table 7-1). Dietary interventions included a cow's milk and egg avoidance diet from 28 weeks gestation (33), a low milk and low egg diet during the third trimester (34), and a milk-free diet from 36 weeks gestation and during lactation (35). No significant effect was reported for fetal or infant sensitization as indicated by cord blood IgE and infant skin-prick testing. Meta-analysis of the three trials (32) found no evidence of a protective effect of maternal dietary antigen avoidance during pregnancy for atopic eczema, asthma, urticaria or any atopic condition in the first 18 months (Table 7-2). The restricted diet during pregnancy was associated with a slight but statistically significant lower maternal mean gestational weight gain and non-significant trends to higher risks of preterm birth and reduced mean birth weight in the infants.

Maternal dietary allergen avoidance during pregnancy has also been a component of the intervention strategies in other randomized trials (18, 36–38). However, as those trials examined the effects of allergen avoidance during both pregnancy and lactation, with other allergen avoidance strategies for the infant, no conclusions can be drawn from these studies pertaining to allergen avoidance during pregnancy. Larger trials of maternal dietary antigen avoidance during pregnancy are required to detect whether there are even modest reductions in risk of allergy in infants and children. Adverse effects of maternal antigen avoidance on gestational weight gain, fetal growth, and preterm birth should be reported. A better understanding of the

Table 7-2   Meta-Analyses of Randomized Trials of Maternal Dietary Allergen Avoidance During Pregnancy for Prevention of Allergy in Infants (32)

Outcome	Studies/participants	RR	95% CI
Atopic eczema (first 18 months)	2/334	1.01	0.57, 1.79
Asthma (first 18 months)	2/334	2.22	0.39, 12.67
Any atopic condition (first 18 months)	1/163	0.76	0.42, 1.38
Urticaria (first 18 months)	1/163	1.01	0.21, 4.87
Preterm birth	2/236	10.06	0.53, 192.2
Pregnancy weight gain (%)	1/164	−3.00	−5.21, −0.79
Birth weight (g)	2/236	−83.45	221.87, 54.97

mechanisms for development of food tolerance and sensitization will facilitate efforts to develop effective allergy prevention strategies.

Breast-feeding

Breast-feeding is the natural and recommended method of infant nutrition for the first months after birth. Few data are available from randomized controlled trials to determine the effect of breast-feeding for prevention of food intolerance and allergy in children. Lucas et al. (39) randomized preterm infants < 1850 g to expressed human milk versus sole or supplemental preterm cow's milk formula feeds, up until hospital discharge. At 18 months, there was no significant difference in incidence of eczema (human milk 20% versus preterm formula 20%), reactions to cow's milk (4% vs. 3%), all food reactions (10% vs. 11%) and asthma and/or wheezing (23% vs. 23%). In subgroup analysis restricted to a small number of infants with a family history of allergy, there was a significant reduction in the incidence of eczema (RR 0.3, 95% CI 0.1–0.8) in infants fed human milk. In a cluster randomized trial of an intervention modeled on the Baby Friendly Hospital Initiative of the World Health Organization and United Nations Children's Fund (40), infants from intervention sites were significantly more likely to be breast-fed, and had significantly reduced incidence of atopic eczema at 1 year (3.3% vs. 6.3%; adjusted OR 0.54; 95% CI, 0.31, 0.95).

Two trials (41, 42) have compared use of human milk with cow's milk formula for early supplemental or sole feeding of infants prior to hospital discharge. Both trials had inadequate methods of infant allocation to feeds, using alternate periods. Juvonen et al. (41) enrolled 92 infants and reported no significant differences in any childhood allergy, or specific allergy including asthma, eczema and food allergy. Saarinen et al. (42), who allocated 3602 infants to treatment, reported no significant difference in cow's milk allergy (RR 0.80, 95% CI 0.51, 1.53) in infants fed human milk compared to a cow's milk formula. Both trials also enrolled a group fed a hydrolyzed infant formula. Systematic review (43) of these two trials also found no significant difference between the use of a hydrolyzed infant formula and human milk. Again, Juvonen et al. (41) reported no significant difference in any childhood allergy, or specific allergy including asthma, eczema and food allergy. Saarinen et al. (42) reported no significant difference in cow's milk allergy (RR 0.71, 95% CI 0.45, 1.12) in infants a hydrolyzed formula compared to human milk.

In observational studies, conflicting results have been reported for the association between breast-feeding and development of clinical allergy, even to adulthood. Several studies (44–50) have reported an increase in allergy in association with breast-feeding but have been criticized methodologically (51), especially regarding the potential for recall bias and lack of a dose-response relationship. It is likely that some of these findings may be the result of "reverse causality"; high-risk infants are more likely to be breast-fed, and more likely to develop allergy. Several reviews (52–56) have attempted to meta-analyse study data associating breast-feeding and clinical allergy. There is considerable difficulty in appraising the results of these reviews given the lack of comparable groups resulting from the inclusion of observational studies in all reviews. However, attempts were made to determine whether results were sensitive to study quality, with the conclusions robust to the exclusion of studies with greatest methodological concern (53, 54). Overall, in high-risk infants, the meta-analyses reported benefits in infancy from exclusive breast-feeding for the first few months for reduced atopic dermatitis (OR 0.58, 95% CI 0.41, 0.92) (53) and asthma (OR 0.52, 95% CI 0.35, 0.79) (54), but not for allergic rhinitis (53). In low-risk infants, there was no evidence of benefit for any manifestation of allergy (52–54).

Several studies have reported that longer, rather than shorter, duration of exclusive breast-feeding offers additional protective effects against allergy. Several of these studies (57–60) have led the American Academy of Pediatrics (AAP)(29) and the European Society for Pediatric Allergy and Clinical Immunology Committee on Hypoallergenic Formulas and the European Society for Paediatric Gastroenterology, Hepatology and Nutrition (ESPACI/ESPGHAN) (61) to recommend at least 6 months and 4–6 months of exclusive breast-feeding, respectively. In contrast, in a systematic review to determine the optimal duration of breast-feeding, Kramer and Kakuma (56) reported no significant reduction in risk of atopic eczema, asthma, or other atopic outcomes in infants exclusively breast-fed for 6 months compared to a shorter duration. However, the data from this review mainly accrue from observational studies, including the use of non-randomized groups from the Belarus cluster randomized trial of the Baby Friendly Hospital Initiative (40). A reduction in clinical but not food-challenge-confirmed allergy at 1 year was reported by one included cohort study (57).

In summary, there is evidence from observational studies that exclusive breast-feeding may prevent infant allergy, particularly eczema and possibly asthma. However, the evidence from observational studies is heterogeneous, with not all population-based studies finding a beneficial significant effect (44–50). Observational studies are unable to account for all confounding, either through bias in study design, measurement error or the failure to measure potential confounders. Meta-analysis of observational studies does not account for this bias, but merely increases the power of the analysis to detect a biased outcome. Most evidence supporting exclusive breast-feeding for allergy prevention points to durations of at least 4–6 months before the introduction of other foods (56–60). It is difficult to see whether this question will ever be adequately answered given the other potential benefits of breast-feeding, particularly reduced infectious morbidity (56), and, in preterm infants, necrotizing enterocolitis (62). Currently, the AAP (29) recommends exclusive breast-feeding for 6 months and ESPACI/ESPGHAN (61) and the Australasian Society of Clinical Immunology and Allergy (ASCIA) (1) for 4–6 months for prevention of cow's milk hypersensitivity and infant allergy.

Maternal Dietary Allergy Avoidance During Lactation

A systematic review found insufficient data from controlled trials to determine the role for allergen avoidance in lactating women (32). One trial of antigen avoidance during lactation enrolled only 26 lactating women (35). No significant protective effect of maternal antigen avoidance on the incidence of atopic eczema up to 18 months (RR 0.73, 95% CI 0.32, 1.64) was reported. Two trials (63, 64) included in previous versions of the review were excluded due to data validity concerns.

For infants with a family history of food-related anaphylaxis (e.g., peanuts, nuts and seafood), there are also insufficient data to recommend any specific maternal dietary interventions to prevent infant sensitization. Currently, for high-risk infants, only the AAP (29) makes a recommendation for maternal allergen avoidance, recommending the elimination of peanuts and nuts from the diets of lactating (and possibly pregnant) women. Both AAP (29) and ASCIA (1) recommend considering avoidance of peanut, nuts and shellfish from the infant's diets until 3 years, although there is no evidence to support this.

Infant Formula

A substantial proportion of the world's infants are not exclusively breast-fed (65). Until health interventions redress this issue, to provide for infants not exclusively breast-fed due to maternal or infant illness, maternal or infant inability, or parental preference, humanized infant formulas are available. Formulas prescribed to infants with the intention of preventing allergy and food intolerance have included hydrolyzed cow's milk, elemental, and adapted soy or hydrolyzed soy formulas. Hydrolyzed formulas are designed to change the allergenic milk protein with the aim of preventing sensitization. They may be produced from cow's milk or soy, be derived from predominately whey or casein proteins, and be partially or extensively hydrolyzed. The process of producing a hydrolyzed formula is individual to the formula, and in general the methods are commercially protected. They involve processes of enzyme-induced cleavage of protein and subsequent purification. Extensively hydrolyzed infant formulas have a majority of milk proteins < 1500 kDa and require clinical testing in infants with demonstrated cow's milk or cow's milk-based formula hypersensitivity (29). The extensively hydrolyzed formula should be tolerated by a minimum of 90% of infants in double-blind placebo-controlled conditions, with 95% confidence. Extensively hydrolyzed formula, or elemental equivalents with amino-acid-only protein fractions, are used for treatment of infants with cow's milk hypersensitivity. In Australia, prescription requires documented cow's milk hypersensitivity. Formulas based on partially hydrolyzed cow's milk protein have 10^3–10^5-times the concentrations of intact cow's milk protein compared to extensively hydrolyzed formulas, and are not used for treatment of hypersensitive infants. This review summarizes the evidence for extensive and partially hydrolyzed infant formula, and the role of soy formula. The systematic reviews of hydrolyzed formula were performed using Cochrane Collaboration methodology and only include controlled clinical trials with = 20% losses and no allergy-preventing co-interventions that were performed differently in treatment and control groups. Treatment groups were analyzed as "intention to treat" – that is, in the group of initial patient allocation. For outcomes, infants are defined as up to 2 years and childhood as 2–10 years.

Early Short-Term Use of a Hydrolyzed Infant Formula

A systematic review of controlled trials (43) found two studies (41, 42) that compared a short duration of early supplemental or sole hydrolyzed formula versus donor human milk feeds or a cow's milk formula in infants who were subsequently encouraged to breast-feed. Both had inadequate methods of treatment allocation. Both studies enrolled unselected infants, not on the basis of allergic heredity. Neither study reported a significant benefit from use of a hydrolyzed compared to donor human milk. One study (42) reported a reduction in infant cow's milk allergy of borderline significance (RR 0.62, 95% CI 0.38, 1.00) from use of an extensively hydrolyzed formula compared to a cow's milk formula, with subgroup analysis suggesting the benefit was only seen in infants at high risk of allergy. The role of early short-term use of a hydrolyzed infant formula for prevention of food hypersensitivity and allergy remains unclear. There is no evidence of benefit that a hydrolyzed formula should be advised in preference to exclusive breast-feeding. Where exclusive breast-feeding is not possible, further large trials are required to define the role of hydrolyzed formula for early short-term infant feeding.

Prolonged Feeding with a Hydrolyzed Infant Formula

A systematic review of controlled trials (43) found 10 eligible studies that compared prolonged feeding with hydrolyzed (extensively or partially hydrolyzed) formula versus cow's milk formula (Table 7-3). Almost all trials enrolled infants at high risk of allergy based on first degree heredity, with some studies including additional screening with cord blood IgE levels. Meta-analysis (Table 7-4) found a significant reduction in infant allergy (seven studies, 2514 infants; typical RR 0.79, 95% CI 0.66, 0.94), but not allergy in later childhood (two studies, 950 infants; typical RR 0.85, 95% CI 0.69, 1.05). There was no significant difference in any specific allergy, including eczema, asthma, rhinitis, or food allergy. However, the significant

Table 7-3   Included Studies In Meta-Analysis of Trials of Hydrolyzed Infant Formula Versus Cow's Milk Formula for Prevention of Food Hypersensitivity and Allergy (43)

Reference	Infants	Indication	Methods	Treatments
Chiroco et al. (96)	Infants of mothers with atopy	Prolonged supplemental or sole formula feeds	Random; blinding not reported; losses unclear	PHWF vs. CMF
De Seta et al. (97)	Infants with ≥1 first-degree relative with allergy	Prolonged supplemental or sole formula feeds	Random, method not reported; blinding not reported; losses not reported	PHWF vs. CMF
Halken et al. (68)	Infants with biparental atopy or uniparental atopy and cord IgE ≥0.3 kU/L	Prolonged supplemental or sole formula feeds	Quasi-random; blinded treatment; losses 20%	EHCF vs. EHWF vs. PHWF
Juvonen et al. (41)	Healthy infants; 62% had family history of atopy	Early, short-term (first 3 days) sole formula feeds in hospital	Quasi-random; blinding not reported; losses 10%	HM vs. EHCF vs. CMF
Lam et al. (98)	High-risk – criteria not reported	Prolonged supplemental or sole formula feeds	Random, method not reported; blinding not reported; losses 8%	PHW vs. CMF
Maggio et al. (99)	Preterm infants, birth weight ≤1750 g and ≤34 weeks	Prolonged supplemental or sole formula feeds identical in calories and nitrogen	Random; blinded; no losses	Preterm HWF vs. Preterm CMF
Mallett et al. (100)	Infants with first-degree family history of allergy	Prolonged supplemental or sole formula feeds	Random, method not reported; not blinded; losses 7% at 4 months; >20% later	EHWF vs. CMF
Marini et al. (101)	Infants with definite family history of allergy	Prolonged supplemental or sole formula feeds	Random, method not reported; unblinded; losses 19% at 3 years	PHWF vs. CMF
Nentwich et al. (70)	Infants with family history of atopy in first-degree relative	Prolonged supplemental or sole formula feeds	Quasi-random; unblended; losses 1% (further 18% not reported in allocated group)	PHWF vs. EHWF
Oldaeus et al. (69)	Infants with two allergic family members or one allergic family member and cord IgE ≥ 0.5 kU/L	Infants weaning from breast	Random; blinded; losses 9%	EHCF vs. PHWCF vs. CMF
Picaud et al. (102)	Low birth weight infants < 1500 g	Preterm infants with prolonged sole formula feeds	Random, method not reported; blinded; losses 11%	Preterm PHWF vs. preterm CMF
Saarinen et al. (42)	Term infants	Early short-term (4 days) supplemental formula feeding in hospital	Quasi-random; blinded; losses unclear	HM vs. EHWF vs. CMF
Szajewska et al. (103)	Low birth weight < 2000 g, appropriate for gestational age	Prolonged sole formula feeds	Random, method not reported; blinded; no losses	Preterm EHWCF vs. preterm CMF

Table 7-3   Included Studies In Meta-Analysis of Trials of Hydrolyzed Infant Formula Versus Cow's Milk Formula for Prevention of Food Hypersensitivity and Allergy (43)—cont'd

Reference	Infants	Indication	Methods	Treatments
Tsai et al. (104)	Infants enrolled according to Family History of Allergy Score	Prolonged supplemental or sole formula feeds	Random, method not reported; unblended; losses unclear	PHWF vs. CMF
Vandenplas et al. (66)	Infants with ≥ 2 first-degree allergic relatives	Prolonged sole formula feeds	Random, method not reported; blinded; losses 11%	PHWF vs. CMF
Vandenplas et al. (105)	Term newborn infants with no family history of atopy	Prolonged sole formula feeds	Random, method not reported; blinded; losses 9%	PHWF vs. CMF
von Berg et al. (67)	Infants with family history of atopy in first-degree relative	Prolonged supplemental or sole formula feeds	Random; blinded; losses in "intention to treat" analysis: 1 year 14.7%; 3 years 19%	PHWF vs. EHWF vs. EHCF vs. CMF
Willems et al. (106)	Infants with family history allergy and cord IgE ≥ 0.5 kU/l	Prolonged sole formula feeds	Quasi-random; unblended; losses 13%	PHWF vs. CMF

CMF, cow's milk formula; PHWF, partially hydrolyzed whey formula; PHWCF, partially hydrolyzed whey casein formula; EHWCF, extensively hydrolyzed whey casein formula; EHWF, extensively hydrolyzed whey formula.

reduction in infant allergy did not persist when the analysis was restricted to trials that blinded investigators and participants to formula type, or to trials with adequate methods of infant allocation and < 10% losses to follow up. In addition, no eligible trial examined the effect of prolonged hydrolyzed formula feeding on allergy beyond early childhood. Meta-analysis of three trials also found that preterm or low birth weight infants fed a hydrolyzed preterm formula versus a preterm cow's milk formula had significantly reduced weight gain, but not reduced growth in head circumference or length. Studies in term infants report no adverse effects on growth.

Prolonged Feeding with Partially Hydrolyzed Formula versus Extensively Hydrolyzed Formula

Three sets of analyses contribute to this comparison in a systematic review (43): those comparing partially hydrolyzed or extensively hydrolyzed formula versus

Table 7-4   Meta-Analysis of Trials of Hydrolyzed Formula versus Cow's Milk Formula for Prevention of Food Hypersensitivity and Allergy (43)

Outcome	Studies/Participants	RR	95% CI
Infant allergy	7/2514	0.79	0.66, 0.94
Childhood allergy	2/950	0.85	0.69, 1.05
Infant asthma	4/318	0.57	0.31, 1.04
Childhood asthma incidence	1/78	0.38	0.08, 1.84
Childhood asthma prevalence	1/872	1.06	0.70, 1.61
Infant eczema	8/2558	0.84	0.68, 1.04
Childhood eczema incidence	2/950	0.83	0.63, 1.10
Childhood eczema prevalence	1/872	0.66	0.43, 1.02
Infant rhinitis	2/256	0.52	0.14, 1.85
Food allergy	1/141	1.82	0.64, 5.16
Cow's milk allergy	1/67	0.36	0.15, 0.89

cow's milk formula, and analysis of trials comparing partially hydrolyzed versus extensively hydrolyzed formula. In studies of partially hydrolyzed formula versus cow's milk formula, meta-analysis (seven studies, 1482 infants) found a significant reduction in infant allergy (seven studies, 1482 infants; RR 0.79, 95% CI 0.65, 0.97), which did not persist to childhood. For specific allergies, no significant differences were reported in infant or childhood asthma, eczema or rhinitis. There were data from one small study (66) showing that use of a partially hydrolyzed whey formula resulted in a significant reduction in cow's milk allergy, confirmed by testing for atopy (RR 0.36, 95% CI 0.15, 0.89). Studies demonstrating benefit used a partially hydrolyzed 100% whey formula, with meta-analysis of six studies including 1391 infants finding a significant reduction in infant allergy (RR 0.73, 95% CI 0.59, 0.90), but not allergy into childhood or for any specific allergy or food hypersensitivity.

Four studies compared extensively hydrolyzed formula with cow's milk formula. No individual study reported a significant reduction in allergy or any specific allergy or food hypersensitivity from use of extensively hydrolyzed formula. Meta-analysis found no significant difference in infant allergy (two studies, 1561 infants; RR 0.87, 95% CI 0.68, 1.13), or childhood allergy (one study, 651 infants; RR 0.89, 95% CI 0.71, 1.13). No significant difference was found in infant or childhood asthma, eczema, or rhinitis or food allergy. Comparing extensively hydrolyzed casein containing formula with cow's milk formula, the German Infant Nutritional Intervention (GINI) Study (67) in 431 infants reported (intention to treat data obtained from authors) a significant reduction in childhood allergy (RR 0.72, 95% CI 0.53, 0.97). Meta-analysis of three studies including 1237 infants found a significant reduction in infant eczema (RR 0.71, 95% CI 0.51, 0.97), with the GINI study reporting a significant reduction in childhood eczema incidence (RR 0.66, 95% CI 0.44, 0.98) and prevalence (RR 0.50, 95% CI 0.27, 0.92) at 3 years.

Four studies (67–70) compared prolonged feeding with extensively hydrolyzed formula to partially hydrolyzed formula in infants at high risk of allergy. No individual study reported any significant differences in allergy or food hypersensitivity. Meta-analysis (three studies, 1806 infants) found no significant difference in infant allergy (RR 0.93, 95% CI 0.75, 1.16). Von Berg (67) reported no significant difference in childhood allergy incidence (RR 0.93, 95% CI 0.74, 1.18). Meta-analysis of two studies (68, 69) found a significant reduction in infant food allergy (RR 0.43, 95% CI 0.19, 0.99), although one of these studies reported no significant difference in infant cow's milk allergy (68).

In summary, evidence for benefit from the use of hydrolyzed infant formula for the prevention of food hypersensitivity and allergy is inconclusive. There is some evidence for use of both a partially hydrolyzed 100% whey formula and an extensively hydrolyzed casein formula in infants at high risk of allergy. Extensively hydrolyzed formula may be better than partially hydrolyzed formula at preventing food allergy. There is no evidence that hydrolyzed formulas should be used in preference to exclusive breast-feeding, and no evidence of benefit for use in infants without a first-degree family history of allergy. There are concerns about the adequacy of growth of preterm or low birth weight infants fed hydrolyzed preterm infant formula. Further large, rigorous trials comparing partially hydrolyzed whey and extensively hydrolyzed casein to cow's milk formula are needed in infants at high risk of allergy. All hydrolyzed formulas should have their ability to support adequate nutrition and growth assessed in appropriately designed controlled clinical trials.

Soy-Based Infant Formula (SBIF)

Current SBIFs are derived from soy protein isolate (SPI), purified modified soy protein isolate with lower levels of phytoestrogens than soy flour, and are iodine-supplemented. Nutritional modifications include methionine fortification, reduction of phytate content and improvement of the mineral suspension resulting in increased absorption of micronutrients (71, 72). A review (73) of the effects of SBIF on growth and development, including both randomized and observational studies, reported that modern SBIFs support normal growth and nutritional status in healthy full-term infants in the first year and current data do not suggest effects on sexual or reproductive development. However, there are insufficient long-term data regarding reproductive development, immune function, visual acuity, cognitive development and thyroid function.

A systematic review of studies of SBIF (74) found three eligible studies enrolling high-risk infants with a history of allergy in a first-degree relative (Table 7-5). No eligible study enrolled infants fed human milk. No study examined the effect of early, short-term soy formula feeding. All compared prolonged soy formula to cow's milk formula feeding. One study (75) was of adequate methodology and without unbalanced allergy-preventing co-interventions in treatment groups. Meta-analysis (Table 7-6) found no significant difference in childhood allergy (two studies; typical RR 0.73, 95% CI 0.37, 1.44), or specific allergy, including asthma, eczema and rhinitis. No significant difference in cow's milk hypersensitivity or allergy was reported. No study compared soy formula to hydrolyzed protein formula. Feeding with a soy formula cannot be recommended for prevention of allergy or food hypersensitivity in high-risk infants. Given the lack of high-quality studies, further research may be warranted to determine the role of soy formula for prevention of allergy or food hypersensitivity in infants unable to be breast-fed with a strong family history of allergy or cow's milk protein hypersensitivity.

Prebiotics and Probiotics

Differences in intestinal microflora are found in infants delivered by cesarean section compared to those delivered vaginally, and in breast-fed versus formula-fed infants (76). Colonizing bifidobacteria and lactobacilli inhibit growth of pathogenic microorganisms through the production of lactic, acetic and other organic acids, with a consequent decrease of intraluminal pH that inhibits the growth of some bacterial pathogens. The composition of the intestinal microflora may be different

Table 7-5   Characteristics of Included Studies Comparing Soy-Based Infant Formulas to Cow's Milk and Hydrolyzed Formulas for Infant Feeding

Study	Population	Methods	Formulas	Criteria for diagnosis
Johnstone et al. (107)	Infants not breast-fed with history of allergy in first-degree relative	Random, method not reported; unblinded; lost 19.5%	SBIF versus evaporated CMF for at least 7 months	Unblinded pediatrician assessment
Kjellman et al. (75)	Infants weaning from breast with history of allergy in both parents	Random, method not reported; unblinded; lost 4%	SBIF versus CMF for at least 9 months	Unblinded pediatrician assessment
Miskelly et al. (108)	Breast-fed infants with supplemental feeds if required; history of allergy in first-degree relative	Random; unblinded; lost: 1 year 9%; 7 years 16%	Supplemental SBIF versus "normal diet" (99% cow's milk exposed) for at least 4 months	Blinded physician assessment; skin-prick tests 6, 12 months; specific and total IgE 3, 12 months

SBIF, soy-based infant formula; CMF, cow's milk formula.

Table 7-6   Meta-Analysis of Trials of Soy-Based Infant Formula versus Cow's Milk Formula for Prevention of Food Hypersensitivity and Allergy (74)

Outcome	Studies/Participants	RR	95% CI
All allergy up to childhood	2/283	0.67	0.18, 2.46
Infant asthma	1/474	1.10	0.86, 1.40
Childhood asthma	3/729	0.71	0.26, 1.92
Infant eczema	1/461	1.20	0.95, 1.52
Childhood eczema	2/283	1.57	0.90, 2.75
Infant rhinitis	1/460	0.94	0.76, 1.16
Childhood rhinitis	1/283	0.69	0.06, 8.00
Cow's milk allergy	1/48	1.09	0.24, 4.86
Soy allergy	1/48	3.26	0.36, 29.17

in those with atopic eczema, and such differences may precede the development of eczema. The most consistent finding in such studies is a reduced proportion of bifidobacteria species in the feces of infants with eczema (77, 78) and atopic sensitization (79), but not wheezy children (78). The recognition of the importance of intestinal flora has led to the development of strategies aimed at manipulating bacterial colonization in formula-fed infants, including the use of prebiotics and probiotics. Prebiotics are nondigestible food components that beneficially affect the host by selectively stimulating the growth or activity of bacteria in the colon. They have frequently been added to infant formula. To be effective, prebiotics should escape digestion and absorption in the upper gastrointestinal tract, reach the large bowel and be used selectively by microorganisms that have been identified to have health-promoting properties. Studies to date in infants have demonstrated significant increases in fecal bifidobacteria in response to formula supplementation with oligosaccharides (80–84), one also demonstrating an increase in lactobacilli (81), but none demonstrating an effect on potentially pathogenic bacteria. In a recent randomized trial, 259 infants at high risk of allergy (parental history of asthma, eczema or rhinitis) were randomized to galacto- and long-chain fructo-oligosaccharides or placebo added to an extensively hydrolyzed whey formula. There were in excess of 20% losses from the trial, and in a subgroup of infants with fecal bacterial counts there were differences at baseline in lactobacilli counts between groups. Fecal bifidobacteria counts increased significantly in the prebiotic group. In 206 infants followed up to 6 months, infants receiving oligosaccharide supplementation had significantly reduced clinical eczema (RR 0.42, 95% CI 0.21, 0.84), although eczema severity scores were not significantly different. No adverse effects were reported. Further research is required to determine whether prebiotics are effective at preventing eczema.

Probiotics are live bacteria that colonize the gut and provide a health benefit to the host. Benefits from use of probiotic bacteria have been found in a systematic review of randomized trials (85) for the treatment of infectious diarrhea, with use of probiotics reducing diarrhea at 3 days (RR 0.66, 95% CI 0.55, 0.77) and mean duration of diarrhea by 30 h (95% CI 18–42 h). Several randomized studies have now demonstrated the efficacy of the use of probiotics in infants with active eczema (86–89), although not all studies have shown conclusive benefits (89). For prevention of allergy, one randomized, placebo-controlled trial (90) reported that supplementation with lactobacillus given prenatally to mothers who had at least one first-degree relative with atopic eczema, rhinitis or asthma, and postnatally for 6 months to their infants, reduced the incidence of atopic eczema up to 2 years (from 46% to 23%; RR 0.51, 95% CI 0.32, 0.84). No significant effect was reported on total or specific serum IgE or skin-prick tests over this period. Excess (17%)

post-randomization losses prevent strong conclusions being drawn from this study. Further studies are needed before probiotics can be recommended in high-risk infants for the prevention of allergy. To date, the most promising data for both prebiotics (84) and probiotics (90) are in infants with or at risk of atopic eczema.

FUTURE DIRECTIONS

To date, dietary primary prevention strategies for food hypersensitivity and allergy have yielded largely unconvincing results. A greater understanding of genetic, physiologic and environmental factors resulting in immune tolerance and sensitization would no doubt facilitate future efforts, and particularly of how the fetus and immature newborn are exposed to and process antigens, and the genetic and immune developmental mechanisms that program sensitization and tolerance. The identification of genetic markers for allergic sensitization will facilitate the identification of infants likely to benefit from primary prevention strategies.

Low rates of exclusive breast-feeding have the potential to contribute substantially to the burden of infant allergy and early food hypersensitivity. In the government and public health domain, greater efforts are required, including in developed countries, to facilitate and encourage exclusive breast-feeding. A reasonable goal of all maternity and infant health care providers is the implementation of the Baby Friendly Hospital Initiative (40).

For specific approaches to infant feeding designed to reduce the incidence of allergy and early food hypersensitivity, adequately powered and rigorous trials of prebiotics and probiotics in high-risk infants are needed, particularly those with the goal of preventing infant atopic eczema. Although there is some evidence for the use of both partially and extensively hydrolyzed formula, in view of methodological concerns and inconsistency of findings further large, well-designed trials comparing partially hydrolyzed whey and extensively hydrolyzed casein to cow's milk formula are needed.

It should be noted that although sensitization is common, clinical reactions to foods are relatively uncommon, and substantial numbers of infants will be required to detect benefits in terms of reduced cow's milk allergy or food allergy in the context of randomized controlled trials. As such, other more prevalent clinical allergic manifestations, particularly infant eczema and wheezing, and subsequent childhood asthma and rhinitis, become more appropriate goals of primary prevention, especially in view of their potential public health benefit. It is also important that trials focused on prevention address clinical manifestations of allergy, and not just sensitization.

CONCLUSIONS

For primary prevention of allergy and early food hypersensitivity, current data support the implementation of public health policies designed to facilitate exclusive breast-feeding in all infants up to the first 6 months. Evidence of benefit for other specific maternal and infant dietary recommendations is found only in infants at high risk of allergy. There is as yet no consensus for definition of high-risk infants, although the addition of cord blood IgE testing is not adequately predictive to warrant use outside clinical trials. The predictive value of family history for clinical allergy is greatest for allergy in first-degree relatives, maternal or sibling allergy as opposed to paternal allergy, and double as opposed to single allergic heredity. Despite identifying allergic heredity, only around half of those infants who subsequently develop clinical allergies are identified at birth.

Where exclusive breast-feeding is not possible in the first 6 months, there is some evidence for use of hydrolyzed formula for prevention of allergy in high-risk infants. For specific types of hydrolyzed formula, there is some evidence for use of both partially hydrolyzed 100% whey formula and extensively hydrolyzed casein formula in infants at high risk of allergy. An extensively hydrolyzed formula may be better than a partially hydrolyzed formula at preventing food hypersensitivity, but is likely to have higher cost. Further rigorous, adequately powered trials are needed to confirm these findings. There is concern regarding the nutritional adequacy of specialized preterm hydrolyzed formula in terms of adequacy of weight gain in low birth weight infants.

There is no evidence to support the use of maternal dietary avoidance measures during lactation and/or breast-feeding, and there are concerns regarding the nutritional impacts of these measures, particularly during pregnancy. There is no evidence to support recommending soy formulas in preference to cow's milk formulas for prevention of allergy and food hypersensitivity. Further trials of both prebiotics and probiotics are needed before they can be recommended in high-risk infants for prevention of atopic eczema.

REFERENCES

1. Prescott SL, Tang ML. The Australasian Society of Clinical Immunology and Allergy position statement: Summary of allergy prevention in children. Med J Aust 182:464–467, 2005.
2. Halken S. Prevention of allergic disease in childhood: clinical and epidemiological aspects of primary and secondary allergy prevention. Pediatr Allergy Immunol 15 (Supp 16):4–5, 2004.
3. Johansson SG, Bieber T, Dahl R, et al. Revised nomenclature for allergy for global use: Report of the Nomenclature Review Committee of the World Allergy Organization, October 2003. J Allergy Clin Immunol 113:832–836, 2004.
4. Burr ML, Butland BK, King S, Vaughan-Williams E. Changes in asthma prevalence: two surveys 15 years apart. Arch Dis Child 64:1452–1456, 1989.
5. Schultz Larsen F. Atopic dermatitis: an increasing problem. Pediatr Allergy Immunol 7:51–53, 1996.
6. Sampson HA. Update on food allergy. J Allergy Clin Immunol 113:805–819; quiz 20; 2004.
7. Osterballe M, Hansen TK, Mortz CG, et al. The prevalence of food hypersensitivity in an unselected population of children and adults. Pediatr Allergy Immunol 16:567–573, 2005.
8. Natale M, Bisson C, Monti G, et al. Cow's milk allergens identification by two-dimensional immunoblotting and mass spectrometry. Mol Nutr Food Res 48:363–369, 2004.
9. Skolnick HS, Conover-Walker MK, Koerner CB, et al. The natural history of peanut allergy. J Allergy Clin Immunol 107:367–374, 2001.
10. Warner JO. The early life origins of asthma and related allergic disorders. Arch Dis Child 89:97–102, 2004.
11. Jones CA, Vance GH, Power LL, et al. Costimulatory molecules in the developing human gastrointestinal tract: a pathway for fetal allergen priming. J Allergy Clin Immunol 108:235–241, 2001.
12. Thornton CA, Vance GH. The placenta: a portal of fetal allergen exposure. Clin Exp Allergy 32:1537–1539, 2002.
13. Bernsen RM, de Jongste JC, Koes BW, et al. Perinatal characteristics and obstetric complications as risk factors for asthma, allergy and eczema at the age of 6 years. Clin Exp Allergy 35:1135–1140, 2005.
14. Jaakkola JJ, Gissler M. Maternal smoking in pregnancy, fetal development, and childhood asthma. Am J Public Health 94:136–140, 2004.
15. Raby BA, Celedon JC, Litonjua AA, et al. Low-normal gestational age as a predictor of asthma at 6 years of age. Pediatrics 114:e327–332, 2004.
16. Kurukulaaratchy RJ, Matthews S, Arshad SH. Defining childhood atopic phenotypes to investigate the association of atopic sensitization with allergic disease. Allergy 60:1280–1286, 2005.
17. Moffatt MF, Cookson WO. Gene identification in asthma and allergy. Int Arch Allergy Immunol 116:247–252, 1998.
18. Arshad SH, Kurukulaaratchy RJ, Fenn M, Matthews S. Early life risk factors for current wheeze, asthma, and bronchial hyperresponsiveness at 10 years of age. Chest 127:502–508, 2005.
19. Sunyer J, Mendendez C, Ventura PJ, et al. Prenatal risk factors of wheezing at the age of four years in Tanzania. Thorax 56:290–295, 2001.
20. Devereux G, Barker RN, Seaton A. Antenatal determinants of neonatal immune responses to allergens. Clin Exp Allergy 32:43–50, 2002.
21. Tariq SM, Matthews SM, Hakim EA, et al. The prevalence of and risk factors for atopy in early childhood: a whole population birth cohort study. J Allergy Clin Immunol 101:587–593, 1998.
22. Dunstan JA, Mori TA, Barden A, et al. Fish oil supplementation in pregnancy modifies neonatal allergen-specific immune responses and clinical outcomes in infants at high risk of atopy: a randomized, controlled trial. J Allergy Clin Immunol 112:1178–1184, 2003.
23. Arshad SH, Stevens M, Hide DW. The effect of genetic and environmental factors on the prevalence of allergic disorders at the age of two years. Clin Exp Allergy 23:504–511, 1993.

24. Peat JK, Li J. Reversing the trend: reducing the prevalence of asthma. J Allergy Clin Immunol 103:1–10, 1999.
25. Bergmann RL, Edenharter G, Bergmann KE, et al. Predictability of early atopy by cord blood-IgE and parental history. Clin Exp Allergy 27:752–760, 1997.
26. Hansen LG, Halken S, Host A, Moller K, Osterballe O. Prediction of allergy from family history and cord blood IgE levels. A follow-up at the age of 5 years. Cord blood IgE. IV. Pediatr Allergy Immunol 4:34–40, 1993.
27. Kjellman NI. Atopic disease in seven-year-old children. Incidence in relation to family history. Acta Paediatr Scand 66:465–471, 1977.
28. Croner S. Prediction and detection of allergy development: influence of genetic and environmental factors. J Pediatr 121:S58–S63, 1992.
29. AAP. American Academy of Pediatrics. Committee on Nutrition. Hypoallergenic infant formulas. Pediatrics 106:346–349, 2000.
30. Asher I, Baena-Cagnani C, Boner A, et al. World Allergy Organization guidelines for prevention of allergy and allergic asthma. Int Arch Allergy Immunol 135:83–92, 2004.
31. Host A, Halken S. Primary prevention of food allergy in infants who are at risk. Curr Opin Allergy Clin Immunol 5:255–259, 2005.
32. Kramer MS, Kakuma R. Maternal dietary antigen avoidance during pregnancy or lactation, or both, for preventing or treating atopic disease in the child. Cochrane Database Syst Rev 3:CD000133, 2006.
33. Falth-Magnusson K, Kjellman NI. Development of atopic disease in babies whose mothers were receiving exclusion diet during pregnancy—a randomized study. J Allergy Clin Immunol 80:868–875, 1987.
34. Lilja G, Dannaeus A, Falth-Magnusson K, et al. Immune response of the atopic woman and foetus: effects of high- and low-dose food allergen intake during late pregnancy. Clin Allergy 18:131–142, 1988.
35. Lovegrove JA, Hampton SM, Morgan JB. The immunological and long-term atopic outcome of infants born to women following a milk-free diet during late pregnancy and lactation: a pilot study. BritJ Nutr 71:223–238, 1994.
36. Appelt GK, Chan-Yeung M, Watson WTA, et al. Breastfeeding and food avoidance are ineffective in preventing sensitization in high risk children. J Allergy Clin Immunol 113:S99, 2004.
37. Hide DW, Matthews S, Tariq S, Arshad SH. Allergen avoidance in infancy and allergy at 4 years of age. Allergy 51:89–93, 1996.
38. Zeiger RS. Food allergen avoidance in the prevention of food allergy in infants and children. Pediatrics 111:1662–1671, 2003.
39. Lucas A, Brooke OG, Morley R, et al. Early diet of preterm infants and development of allergic or atopic disease: randomised prospective study. BMJ 300:837–840, 1990.
40. Kramer MS, Chalmers B, Hodnett ED, et al. Promotion of Breastfeeding Intervention Trial (PROBIT): a randomized trial in the Republic of Belarus. JAMA 285:413–420, 2001.
41. Juvonen P, Mansson M, Andersson C, Jakobsson I. Allergy development and macromolecular absorption in infants with different feeding regimens during the first three days of life. A three-year prospective follow-up. Acta Paediatr 85:1047–1052, 1996.
42. Saarinen KM, Juntunen-Backman K, Jarvenpaa AL, et al. Supplementary feeding in maternity hospitals and the risk of cow's milk allergy: A prospective study of 6209 infants. J Allergy Clin Immunol 104:457–461, 1999.
43. Osborn DA, Sinn J. Formulas containing hydrolysed protein for prevention of allergy and food intolerance in infants. Cochrane Database Syst Rev CD003664, 2006.
44. Taylor B, Wadsworth J, Golding J, Butler N. Breast feeding, eczema, asthma, and hayfever. J Epidemiol Community Health 37:95–99, 1983.
45. Kaplan BA, Mascie-Taylor CG. Biosocial factors in the epidemiology of childhood asthma in a British national sample. J Epidemiol Community Health 39:152–156, 1985.
46. Rusconi F, Galassi C, Corbo GM, et al. Risk factors for early, persistent, and late-onset wheezing in young children. SIDRIA Collaborative Group. Am J Respir Crit Care Med 160:1617–1622, 1999.
47. Wright AL, Holberg CJ, Taussig LM, Martinez FD. Factors influencing the relation of infant feeding to asthma and recurrent wheeze in childhood. Thorax 56:192–197, 2001.
48. Bergmann RL, Diepgen TL, Kuss O, et al. Breastfeeding duration is a risk factor for atopic eczema. Clin Exp Allergy 32:205–209, 2002.
49. Miyake Y, Yura A, Iki M. Breastfeeding and the prevalence of symptoms of allergic disorders in Japanese adolescents. Clin Exp Allergy 33:312–316, 2003.
50. Sears MR, Greene JM, Willan AR, et al. Long-term relation between breastfeeding and development of atopy and asthma in children and young adults: a longitudinal study. Lancet 360:901–907, 2002.
51. Friedman NJ, Zeiger RS. The role of breast-feeding in the development of allergies and asthma. J Allergy Clin Immunol 115:1238–1248, 2005.
52. Mimouni Bloch A, Mimouni D, Mimouni M, Gdalevich M. Does breastfeeding protect against allergic rhinitis during childhood? A meta-analysis of prospective studies. Acta Paediatr 91:275–279, 2002.
53. Gdalevich M, Mimouni D, David M, Mimouni M. Breast-feeding and the onset of atopic dermatitis in childhood: a systematic review and meta-analysis of prospective studies. J Am Acad Dermatol 45:520–527, 2001.
54. Gdalevich M, Mimouni D, Mimouni M. Breast-feeding and the risk of bronchial asthma in childhood: a systematic review with meta-analysis of prospective studies. J Pediatr 139:261–266, 2001.

55. van Odijk J, Kull I, Borres MP, et al. Breastfeeding and allergic disease: a multidisciplinary review of the literature (1966–2001) on the mode of early feeding in infancy and its impact on later atopic manifestations. Allergy 58:833–843, 2003.

56. Kramer MS, Kakuma R. Optimal duration of exclusive breastfeeding. Cochrane Database Syst Rev CD003517, 2002.

57. Kajosaari M, Saarinen UM. Prophylaxis of atopic disease by six months' total solid food elimination. Evaluation of 135 exclusively breast-fed infants of atopic families. Acta Paediatr Scand 72:411–414, 1983.

58. Kull I, Almqvist C, Lilja G, et al. Breast-feeding reduces the risk of asthma during the first 4 years of life. J Allergy Clin Immunol 114:755–760, 2004.

59. Kull I, Wickman M, Lilja G, et al. Breast feeding and allergic diseases in infants—a prospective birth cohort study. Arch Dis Child 87:478–481, 2002.

60. Oddy WH, Holt PG, Sly PD, et al. Association between breast feeding and asthma in 6 year old children: findings of a prospective birth cohort study. BMJ 319:815–819, 1999.

61. Host A, Koletzko B, Dreborg S, et al. Dietary products used in infants for treatment and prevention of food allergy. Joint Statement of the European Society for Pediatric Allergy and Clinical Immunology (ESPACI) Committee on Hypoallergenic Formulas and the European Society for Pediatric Gastroenterology, Hepatology and Nutrition (ESPGHAN) Committee on Nutrition. Arch Dis Child 81:80–84, 1999.

62. McGuire W, Anthony MY. Donor human milk versus formula for preventing necrotising enterocolitis in preterm infants: systematic review. Arch Dis Child Fetal Neonatal Ed 88:F11–14, 2003.

63. Chandra RK, Puri S, Suraiya C, Cheema PS. Influence of maternal food antigen avoidance during pregnancy and lactation on incidence of atopic eczema in infants. Clin Allergy 16:563–569, 1986.

64. Chandra RK, Puri S, Hamed A. Influence of maternal diet during lactation and use of formula feeds on development of atopic eczema in high risk infants. BMJ 299:228–230, 1989.

65. UNICEF. Progress for Children: A Report Card on Nutrition (No. 4): UNICEF; 2006.

66. Vandenplas Y, Hauser B, Van den Borre C, et al. Effect of a whey hydrolysate prophylaxis of atopic disease. Ann Allergy 68:419–424, 1992.

67. von Berg A, Koletzko S, Grubl A, et al. The effect of hydrolyzed cow's milk formula for allergy prevention in the first year of life: the German Infant Nutritional Intervention Study, a randomized double-blind trial. J Allergy Clin Immunol 111:533–540, 2003.

68. Halken S, Hansen KS, Jacobsen HP, et al. Comparison of a partially hydrolyzed infant formula with two extensively hydrolyzed formulas for allergy prevention: a prospective, randomized study. Pediatr Allergy Immunol 11:149–161, 2000.

69. Oldaeus G, Anjou K, Bjorksten B, et al. Extensively and partially hydrolysed infant formulas for allergy prophylaxis. Arch Dis Child 77:4–10, 1997.

70. Nentwich I, Michkova E, Nevoral J, et al. Cow's milk-specific cellular and humoral immune responses and atopy skin symptoms in infants from atopic families fed a partially (pHF) or extensively (eHF) hydrolyzed infant formula. Allergy 56:1144–1156, 2001.

71. Merritt RJ, Jenks BH. Safety of soy-based infant formulas containing isoflavones: the clinical evidence. J Nutr 134:1220S–1224S, 2004.

72. AAP. Committee on Nutrition. Soy protein-based formulas: recommendations for use in infant feeding. Pediatrics 101:148–153, 1998.

73. Mendez MA, Anthony MS, Arab L. Soy-based formulae and infant growth and development: a review. J Nutr 132:2127–2130, 2002.

74. Osborn DA, Sinn J. Soy formula for prevention of allergy and food intolerance in infants. Cochrane Database Syst Rev CD003741, 2006.

75. Kjellman NI, Johansson SG. Soy versus cow's milk in infants with a biparental history of atopic disease: development of atopic disease and immunoglobulins from birth to 4 years of age. Clin Allergy 9:347–358, 1979.

76. Agostoni C, Axelsson I, Goulet O, et al. Prebiotic oligosaccharides in dietetic products for infants: a commentary by the ESPGHAN Committee on Nutrition. J Pediatr Gastroenterol Nutr 39:465–473, 2004.

77. Bjorksten B, Sepp E, Julge K, et al. Allergy development and the intestinal microflora during the first year of life. J Allergy Clin Immunol 108:516–520, 2001.

78. Murray CS, Tannock GW, Simon MA, et al. Fecal microbiota in sensitized wheezy and non-sensitized non-wheezy children: a nested case-control study. Clin Exp Allergy 35:741–745, 2005.

79. Kalliomaki M, Kirjavainen P, Eerola E, et al. Distinct patterns of neonatal gut microflora in infants in whom atopy was and was not developing. J Allergy Clin Immunol 107:129–134, 2001.

80. Boehm G, Lidestri M, Casetta P, et al. Supplementation of a bovine milk formula with an oligosaccharide mixture increases counts of faecal bifidobacteria in preterm infants. Arch Dis Child Fetal Neonatal Ed 86:F178–181, 2002.

81. Moro G, Minoli I, Mosca M, et al. Dosage-related bifidogenic effects of galacto- and fructooligosaccharides in formula-fed term infants. J Pediatr Gastroenterol Nutr 34:291–295, 2002.

82. Schmelzle H, Wirth S, Skopnik H, et al. Randomized double-blind study of the nutritional efficacy and bifidogenicity of a new infant formula containing partially hydrolyzed protein, a high beta-palmitic acid level, and nondigestible oligosaccharides. J Pediatr Gastroenterol Nutr 36:343–351, 2003.

83. Decsi T, Arato A, Balogh M, et al. Prebiotikus hatasu oligoszacharidok egeszseges csecsemok szekletflorajara gyakorolt hatasanak randomizalt, placeboval kontrollalt vizsgalata. Orvosi Hetilap 146:2445–2450, 2005.

84. Moro G, Arslanoglu S, Stahl B, et al. A mixture of prebiotic oligosaccharides reduces the incidence of atopic dermatitis during the first six months of age. Arch Dis Child 91:814–819, 2006.

85. Allen SJ, Okoko B, Martinez E, etal. Probiotics for treating infectious diarrhoea. Cochrane Database Syst Rev CD003048, 2004.

86. Majamaa H, Isolauri E. Probiotics: a novel approach in the management of food allergy. J Allergy Clin Immunol 99:179–185, 1997.

87. Isolauri E, Arvola T, Sutas Y, et al. Probiotics in the management of atopic eczema. Clin Exp Allergy 30:1604–1610, 2000.

88. Rosenfeldt V, Benfeldt E, Nielsen SD, et al. Effect of probiotic Lactobacillus strains in children with atopic dermatitis. J Allergy Clin Immunol 111:389–395, 2003.

89. Viljanen M, Savilahti E, Haahtela T, et al. Probiotics in the treatment of atopic eczema/dermatitis syndrome in infants: a double-blind placebo-controlled trial. Allergy 60:494–500, 2005.

90. Kalliomaki M, Salminen S, Arvilommi H, et al. Probiotics in primary prevention of atopic disease: a randomised placebo-controlled trial. Lancet 357:1076–1079, 2001.

91. Falth-Magnusson K, Kjellman NI. Allergy prevention by maternal elimination diet during late pregnancy—a 5-year follow-up of a randomized study. J Allergy Clin Immunol 89:709–713, 1992.

92. Falth-Magnusson K, Oman H, Kjellman NI. Maternal abstention from cow milk and egg in allergy risk pregnancies. Effect on antibody production in the mother and the newborn. Allergy 42:64–73, 1987.

93. Kjellman NI, Bjorksten B, Hattevig G, Falth-Magnusson K. Natural history of food allergy. Ann Allergy 61:83–87, 1988.

94. Lilja G, Dannaeus A, Foucard T, et al. Effects of maternal diet during late pregnancy and lactation on the development of atopic diseases in infants up to 18 months of age—in-vivo results. Clin Exp Allergy 19:473–479, 1989.

95. Lilja G, Dannaeus A, Foucard T, et al. Effects of maternal diet during late pregnancy and lactation on the development of IgE and egg- and milk-specific IgE and IgG antibodies in infants. Clin Exp Allergy 21:195–202, 1991.

96. Chirico G, Gasparoni A, Ciardelli L, et al. Immunogenicity and antigenicity of a partially hydrolyzed cow's milk infant formula. Allergy 52:82–88, 1997.

97. de Seta L, Siani P, Cirillo G, et al. La prevenzione delle malattie allergiche con formula H.A.: follow-up a 24 mesi. Pediatr Med Chir 16:251–254, 1994.

98. Lam BC, Yeung CY. The effect of breast milk, infant formula and hypoallergenic formula on incidence of atopic manifestation in high risk infants. Nestle Internal Report 1992.

99. Maggio L, Zuppa AA, Sawatzki G, et al. Higher urinary excretion of essential amino acids in preterm infants fed protein hydrolysates. Acta Paediatr 94:75–84, 2005.

100. Mallet E, Henocq A. Long-term prevention of allergic diseases by using protein hydrolysate formula in at-risk infants. J Pediatr 121:S95–100, 1992.

101. Marini A, Agosti M, Motta G, Mosca F. Effects of a dietary and environmental prevention programme on the incidence of allergic symptoms in high atopic risk infants: three years' follow-up. Acta Paediatr Suppl 414:1–21, 1996.

102. Picaud JC, Rigo J, Normand SL, et al. Nutritional efficacy of preterm formula with a partially hydrolyzed protein source: a randomized pilot study. J Pediatr Gastroenterol Nutr 32:555–561, 2001.

103. Szajewska H, Albrecht P, Stoitiska BP, et al. Extensive and partial protein hydrolysate preterm formulas: the effect on growth rate, protein metabolism indices, and plasma amino acid concentrations. J Pediatr Gastroenterol Nutr 32:303–309, 2001.

104. Tsai YT, Chou CC, Hsieh KH. The effect of hypoallergenic formula on the occurrence of allergic diseases in high risk infants. Zhonghua Min Guo Xiao Er Ke Yi Xue Hui Za Zhi 32:137–144, 1991.

105. Vandenplas Y, Hauser B, Blecker U, et al. The nutritional value of a whey hydrolysate formula compared with a whey-predominant formula in healthy infants. J Pediatr Gastroenterol Nutr 17:92–96, 1993.

106. Willems R, Duchateau J, Magrez P, et al. Influence of hypoallergenic milk formula on the incidence of early allergic manifestations in infants predisposed to atopic diseases. Ann Allergy 71:147–150, 1993.

107. Johnstone DE, Dutton AM. Dietary prophylaxis of allergic disease in children. N Engl J Med 274:715–719, 1966.

108. Miskelly FG, Burr ML, Vaughan-Williams E, et al. Infant feeding and allergy. Arch Dis Child 63:388–393, 1988.

Chapter 8

Toll-like Receptor Responses in Neonatal Dendritic Cells

Stanislas Goriely, MD, PhD, FNRS • Ezra Aksoy, PhD • Dominique De Wit, PhD • Michel Goldman, MD, PhD • Fabienne Willems, PhD

Toll-like Receptors and Pathogen Recognition

Study of Neonatal APC: Whole Blood, CBMC, Isolated Cells, Monocyte-Derived DC: Which System can we Trust?

Subsets and Phenotypes of Neonatal DCs

Early Inflammatory Response by Neonatal APCs

Production of Th1-Driving Cytokines by Neonatal APCs

Type I IFN Production by Neonatal APCs

Neonatal DC Function and Clinical Implications

Neonatal immune responses are considered to be immature, as witnessed by increased susceptibility to infectious pathogens or suboptimal responses to vaccine administration. Many studies have focused on T and B cell adaptive responses in newborns. More recently, the function of neonatal antigen-presenting cells (APC) and their potential role in immune immaturity have also been explored. In order to respond to invading pathogens, the "innate immune response", initiated by germline-encoded pattern recognition molecules, directly leads to microbicidal pathways and inflammation. It is now clear, however, that they are also required for the development of adequate "adaptive immunity" (1). The discovery and characterization of Toll-like receptors (TLRs) have considerably increased our understanding of how the innate and adaptive responses operate in concert to achieve systemic immunity and protection of the host against a diverse range of pathogens. The critical players of the process of linking the two arms of the immune response are dendritic cells (DC) (2). In this chapter, we will first review some of the most important advances toward understanding the molecular and cellular mechanisms underlying TLR-mediated pathogen recognition. We will then describe what is known on DC and APC functions in early life, focusing on TLR responses. Finally, we will discuss potential clinical implications of these studies, in terms of infectious and allergic diseases and immunization strategies.

TOLL-LIKE RECEPTORS AND PATHOGEN RECOGNITION

The innate immune system uses non-clonal, evolutionarily conserved, germline-encoded sets of molecules referred to as pathogen recognition receptors (PRRs) that sense and respond to pathogenic infections, mostly but not all of microbial origin, including bacteria, viruses, protozoa and fungi. PRRs are either secreted, cell-surface expressed, or reside in the intracellular compartments of the host and they recognize evolutionarily conserved molecular structures from diverse pathogens, referred to as pathogen-associated molecular patterns (PAMPs).

The Toll-like receptor (TLR) family has emerged as the key sensors of microbial infections that play an instructive role in innate immune responses against microbial pathogens as well as the subsequent induction of adaptive immune responses. TLRs are archetypal PRR family members, recognizing diverse PAMPs from microbial pathogens, triggering inflammatory and antiviral responses and DC maturation, which finally result in the eradication of invading pathogens. TLRs are evolutionarily conserved molecules and are characterized by an extracellular leucine-rich repeat (LRR) domain and an intracellular Toll/IL-1 receptor (TIR) domain (also present in the IL-1 receptor family) (3).

LRRs are found in the cytoplasmic and transmembrane proteins, which are involved in PAMP recognition and signal transduction (4). The intracellular domain of TLRs, the TIR domain, is a conserved protein-protein interaction module, which is found in a number of transmembrane and cytoplasmic proteins in plants and arthropods as well as in humans. Essentially, all the TIR-containing molecules have important functions in host defense, thus making the TIR domain one of the earliest motifs evolved (5). There are 10 functional TLRs identified in human and 13 in mouse, which can recognize distinct PAMPs from a number of microbial organisms. Here, we review some of the most important recent advances toward understanding the molecular and cellular mechanisms underlying TLR-mediated recognition of PAMPs and the downstream signaling cascades that initiate innate immune responses.

TLRs and their Ligands

TLR-4

LPS is the outer component of the membrane of Gram-negative (−) bacteria and is the causative agent of endotoxin shock. Both positional cloning of the locus responsible for LPS hyporesponsiveness in C3H/HeJ mice strain (generated by a missense mutation in the *Tlr*4 gene) and the generation of TLR-4$^{-/-}$ mice have established that TLR-4 is required for LPS responsiveness (6–9). TLR-4$^{-/-}$ DCs and macrophages exhibit diminished production of cytokines and phenotypic maturation (in terms of upregulation of co-stimulatory molecules) in response to LPS. In humans, co-segregating missense mutations (Asp299Gly and Thr399Ile) in the extracellular domain of the TLR-4 receptor are associated with blunted responses to inhaled LPS and with a higher risk for developing severe sepsis (10). Furthermore, the reported mutations in the *Tlr*4 gene confer a lower risk for artherosclerosis but increased development of chronic periodontitis (11, 12). LPS binding and activation of TLR-4 requires several additional molecules. One of such molecules is glycosyl-phosphatidylinositol-anchored protein, CD14, required for LPS responsiveness. It was proposed that LPS is captured by the plasma LPS binding protein (LBP) and transferred to CD14, abundantly expressed on mononuclear phagocytes (i.e. monocytes and macrophages) (13, 14). Notably, partial deletion or complete deficiency in the gene encoding CD14 results in LPS hyporesponsiveness (15). Other molecules include myeloid differentiation (MD)-2 protein, which associates with the extracellular domain of TLR-4 and is required for LPS signaling. Notably, gene-targeting studies have provided evidence that MD-2 is indispensable and unique to TLR-4 (16, 17). Overall, these findings draw a model mechanism by which LPS is recognized by distinct soluble proteins and clusters of receptors, associated within lipid rafts (reviewed in refs 18 and 19).

TLR-2 (TLR-1, TLR-6)

TLR-2 recognizes numerous microbial components, including peptidoglycan from the cell-wall component of Gram-positive (+) bacteria such as *Staphylococcus aureus*, lipoproteins and lipopeptides from diverse bacterial species, glyco-phosphatidylinositol anchors from *Trypanosoma cruzi*, lipoarabinomannan from *Mycobacterium tuberculosis*, porins of *Neisseria meningitides*, and finally the yeast cell-wall component zymosan (9, 20–22). Targeted deletion of the *Tlr2* gene revealed that TLR-2 is an important molecule in resistance to *Staphylococcus aureus* (23).

TLR-2 ligands form heterodimers between TLR-2 and TLR-6 or -1. Neither TLR-2$^{-/-}$ nor TLR-6$^{-/-}$ macrophages respond to synthetic mycoplasmal lipopeptide macrophage-activating lipopeptide 2 (MALP-2), whereas TLR-6$^{-/-}$ but not TLR-2$^{-/-}$ macrophages respond normally to synthetic lipopeptide PAM$_3$CSK$_4$ and peptidoglycan (9, 22, 24, 25). A probable consequence of cooperation of TLR-2 with other TLRs is to increase the repertoire of ligand specifications.

TLR-3

Viral replication often results in the generation of double-stranded (ds)RNA that possesses immunostimulatory potential to activate immune cells. Synthetic dsRNA mimics polyinosinic-polycytidylic acid (poly(I:C)); certain mRNA structures from apoptotic cells or silencing (si)RNAs can induce activation of TLR-3 (26–28). TLR-3$^{-/-}$ mice exhibit reduced inflammatory responses mediated by reovirus genomic dsRNA, or by poly(I:C) stimulation (26). However, TLR-3 is not the only requisite for generation of effective antiviral responses against infections to viruses, including lymphocytic choriomeningitis virus (LCMV), vesicular stomatitis virus (VSV) and murine cytomegalovirus (MCMV) (29–31). Importantly, recent studies propose that TLR-3 may have evolved to permit cross-priming of cytotoxic T lymphocyte (CTL)s against viruses that do not directly infect DCs (32).

TLR-5

Flagellated bacteria cause a broad range of serious gastrointestinal, urinary tract and respiratory tract infections. Flagellin is a 55 kDa monomer that is obtained from bacterial flagella, polymeric rod-like structures from the outer membrane of Gram$^-$ bacteria used for motility (33). It is the principal stimulant of inflammatory cytokine production in lung epithelial cells and is expressed on the basolateral but not apical surface of the intestinal epithelia (34, 35). TLR-5 recognizes a highly conserved structure that is particular to bacterial flagellin (33).

TLR-7 and TLR-8

Mouse TLR-7 and human TLR-7 and -8 were demonstrated to recognize distinct single stranded (ss)RNA structures mainly of viral origin, including human immunodeficiency virus type I (HIV-1), VSV and influenza virus (36–38). TLR-7 can also recognize several types of synthetic imidazoquinoline and guanine ribonucleoside (e.g., loxorubin) analogues (39, 40). These guanosine analogues possess antiviral properties and they induce type I IFNs to activate both humoral and cellular responses (41–43). The potent antiviral agent Resiquimod mainly depends on its potency to induce cytokines, including type I IFNs and IL-12 in plasmacytoid DCs (pDCs) and myeloid DCs (mDCs), respectively. Particularly, ssRNA and R-848 (a potent imiquimod analogue) can induce production of large quantities of type I IFNs from pDCs through TLR-7 engagement (36, 40, 44–46). In contrast, TLR-7 engagement on mDCs results in the production of IL-12p40 but not IFN-α (44). TLR-7$^{-/-}$ mice exhibit impaired immunity against ssRNA viruses such as VSV and influenza, which further highlights the importance of this receptor in host antiviral defense (47).

TLR-9

Unmethylated CpG motifs are common in bacterial and viral DNA, while CpG motifs in vertebrate DNA are methylated, endowing the microbial DNA immunogenicity/adjuvanticity (48). TLR-9 is essential for immune responses to bacterial DNA and synthetic oligodeoxynucleotides containing unmethylated CpG dinucleotides (CpG-DNA) (48, 49). The optimal immunostimulatory CpG sequences in human and mouse differ mainly due to the differences in the amino acid sequences between the extracellular regions of human and mouse TLR-9 (48, 50). Bacterial DNA and CpG oligonucleotides stimulate the proliferation of B cells and activate human pDCs and murine DCs (both mDCs and pDCs) to produce type I IFNs (particularly, IFN-α) (44, 51–54). CpG-stimulated pDCs induce plasma cell differentiation in naive and memory B cells in the absence of T-cell help, providing an effective humoral vaccine adjuvant (55). In addition CpG is a potent stimulator of Th1 responses (56–59). TLR-9$^{-/-}$ DCs are unresponsive to CpG-DNA in terms of phenotypic maturation and production of cytokines including type I IFNs. Notably, these mice exhibit defects in clearing MCMV infections (30, 60). Recognition of herpes simplex virus (HSV-1 or HSV-2) by pDCs can be achieved by functional TLR-9 in vitro (61, 62). Finally, it was also found that hemozoin (a hydrophobic heme polymer) purified from *Plasmodium falciparum* is a novel non-DNA ligand for TLR-9 (63).

TLR-11

TLR-11, a TLR member present in mice, but not humans, displays a distinct pattern of expression in mouse macrophages and liver, kidney, and bladder epithelial cells. Cells expressing TLR-11 do not respond to known TLR ligands but instead respond to uropathogenic bacteria (i.e. *Escherichia coli*). Notably, TLR-11$^{-/-}$ mice exhibit high susceptibility to uropathogenic bacteria, pointing out an important role for TLR-11 in preventing infection of internal organs of the urogenital system (64). Finally, a profilin-like molecule from the protozoan parasite *Toxoplasma gondii* was shown to trigger interleukin IL-12 through TLR-11 (only in mouse) and optimal resistance to *T. gondii* infection, which overall establishes a role for TLR11 in host recognition of protozoan pathogens (65).

TLR-independent Pathogen Recognition Receptors

Viruses and certain bacterial pathogens can gain access to the intracellular compartments such as the cytosol. In order to detect microbial presence to block microbial replication, the host defense has evolved several mechanisms, including cytosolic molecules acting as intracellular PRRs that are restricted to the vertebrates. Here we review some of the intracellular PRRs and/or molecules, particularly focusing on the dsRNA-activated protein kinase PKR, RNA helicase RIG-1 and Nod family of proteins.

Double-Stranded RNA-Activated Protein Kinase PKR

The dsRNA-dependent protein kinase PKR is the first molecule that was identified as a dsRNA sensor (66). PKR catalytic activity is stimulated by PKR binding to dsRNA produced during viral infection. The single-stranded tails flanking the dsRNA core provide the critical determinant for PKR activity (66, 67). PKR primarily prevents virus replication by inhibiting the translation of viral mRNAs while concomitantly participating in the production of type I IFNs and the establishment of an antiviral state (68). Mice deficient in *Pkr* gene are susceptible to viral infections owing to increased viral replication (68). Particularly, $PKR^{-/-}$ DCs and fibroblasts display decreased IFN type I IFN production mediated by dsRNA encounter (31, 69). PKR was also reported to be involved in NF-κB activation by poly(I:C) and LPS (70, 71). Overall, although PKR contributes to limit viral replication and type I IFN induction by viral or synthetic dsRNA encounter, it is not the only requirement for type I IFN induction to viral infection (72).

RNA Helicase RIG-1

Among more than 100 helicases in the human genome, DExD/H box helicases have the potential to unwind dsRNA by their intrinsic ATPase activity. These helicases can be found in most organisms and are involved in important cellular processes, including mRNA splicing and RNA interference (RNAi) (73). DExD/H box-containing RNA helicase retinoic acid inducible gene-1 (RIG-1) is important in virus-induced activation of type I IFN. RIG-1 exhibits unusual features: its N-(amino) terminus contains two tandem CARD motifs and the C-(carboxyl)-terminus has a helicase domain (73). Recently, RIG-1 was demonstrated to interact with dsRNA and augment type I IFN production in response to viruses using an ATPase-dependent pathway. In addition, the CARD motif of RIG-1 transduces signals resulting in the activation of two important transcription factors, IRF-3 and NF-κB (74).

Nod Family of Proteins

The other class of proteins involved in intracellular recognition of microbes and PAMPs are nucleotide-binding oligomerization domain (Nod) proteins. Nods are members of the nucleotide-binding site and leucine-rich repeat (NBS-LRR) family that possess N-terminal caspase recruitment domain (CARD) and a LRR domain (similar to that found in TLR family). They play important functions in mediating recognition of intracellular bacteria (reviewed in refs 75 and 76). Nod1/CARD4 detects bacterial peptidoglycan from Gram⁻ bacteria in the cytosol (77). It has a CARD, NACHT and an LRR domain. The synthetic component of Gram⁻ peptidoglycan, γ-D-glutamyl-mesoDAP, is the minimal structure recognized by Nod1 (77, 78). It is suggested that basal-state epithelial cells (e.g., in the intestinal tract) possess a Nod1-dependent Gram⁻ bacterial sensing system. Nod2 is predominantly expressed in the cells of myeloid origin and recognizes Gram⁻ and Gram⁺ bacteria. Nod2 shares significant homology to Nod1 but has two CARD domains. The muramyl dipeptide (the active component of Freund's adjuvant) from peptidoglycan fractions is the specific bacterial ligand for Nod2 (76). Nod2 mutant mice display enhanced TLR2-mediated NF-κB activation and Th1 responses, indicating an anti-inflammatory function of this molecule in innate immunity (79). Taken together, Nods are important intracellular PRRs involved in innate defense against bacteria.

TLR Signaling Pathways

During infections, the signal transduction pathway activated by TLRs is critical for the initiation of innate immune responses and for the induction of inflammatory cytokines and type I IFNs. TLRs, upon ligand binding, dimerize and undergo conformational change that is required for the recruitment of downstream molecules involved in TLR signaling. A multiplicity of adaptor molecules generates the basis for specificity in the signaling processes activated by each TLR.

Broadly speaking, two major pathways are activated by TLRs (Fig. 8-1). The first of these culminates in the activation of the transcription factor NF-κB, which acts as a master switch for inflammation, regulating the transcription of many genes that encode proteins involved in immunity and inflammation. The second leads to activation of the MAP kinases p38 and Jun amino-terminal kinase (JNK), which

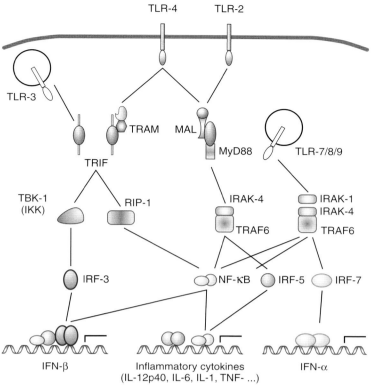

Figure 8-1 TLR signaling pathways. Stimulation of TLRs (with the exception of TLR-3) triggers the association of MyD88, the universal adapter molecule, which in turn recruits IRAK (IL-1R-associated kinase) family and TRAF6 (TNF-receptor-associated factor 6) to the receptor complex. The signalosome complex then dissociates from the receptor and activates NF-κB, IRF-5 and MAP kinases (not shown). In addition, TLR-2 and TLR-4 also utilize MAL (TIRAP) adaptor molecule. The "MyD88-dependent" pathway leads to the production of inflammatory cytokines. The "MyD88-independent pathway", triggered by TLR-3 and TLR-4, utilizes TRIF and TRAM (TLR4 only) adapter molecules, which in turn activate TBK-1 and IKKϵ to induce IRF-3 activation. This pathway also involves RIP-1 (receptor-interacting serine-threonine kinase I), which is responsible for the late phase of NF-κB activation. This pathway leads to the production of IFN-β and the expression of IFN-responsive genes. Finally, TLR-7/8/9 subfamily can also activate IRF-7 in a "MyD88-dependent" manner, leading to type I IFN production, for example in plasmacytoid DCs.

also participate in increased transcription and regulate the stability of mRNAs that contain AU repeats. Much effort has been directed towards deciphering the protein components that participate in TLR signaling pathways, and novel protein kinases have been found, most notably the IL-1 receptor associated kinase (IRAK) family. With the exception of TLR-3, it appears that all TLRs activate NF-κB and MAP kinases via a pathway that involves IRAK-4 and IRAK-1. The discovery of a set of adaptor proteins that are differentially recruited to TLRs has provided the first indication of the molecular basis of the specificity of TLR signaling and the existence of MyD88-independent pathways (80).

MyD88

The myeloid differentiation primary-response protein 88 (MyD88) is the first adaptor molecule described and, similar to TLRs, it has a Toll-IL-1 receptor (TIR) domain. MyD88 links almost all TLR members, with the exception of TLR-3, to the downstream NF-κB and MAP kinase pathways (81). Upon TLR ligand-induced dimerization, MyD88 is recruited through TIR domain interaction, leading in turn to the recruitment of IL-1 receptor associated kinase 4 (IRAK-4) (whose death domain interacts with the death domain of MyD88). IRAK-4 becomes activated and phosphorylates IRAK-1, which in turn activates TNF-associated factor 6 (TRAF6). A series of ubiquitinylation reactions then occur on TRAF6 and on the protein kinase TGF-b-activated kinase (TAK)-1, which is a candidate kinase for the activation of the inhibitor of NF-κB kinase (IKK) complex, leading to NF-κB activation, and p38 and JNK.

MyD88$^{-/-}$ innate cell populations do not respond to stimulation by IL-1, TLR-2,-7,-8 and -9 ligands and are hyporesponsive to TLR-4 activation by LPS and lipid A (82, 83). Particularly, DCs and macrophages from MyD88$^{-/-}$ mice exhibit a loss of production of inflammatory cytokines such as IL-1, TNF-α and immunomodulatory cytokine IL-12p40 mediated by almost all known TLR ligands. Furthermore, MyD88$^{-/-}$ mice are highly resistant to LPS-induced endotoxin shock but are highly susceptible to bacterial infections and have to be maintained in pathogen-free conditions (83). Strikingly, MyD88$^{-/-}$ DCs display normal phenotypic maturation (observed by upregulation of co-stimulatory molecules) comparable to wild-type DCs and produce type I IFN-β in response to LPS and poly(I:C). Moreover, LPS or poly(I:C) mediated activation of NF-κB and MAPKs is delayed in these DCs (reviewed in refs 84–88).

Additional studies carried out in MyD88$^{-/-}$ mice demonstrated that MyD88 not only triggers innate immune responses but also controls activation of adaptive immune responses (89–91). Although MyD88$^{-/-}$ DCs appear normal in terms of their T cell-stimulatory capacity, their Th1-polarizing ability is diminished (89). In addition, MyD88$^{-/-}$ mice show general defects in clearing *Staphylococcus aureus*, *Toxoplasma gondii* and mycobacterial infections (23, 92, 93).

MAL

Identification of the MyD88-independent pathway led to the discovery of a second novel TIR-domain-containing adaptor protein, MyD88 adaptor like (MAL, also referred as TIRAP) (94, 95). The N-terminus of MAL shows no similarity to any known proteins; however, the C-terminus is similar to the TIR domain of MyD88. MAL can homodimerize or heterodimerize with MyD88 to activate NF-κB and MAP kinase pathways (94, 95). Generation of MAL$^{-/-}$ mice and physiological and biochemical analysis of MAL$^{-/-}$ DCs have highlighted the critical role of this molecule being specific for signaling downstream of TLR4 and TLR2. These studies have elucidated that MAL$^{-/-}$ DCs do not produce proinflammatory cytokines (such as TNF-α and IL-1) in response to LPS and TLR2 ligands, and they do not upregulate co-stimulatory molecules mediated by petidoglycan or MALP-2 (96, 97).

TRIF

The third adaptor molecule, TIR-related adaptor protein inducing IFN-β (TRIF), is recruited by both TLR-4 and TLR-3, and is responsible for activation of the transcription factor interferon response factor (IRF)-3 (84, 87) acting via an inhibitor of κB kinase (IKK)-like kinase, termed tank binding kinase (TBK)-1 (98). The discovery of TRIF provided the first molecular basis for why TLR-3 and TLR-4, but not TLR-2, are able to induce IFN-β, since both TLR-3 and TLR-4 can signal via TRIF to the IKK family kinase TBK-1, which phosphorylates IRF-3.

The physiological role of TRIF was revealed by targeted deletion of the *Trif* gene or by generation of the *lps^2* strain that has a random germline mutagenesis leading to a distal frameshift error in the gene encoding TRIF (84, 87, 99). These studies have demonstrated that TRIF is essential for TLR-3- and TLR-4-mediated activation of the MyD88-independent pathway, subsequently resulting in the activation of transcription factor IRF-3. DCs and macrophages from TRIF$^{-/-}$ mice or the *lps^2* mutant strain display impaired LPS- and poly(I:C)-mediated IRF-3 activation that is required for IFN-β production and the expression of IRGs such as IFN inducible protein 10 (IP-10). Furthermore, TRIF$^{-/-}$ mice also exhibit defective production of inflammatory cytokines including TNF-α, IL-1, IL-12p40 in response to LPS and poly(I:C). These mice are highly susceptible to MCMV infections (29, 30). Overall the TRIF-dependent pathway appears to control almost all LPS- and poly(I:C)-mediated inflammatory responses in DCs and macrophages.

TRAM

The fourth TIR-domain-containing adaptor to be described was TRIF-related adaptor molecule (TRAM) (98, 100). TRAM associates only with TRIF and TLR-4 and inhibition of TRAM expression by silencing (si)RNA abolishes TLR4- but not TLR-3-mediated induction of IFN-β and IRGs (98). Further analysis of TRAM$^{-/-}$ mice established that TRAM is specifically involved in only TLR-4 signaling. Similar to TRIF$^{-/-}$ DCs, TRAM$^{-/-}$ DCs exhibit impaired activation of IRF-3 and reduced expression of IRGs in response to TLR-4 ligands (100).

Other Transcription Factors and their Role in TLR Signaling Pathways

More recently, attention has turned to the IRF family of transcription factors that have important roles in the regulation of type I IFN production and a growing list of other genes.

IRF-7 is a key transcription factor required for induction of type I IFNs, and is expressed only following exposure of cells to type I IFNs (101, 102). One exception to this statement is the pDCs, which express copious levels of IRF-3 and IRF-7 constitutively and are considered as "IFN factories" of the host (102). IRF-7$^{-/-}$ mice exhibit increased susceptibility to HSV and MCMV infections(103). IRF-7 activation occurs by both MyD88-dependent pathways (activated by TLR-9 or -7) and TRIF-dependent pathways (activated via TBK-1). Importantly, IRF-7 interacts with MyD88, IRAK-1 and TRAF6 to form a signaling complex (104–106). Notably, IFN-α production and IRF-7 activation in response to TLR-7 and TLR-9 ligands are abolished in IRAK-1-deficient pDCs(106).

Another IRF member, IRF-5, is found downstream of MyD88, and is activated by multiple TLRs. IRF-5 is essential for the induction of a range of pro-inflammatory genes, including IL-6, IL-12 and TNF, but not IFN-α, and is found in a trimeric complex with MyD88 and TRAF6 (107). Importantly, recent data provide strong evidence that IRF-5 is also an essential transducer of the TLR-7-dependent induction of type I IFNs (108).

TLR Expression and DC Subpopulations

DCs are a heterologous cell population with respect to their morphology, phenotype, enzymatic capacity, endocytic and phagocytic capacity as well as their distribution within tissues (109). First originating from CD34$^+$ hematopoietic progenitors and blood DC precursors, they localize into tissues through the bloodstream and give rise to several immature DC subpopulations. Human blood contains at least two distinct DC subtypes: myeloid CD11c$^+$ DCs (mDCs) and plasmacytoid DCs (pDCs) (110). Monocytes can also differentiate into myeloid DCs in the presence of GM-CSF (granulocyte macrophage-colony stimulating factor) and IL-4 (111, 112) or by migrating through the endothelium (113, 114). mDCs produce high amounts of IL-12 in response to certain TLR ligands (115, 116). pDCs, on the other hand, possess a unique ability to secrete large amounts of type I IFN upon TLR triggering or viral infection (44, 60, 117–119).

These DC subsets differentially express TLR repertoires, leading to specialization of their responses towards certain classes of pathogens (120–124). As shown in

Table 8-1   TLR Expression in Human Circulating pDC, mDC and Monocytes assessed by RT-PCR

	pDC	mDC	Monocytes
TLR-1	+	++	++
TLR-2	−	++	++
TLR-3	−	++	−
TLR-4	−	+	++
TLR-5	−	+	++
TLR-6	+	+	+
TLR-7	++	− or +	− or +
TLR-8	−	+	++
TLR-9	++	−	−
TLR-10	+	+	−

mRNA expression of the different TLR members was assessed by RT-PCR (refs 120–124)
−, indetectable; +, weakly expressed; ++, strongly expressed.

Table 8-1, circulating human mDCs express mRNA for most TLRs except TLR-9 (and maybe TLR-7). The TLR expression pattern on human monocytes is comparable except for increased TLR-2 and TLR-4 and absence of TLR-3. In contrast, human pDCs express high levels of TLR-9 and TLR-7 but no TLR-2,-3,-4,-5 or -8. As a consequence, monocytes and mDCs respond to PGN and LPS but are unresponsive to CpG-ODN. PolyI:C preferentially activates mDCs, while pDCs respond to both CpG-ODN and ssRNA but not to LPS or PGN. Interestingly, Imiquimod (R-848) is capable of stimulating both mDC and pDC subsets through recognition of both TLR-7 and TLR-8(125).

STUDY OF NEONATAL APC: WHOLE BLOOD, CBMC, ISOLATED CELLS, MONOCYTE-DERIVED DC: WHICH SYSTEM CAN WE TRUST?

There are several complementary approaches that can be used to compare adult and neonatal APC functions. Understanding the differences between the models can help to reconcile observations that sometimes seem to be conflicting.

There are evident ethical and technical limitations for the study of the human neonatal immune system. Umbilical cord blood represents the most convenient source of neonatal cells. It is easily collected at birth in large amounts (30–150ml) without causing any harm to the neonate or the mother. Birth, however, is a very "stressful" situation which might transiently influence the function of immune cells. The mode of delivery or the type of analgesia, for example, can affect cytokine production by cord blood mononuclear cells (126–129). Peripheral blood can also be collected in infants, for example during elective surgery, but the amount is limited (usually less than 5 ml).

Studies using whole blood samples have several advantages; (i) they allow "ex vivo" assessment of immune cell function, reducing possible isolation artifacts; (ii) they take into account interaction between immune cells and also assess the role of soluble circulating factors present in the plasma; and (iii) they can be performed even with small amounts of blood. There are also some limitations: Ex vivo whole blood is a "closed" system, in which primary and secondary mediators are released and greatly amplified (e.g., by activation of the complement cascade) as compared to in vivo situations where circulating immune cells interact with the endothelium and migrate to the adjacent tissues. It is therefore impossible to discriminate between initial activation and secondary feedback loops. Also, there are marked changes with age in the relative proportions of each cell type in circulating blood.

Hence, comparison of adult and neonatal cells is less biased when mononuclear cells are isolated by density gradient and counted. The comparison of cord blood mononuclear cell (CBMC) vs. peripheral blood mononuclear cell (PBMC) functions also reduces the direct influence of soluble factors present in the plasma.

In order to study intrinsic properties of neonatal APCs, these cells have to be isolated. Indeed, APC function in whole blood or among other mononuclear cells is greatly influenced by soluble mediators (such as TNF-α, IFN-γ or type I IFN) or interaction with other cell types (such as CD4$^+$ or CD8$^+$ T lymphocytes, NK T cells, γδ T cells). In comparison to monocytes (5–15% of mononuclear cells), circulating myeloid and plasmacytoid dendritic cells (less than 1%) are difficult to isolate and to study. Furthermore, the function of these subpopulations in the adult is yet not very well characterized. Romani et al. described a now well-established method for the generation of significant numbers of DCs from human monocytes cultured for several days in the presence of IL-4 and GM-CSF (130). This approach allows functional and molecular analysis of myeloid DC. When applied to cord blood, it also further reduces the influence of soluble mediators (such as corticosteroids) which are released during delivery and of direct activation of monocytes by the isolation procedure. However, variations in the in vitro culture steps and the use of exogenous recombinant cytokines increase the risk of discrepancies in the results generated by this model.

Finally, animal models can also be very beneficial to our understanding of APC function in early life. Murine models have been widely used to study early life immunization (131). The age of the animals (birth vs. 1 week) that reflects best immune function of human neonates is still debated. There are also major differences in dendritic cell biology across species (such as TLR repertoire or cytokines expressed by the different subpopulations), which should be taken into account when comparing results generated from human and murine studies.

SUBSETS AND PHENOTYPES OF NEONATAL DCs

In mice models, several reports indicated that the absolute number of APCs in the first few days of life is strongly reduced in comparison to adult animals (132–134). Moreover, placental macrophages of fetal origin were shown to have reduced antigen-presenting capacity (135). Similarly, it was reported that skin Langerhans cells and splenic DCs express low MHC class II and co-stimulatory molecules in the first few weeks of life (133, 136). A more detailed study of the ontogeny of splenic DC indicated that the distribution of DC subsets differs in neonatal mice. At birth, plasmacytoid CD11c^{low}B220$^+$ DC and CD11c$^+$CD8α$^-$ subsets are predominant in the spleen (132, 134, 137). During the first week of life, the CD11c$^+$CD8α$^+$ subpopulation rapidly increases. Apart from these differences, phenotypic maturation in response to TLR-9 or TLR-4 triggering was found to be comparable to adult cells and neonatal CD11c$^+$ cells were found efficient at presenting antigens.

In rats, colonization of the respiratory tract mucosa by DC happens during the first weeks of life. These cells are functionally immature, expressing low MHC class II molecules and being unable to mature in response to GM-CSF or local inflammation (138).

In humans, low MHC class II molecule expression on cord blood monocytes was reported (139). Their microbicidal activity was also shown to be decreased in comparison to adult cells (140). Initial studies on cord blood dendritic cells, using cell fractions enriched by densitiy gradient, indicated that these cells also express low MHC class II and ICAM-1 (intercellular adhesion molecule-1) molecules (141). They also display lower allogenic stimulatory capacity. It was reported that circulating cord blood DCs were exclusivley composed of immature CD11c$^-$ plasmacytoid DCs (142). Using other isolation procedures, Borras et al. showed that both plasmacytoid and conventional CD11c$^+$ DC subsets were present in cord blood but that the ratio (3:1) was inversed as compared to adults (1:3) (143). Using whole blood assay, we showed that maturation of cord blood mDC induced by LPS or polyI:C was incomplete as compared to adult cells (144). Similar observations were obtained for cord blood pDC in response to CpG oligonucleotides (145). After in vitro differentiation in the presence of IL-4 and GM-CSF, cord blood monocytes expressed the classical surface markers of immature myeloid DC. When compared to adult mDC, HLA-DR, CD80 and CD40 surface expression was found to be reduced in neonatal cells and incomplete maturation was observed upon LPS stimulation (146, 147). We observed that neonatal mDCs are less efficient than adult DC in inducing IFN-γ production by allogenic adult CD4$^+$ T cells. However, importantly, neonatal mDC efficiently prime Melan A-specific CD8$^+$ T cells, leading to IFN-γ production and cytolytic activity (148).

In summary, the different human DC subsets are generally considered to be less mature than adult cells, in terms of expression of surface markers or allostimulatory capacity. This notion is more controversial in mice models, for which age (birth vs. 1 week), isolation procedure and the organ (spleen vs. skin) have to be taken into account.

EARLY INFLAMMATORY RESPONSE BY NEONATAL APCs

When monocytes and other APCs are activated by microbial compounds, large amounts of pro-inflammatory cytokines and chemokines, such as TNF-α, IL-1 or IL-8, are readily produced. Several reports have noted that production of TNF-α is impaired in early life. This defect is observed only in certain experimental conditions. It was initially described in cord blood from preterm infants (149). It was further shown that, in response to LPS, the CD14-independent pathway was affected and that the defect could be restored by a factor present in adult plasma (which is not soluble CD14 or LPS-binding protein) (150). More recently, the production of TNF-α by cord blood in response to various TLR ligands was tested (151). Stimulation of whole cord blood or isolated monocytes (in the presence of neonatal plasma) with TLR-2, TLR-4 or TLR-7 ligands led to decreased TNF-α release. In contrast, R848 (TLR-7/8 ligand) was capable of inducing high levels of this cytokine in both adult and neonatal blood. As previously described, addition of adult plasma can restore TNF-α production in neonatal cells, suggesting that newborn plasma lacks a soluble factor that is required for the activation of certain TLRs. Furthermore, it also indicates that neonatal monocytes are capable of producing TNF-α under appropriate conditions, even if lower MyD88 expression has been reported (152).

It is not clear from these studies whether the TNF-α defect is selective or whether production of other inflammatory cytokines which are usually regulated by the same molecular events is also affected. In particular, LPS-induced NF-κB and MAPK activation seems to be comparable in adult and neonatal cells (152). Furthermore, no major differences in TNF-α mRNA levels were observed between adults and newborns. It is therefore possible that posttranscriptional or posttranslational events are involved in defective TNF-α synthesis.

PRODUCTION OF TH1-DRIVING CYTOKINES BY NEONATAL APCs

IL-12 is the best-defined Th1-driving cytokine (153). Its active form requires synthesis and covalent binding of two independently regulated subunits (p35 and p40: Fig. 8-2). In comparison to inflammatory cytokines such as TNF-α, IL-12 synthesis is tightly regulated, requiring activation of several signaling pathways. Its cellular source is also more restricted. While LPS-stimulated monocytes are capable of

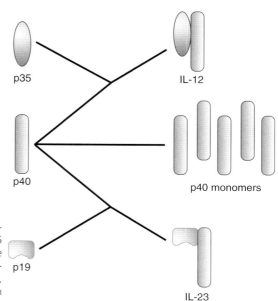

Figure 8-2 Formation of interleukin-12 and -23 heterodimers. The p40 subunit can associate with the p35 molecule to form bioactive IL-12. Association with the p19 molecule leads to the formation of another heterodimeric cytokine known as IL-23. Finally, p40 monomers, with no known biological function, are also secreted in large excess.

secreting IL-12p40 and low levels of IL-12p70 in the presence of IFN-γ, the major producers of bioactive IL-12 are DCs (153). It was shown that IL-12p70 production was strongly reduced in LPS-stimulated CBMCs vs. PBMCs (154). Similar observations were obtained in CBMC or whole blood for other stimulators, including group B streptococcus, *S. aureus*, polyI:C or *B. pertussis* toxin (144, 155–157). Addition of adult or fetal calf serum does not overcome impaired IL-12 synthesis in CBMC as was the case for TNF-α production, suggesting a different mechanism (156). Interestingly, in response to live commensal bacteria, CBMCs are capable of producing significant amounts of IL-12(158).

Neonatal monocyte-derived DCs also produce low levels of IL-12p70 in response to LPS, polyI:C, *B. pertussis* toxin or CD40 ligation (147, 148, 157, 159, 160), suggesting that low IL-12 production is an intrinsic property of neonatal DC. Importantly, addition of recombinant IFN-γ increases IL-12 production by both adult and neonatal LPS-activated DCs (159). Furthermore, Upham et al. observed that in vitro differentiation of cord-blood monocytes into DC restored IL-12 production to adult levels (161). These results indicate that under certain experimental conditions, neonatal mDCs are capable of producing adult-like levels of IL-12. It is not clear whether IFN-γ could also be effective in circulating CBMCs. Indeed, a relative decrease in STAT-1 phosphorylation in response to exogenous IFN-γ was observed in cord blood monocytes (162).

IL-12p40 monomers are secreted in large excess over IL-12p70. The defects in IL-12p70 synthesis in cord blood, CBMCs or neonatal mDCs is much more pronounced than that of IL-12p40. In fact, in response to most stimuli tested, IL-12p40 secretion or mRNA expression is minimally affected. In sharp contrast, we showed a major defect in the expression of the IL-12p35 mRNA in neonatal mDCs (159).

Isolated splenic DCs from neonatal mice are able to produce significant levels of IL-12 in response to CpG oligonucleotides (134). However, in response to a combination of cytokines and TLR ligands, neonatal DC were shown to produce lower IL-12p70 but comparable IL-12p40 levels (132). It was recently suggested that in vivo, IL-12 production by neonatal murine DC was repressed by IL-10-producing B cells (163).

IL-23 is a heterodimeric cytokine structurally related to IL-12, implicated in protective and autoimmune responses (164). The p40 subunit is common to both IL-12 and IL-23 (Fig. 8-2). We recently investigated the capacity of neonatal APCs to express IL-23(p19) mRNA and produce bioactive IL-23 (165). LPS stimulation induced the transcription of IL-23(p19) mRNA in both adult and neonatal mDC. In comparison to adult DC, their neonatal counterparts produced similar levels of IL-23 protein, in reponse to Toll-like receptor (TLR)-2- and TLR-3 ligands, and even higher levels in response to TLR-4 or TLR-8 ligands. The same profile was observed in CBMCs, indicating that it is not a consequence of in vitro differentiation.

Regulation of IL-12 Genes in Neonatal APCs: Increased IL-12p40 mRNA Instability in CBMC

Previous studies have shown that low IL-12 synthesis in CBMC was associated with reduced IL-12p40 mRNA stability (154). IL-12p35 gene expression was not assessed in this report because, until recently, IL-12 synthesis in monocytic cells was thought to be mainly regulated at the level of p40 gene expression (166). A similar mechanism was also shown to be involved in low production by CMBC of other myeloid cytokines such as GM-CSF, M-CSF and IL-15 (167, 168). Post-transcriptional gene regulation involves protein complexes that bind the 3'-untranslated region (3'-UTR) of mRNA. It was shown that the activity of one group of these proteins (AUF-1) was increased in CBMC as compared to adult PBMC, possibly leading to accelerated degradation of mRNA containing AUUUA motifs in their 3'-UTR regions (169).

Regulation of IL-12 Genes in Neonatal APCs: Impaired IL-12p35 Transcriptional Activation in Neonatal mDC

Initiation of transcription involves a large number of transcription factors that bind to cis-acting elements. The IL-12p35 promoter region has recently been studied. As seen in Figure 8-3, a binding site for NF-κB has been identified upstream of the TATA box. NF-κB mediates induction of most pro-inflammatory cytokines. Several Rel family members are recruited to the p35 promoter including p65, p50 and c-Rel. IL-12p35 gene transcription upon TLR-4 engagement was also found to depend on the binding of Sp1 to several critical sites (146, 170, 171). Within the same region, binding of IRF-1 and ICSBP have been implicated in the enhancing effects of IFN-γ on IL-12p35 activation (171, 172). Recently, we showed that IL-12p35 activation in response to TLR-3 and TLR-4 signaling requires recruitment of IRF-3 to this region (173). In addition, other IRF family members (such as IRF-5 and IRF-7) might also be implicated in TLR-mediated p35 gene activation (unpublished results).

In eukaryotes, genomic DNA is incorporated into chromatin, which consists of assembled nucleosomes. Local chromatin structure modulates the access of specific transcription factors to DNA. Remodeling events play an important role in the regulation of immune functions by controling the expression of a number of key cytokine genes (174). Within the p35 promoter region, a single nucleosome (termed nuc-2; see Fig. 8-3) is rapidly and selectively remodeled upon transcriptional activation of the gene (146). Importantly, the critical binding sites for Sp1 and IRF transcription factors are located in the region protected by nuc-2. It is tempting to speculate that recruitment of Sp1, which is constitutively present in the positioned nucleus of DC, is regulated by the remodeling of nuc-2.

In order to define the molecular mechanisms responsible for defective TLR-4-mediated IL-12p35 transcriptional activation in neonatal mDCs, we compared the DNA binding activity of several transcription factors (175). We found that

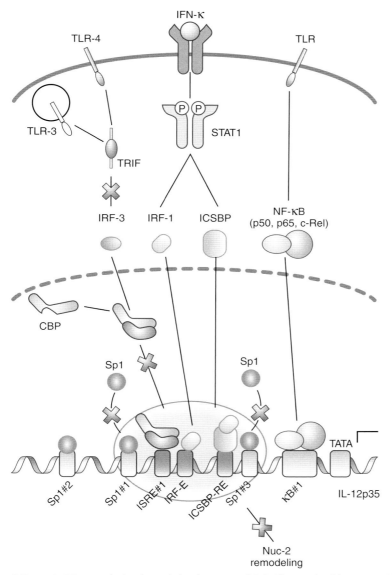

Figure 8-3 IL-12p35 transcriptional regulation in neonatal DC. The proximal human *IL-12 p35* promoter is represented with the major *cis*-elements that have been identified. In response to TLR triggering, both NF-κB and IRF-3 transcription factors are required for efficient IL-12p35 activation. IFN-γ-induced signals, leading to IRF-1 and ICSBP (IRF-8) activation, strongly enhance transcriptional activation of the p35 gene. The position of nuc-2 in resting cells is also depicted. This nucleosome is selectively remodeled upon activation of the gene. The proposed molecular mechanisms leading to impaired IL-12p35 gene expression in human neonatal DCs are summarized.

LPS-induced NF-κB p65 and IRF-1 activation was similar in adult and neonatal mDCs. Likewise, in vitro binding activity to the Sp1 site did not differ in adults and newborns. However, we recently observed that IRF-3 activation was strongly repressed in LPS-treated neonatal mDCs (unpublished data). Likewise, we demonstrated that nuc-2 remodeling in neonatal mDCs was profoundly impaired in response to LPS. Both nuc-2 remodeling and IL-12p35 gene transcription were restored upon addition of recombinant IFN-γ. IRF-3 forms complexes with transcriptional coactivators (such as CBP/p300) which are required for histone acetylation and chromatin remodeling (176). Our results therefore suggest that TLR-4-mediated nuc-2 remodeling involves IRF-3 activation, which is impaired in neonatal DCs. This hypothesis is also compatible with the fact that IL-23 production is maintained as IRF-3 is not implicated in IL-12p40 or IL-23p19 activation.

TYPE I IFN PRODUCTION BY NEONATAL APCs

Type I IFN Production by Plasmacytoid DCs

Five TLRs (TLR-3, -4, -7, -8, -9) have been shown to induce type I IFN (177). Their induction is regulated primarily at the transcriptional level, wherein IRF members play a central role (178). Among the PBMCs, pDCs represent the major source of IFN-α upon exposure to TLR-7 and TLR-9 ligands (179, 180). As previously mentioned, TLR-9 senses the unmethylated CpG DNA of bacteria and viruses (122, 181), whereas TLR-7 is specialized in the recognition of single-stranded viral RNA (182). In addition to ssRNA, the synthetic chemical compounds imidazoquinolines (Imiquimod and Resiquimod (R-848)) activate TLR-7 in both humans and mice (40, 183, 184).

We first analyzed IFN-α/β production by purified pDCs from cord blood upon CpG stimulation. We observed that these cells are intrinsically deficient in CpG-induced type I IFN production at birth (145). This neonatal defect is detected at both protein and mRNA levels and cannot be attributed to a lower expression of TLR-9 in cord blood pDCs.

When stimulated with Resiquimod R-848, neonatal pDCs also present a decreased secretion of type I IFNs, whereas TLR-7 expression is comparable to the adult level (unpublished data).

In addition to this defective type I IFN production, circulating neonatal pDCs present an incomplete maturation in the presence or TLR-7 and -9 ligands. Furthermore, it appears that the default in type I IFN release of cord blood stimulated pDCs can be extended to a larger number of cytokines and chemokines. Neonatal pDCs present a global defect in response to TLR-7 and -9 ligands including chemokine and cytokine production and phenotypical maturation.

Human pDCs present the unique function as professional type I IFN-producing cells for many reasons. As previously mentioned, pDCs, but not other hematopoietic cell types, constitutively express high levels of IRF-7 (185), required for type I IFN production (186). Futhermore, pDCs, but not other cell types, have the unique capacity to retain CpG-ODN in the endosome compartment for a prolonged period, allowing direct signaling through TLR-9 to trigger massive IFN-α production (187). Recent data provide evidence that IRF-5 is also an essential transducer of the TLR-7-dependent induction of type I IFNs (108). Under particular conditions, IRF-5 forms both homodimers as well as heterodimers with IRF-3 or IRF-7. Of note, pDCs also express high constitutive levels of IRF-5. On the other hand, even if this pathway remains to be elucidated in human pDCs, there is strong evidence showing that proinflammatory cytokine and chemokine induction seems to be dependent on NF-κB signaling pathway (108).

We compared the expression of IRF-7 in cord blood pDCs to their adult counterparts. Our results indicate that the basal level of IRF-7 is comparable in both populations. It remains to be determined whether activation and nuclear translocation of IRF-7 are functional in cord blood pDCs. The same questions need to be addressed for other factors regulating cytokine production and maturation of human pDCs, such as IRF-5, TRAF6, IRAK-1/4 and NF-κB.

Type I IFN Production by Myeloid DCs

Myeloid DCs are also able to produce type I IFN in response to TLR activation. Activation of the TRIF-dependent pathway by TLR-3 and TLR-4 ligands leads to

TBK-1/IKKε and IRF-3 activation, which induces transcription at the IFN-β promoter (84, 87, 188). PolyI:C is also capable of inducing IFN-α from circulating mDCs (189). When comparing whole cord vs. adult blood or CBMC vs. adult PBMC, we observed that IFN-α release by neonatal cells upon polyI:C stimulation was significantly lower (144). This defect, however, appears less pronounced after in vitro differentiation of monocytes into mDCs (unpublished data).

We analyzed IFN-β production by adult and neonatal DCs stimulated by LPS. IFN-β protein and mRNA levels were strongly reduced in neonates (unpublished data). This result is consistent with the observation that TLR4-mediated IRF-3 activation is hampered in neonatal DCs (see previous section). In mDCs, IFN-β acts in an autocrine/paracrine fashion to activate a second wave of transcription (190). It is also in part responsible for upregulation of co-stimulatory molecules (191). By comparing LPS-induced gene expression patterns by microarray analysis in adult and neonatal DCs, we observed that expression of a subset of IFN-dependent genes was significantly decreased in neonatal mDCs as compared to their adult counterparts. In sharp contrast, among NF-κB-inducible genes, no significant difference of expression was observed between the two groups, suggesting that TLR-4-triggered events leading to NF-κB activation are functional in neonatal DCs. These data indicate that downstream of TLR-4, TRIF-dependent activation of IRF-3 is compromised in neonatal mDCs. On the other hand, MyD88-dependent events seem to be globally maintained, suggesting a selective signaling defect. It remains to be determined how TLR-4-triggered events are regulated in early life.

NEONATAL DC FUNCTION AND CLINICAL IMPLICATIONS

Susceptibility to Infections

Human newborns are more susceptible than adults to infections with intracellular micro-organisms such as *Mycobacterium tuberculosis*, *Listeria monocytogenes*, *Toxoplasma gondii* or viruses, including human immunodeficiency virus (HIV), respiratory syncytial virus (RSV), herpes simplex virus (HSV) or cytomegalovirus (CMV) (192–195). In most cases, neonatal hepatitis B infection takes a chronic and asymptomatic form that is responsible for cirrhosis and hepatocarcinoma development (196). These clinical observations suggest that T-cell-mediated immune responses offer limited protection in early life (197). However, the neonatal period and early infancy are not associated with global immunodeficiency. Moreover, in utero exposure with *Trypanosoma cruzi* or CMV, neonatal vaccination with BCG or early infection with *Bordetella pertussis* induces detectable adult-like cellular immune responses (198–201).

Are the experimental data on neonatal DC exposed in the previous section compatible with these observations? DCs are required for the initiation of the immune response as they have the capacity for stimulating both CD4[+] and CD8[+] naive T cells. These professional APCs are crucial in mediating polarization of CD4[+] naive T cells into Th1 and Th2 effectors. Impaired DC function in human neonates, such as reduced expression of co-stimulatory or MHC class II molecules or production of immunomodulatory cytokines such as type I IFN or IL-12, could therefore directly impact on the quality and the duration of the immune response. It is also clear that under appropriate stimulation, neonatal DCs are capable of adult-like responses. For example, in vivo, Flt3 ligand, a hematopoietic growth factor, strongly increases DC numbers when administered to neonatal mice (202, 203). This treatment led to an increased capacity of DC to produce IL-12 and IFN-α which was associated with an increased resistance against HSV-1 and *Listeria monocytogenes*. These results indicate that neonatal DC function can be modulated to enhance resistance against intracellular pathogens.

Most observations on neonatal DCs have been performed using purified TLR ligands. It remains to be determined how neonatal DCs respond to live micro-organisms, which can trigger multiple TLR and interact with other pathogen-recognition molecules. In particular, viruses and some bacterial pathogens can gain access to the intracellular compartments and activate cytosolic receptors. For example, it is not known whether activation of RIG-1 or PKR by viruses, unlike engagement of TLR-4, is able to trigger type I IFN secretion by neonatal mDCs. In a similar fashion, could direct activation of pDC with live viruses trigger TLR-independent type I IFN synthesis? These issues remain to be clarified.

Defective IL-12 Synthesis and Intracellular Pathogens

The understanding of the role of IL-12 in infectious diseases has recently evolved. Numerous studies using mouse models indicate that IL-12 plays a major role in the development of protective innate and adaptive immune response against most intracellular pathogens (153). IL-12p40$^{-/-}$ and IL-12p35$^{-/-}$ mice infected with _L. major_ are equally susceptible to this parasite (204). However, for other micro-organisms, such as _Salmonella enteritidis_, _Mycobacterium_ spp. or _T. gondii_, IL-12p35$^{-/-}$ mice are less affected than IL-12p40$^{-/-}$ animals (205–209). These observations are consistent with the implication of the p40 chain in both IL-12 and IL-23 synthesis. Indeed, IL-23p19-deficient mice infected with _K. pneumoniae_ develop normal IFN-γ responses but cannot produce IL-17 and, as a consequence, have increased susceptibility to this pathogen (210). In the absence of IL-23, mice infected by _M. tuberculosis_ are still capable of mounting an adequate and protective Th1-type response (211). Conversely, in the absence of IL-12, IL-23 provides a moderate level of protection through the induction of antigen-specific IFN-γ and IL-17-producing CD4$^+$ T cells. These results indicate that there is a certain degree of redundancy between IL-12 and IL-23 functions. In human neonates, where the IL-12/IFNγ axis is likely to be compromised, functional IL-23/IL-17 responses could be particularly important for the protection against infectious pathogens.

In humans, inherited defects of both IL-12 and IL-23 signaling pathways (such as mutations in IL-12Rβ1 or IL-12p40 genes) have been identified (212). These individuals are susceptible to mycobacteria and salmonella infections. However, in contrast to mice studies, these patients are still capable of responding to a large variety of infectious agents, including intracellular bacteria and viruses. Overall, these findings suggest that, in humans, IL-12/IL-23 and even IFN-γ play a redundant role during natural exposure to most micro-organisms.

Interestingly, two patients with a STAT1 mutation that impairs both type I and type II IFN signaling suffered from both mycobacterial disease and disseminated HSV-1 infections (213). These data suggest that type I IFN probably plays a major role in the protection against HSV.

CD4$^+$ and CD8$^+$ T Cell Responses in Newborns

DCs are required for the initiation of the immune response as they have the capacity for stimulating both CD4$^+$ and CD8$^+$ naive T cells. Following congenital infection by _T. cruzi_ and CMV, newborns develop cytotoxic T cell responses (198, 199). These effector CD8$^+$ T cells are comparable to those generally detected in infected adults. Of note, they are capable of producing large amounts of IFN-γ. Interestingly, this mature cytotoxic response is rarely observed in HIV-infected infants (214–216). More studies are required to define CD4$^+$ T cell responses during these early infections. In young children (< 4 years) CMV-specific CD4$^+$ T cells produce very low levels of IFN-γ as compared to adults, a situation associated with prolonged viral shedding into the urine and saliva (217, 218). In murine models of viral infections, initial activation of CD8$^+$ T cells does not require the help of CD4$^+$ T cells (219–221). However, these cells are required for prolonged effector function and establishment of memory. Differentiation of naive CD4$^+$ and CD8$^+$ T cells into high IFN-γ-producing cells involves different pathways. The IFN-γ gene in CD8$^+$ T cells can be activated independently of T-bet or IL-12-induced STAT-4 activation (222). Importantly, hypermethylation of the IFN-γ promoter is observed in cord blood T CD4$^+$ but not CD8$^+$ T cells (223). In mice, splenic neonatal DC induce efficient CTL responses both in vitro and in vivo (137). Similarly, human cord blood-derived mDCs efficiently prime Melan A-specific CTL in vitro, leading to IFN-γ production and cytolytic activity (148). Overall, these data indicate that under appropriate stimulation, such as prolonged contact with a pathogen, effector CD8$^+$ T cell response can develop in utero, even if the context is globally unfavorable for Th1-type responses.

Defective Type I IFN Synthesis and Viruses

Human newborns are highly susceptible to infections with viruses, including HIV, RSV, CMV and HSV. Detection of viral infection leads to the production of type I IFNs. These cytokines not only directly inhibit viral replication but also activate immune effector cells such as NK cells, cytotoxic T cells and macrophages to eliminate infected cells. Virtually all cell types are capable of producing type I IFNs in response to viral infections; the amount of synthesized IFNs depends on the type of virus and target cells. As already mentioned, plasmacytoid DCs are the major producers of type I IFNs in humans. More precisely, pDCs represent a highly specialized subset of DCs that function as a sentinel for viral infection and are responsible for the vast amount of type I IFNs during viral infection. The molecular mechanisms underlying the ability of pDCs to produce high levels of type I IFNs following viral stimulation are not fully understood. Recent data support the concept that pDCs utilize their TLR machinery to respond to viral products. Indeed, TLR-9 senses unmethylated DNA present in bacteria and viruses (181), whereas TLR-7 can recognize viral single-stranded RNA (182). This process occurs intracellularly in the endosomal compartment and is independent of viral replication. As an example, the recognition of herpes simplex virus (HSV-1 and -2) has been shown to depend on TLR-9 in human pDCs (224) and to strictly require the activation of IRF-7 for massive IFN-α production by the infected cells (185). Murine cytomegalovirus (MCMV) has also been shown to activate directly pDCs through TLR-9 (122). On the other hand, TLR-7 allows pDCs to sense influenza virus and vesicular stomatitis virus (VSV) (36, 180). Upon human immunodeficiency virus (HIV) infection, pDC activation is triggered by the recognition of HIV genomic RNA by TLR-7 (225).

One of the questions arising from the literature today is whether pDCs are capable of detecting ssRNA virus replication via cytolytic double-stranded RNA; or whether other cell types such as myeloid dendritic cells (mDCs) take over responsibility for viruses that escape endosomal recognition. It is interesting to note that TLR-3, which allows mDCs to respond to Poly(I:C)-mimicking viral dsRNA, is absent in pDCs. New concepts for viral recognition by pDCs have recently emerged showing that human pDCs can detect an ssRNA virus (RSV) that directly enters the cytosol via fusion protein (226). This detection leads to the production of vast amounts of IFN-α independently of endosomal acidification. Cytolitic detection of dsRNA extends the repertoire of pDCs for virus detection and instant type I IFN production. Finally, an RNA helicase, RIG-1, has been also suggested to sense viral dsRNA (227). RIG-1 is essential for induction of type I IFNs after infection with RNA viruses in mDC (228). RIG-1 induces type I IFNs by activating IRF-3 (229). At present there is no evidence that human pDCs use the RIG-1 system for viral detection. One could speculate that the RIG-1 and TLR systems exert antiviral responses in a cell-specific manner.

Using specific TLR-7 and -9 ligands as stimulants, we showed that pDCs purified from human cord blood were deficient in their type I IFN production. Direct viral infections of neonatal pDCs will have to be performed, using live wild-type strains. It is indeed crucial to know in this context whether a neonatal pDC exposed to viruses is capable or not of synthesizing normal amounts of type I IFNs. It will be also interesting to analyze the other factors produced during viral infection. If our studies reveal a profound defect of neonatal pDCs in response to entire viruses, one could speculate on the use of those cells as targets for new therapeutic strategies using effective adjuvants which could convert defective responses to more intense and protective immune responses.

Neonatal DC Functions and Allergies

The important rise in prevalence of allergic disorders, which has been observed these last decades in developed countries, clearly manifests itself primarily during infancy (230). Immaturity of the APC compartment and limitation of Th1 responses could contribute to the preferential development of Th2-polarized memory responses towards environmental allergens encountered in early life. It is fundamental to define both genetic and environmental factors that lead to the development of atopy and asthma. It has been suggested that delayed postnatal immune maturation could be a determinant factor (231).

In utero contact with environmental allergens leads to weak Th2-biased responses (232). In vitro IFN-γ production is reduced until the age of 1 year (233, 234). Thereafter, it steadily increases, reaching adult levels between the ages of 3 and 5. This maturation process is slower in children genetically predisposed to atopy (235–237). IL-12 production capacity increases more gradually, reaching adult levels in the course of adolescence (156). Decreased IL-12 production at birth is correlated with development of allergic disorders by the age of 6 (238). Moreover, a polymorphism in the *IL-12(p40)* gene has been associated with increased severity of asthma (239). Environmental factors that regulate the maturation of Th1 responses have not been clearly defined yet. It is highly plausible that microbial signals, either from infections or the gut microflora, are required for appropriate immune maturation (240). For example, polysaccharide A (PSA) from *Bacteroides fragilis* taken up by intestinal DC allows redirection of the Th1/Th2 balance in germ-free mice (241). The Th1-driving capacity of PSA involves direct induction of IL-12 synthesis by DC. It would be interesting to define whether PSA could be active on neonatal DCs. Numerous epidemiological studies have implicated exposure to other microbial compounds, such as endotoxin, in postnatal immune maturation (242, 243). Supporting this hypothesis, polymorphism in the *CD14* gene has been associated with atopic sensitization (244).

Respiratory syncytial virus (RSV)-induced bronchiolitis in early life is an important risk factor for the development of asthma (245). It was suggested that RSV has a direct Th2-driving effect on the immune response (246, 247). Local cytokine production could therefore lead to consolidation of Th2 memory response toward inhaled allergens. However, epidemiological studies showed that atopy and RSV infections were independent risk factors for the development of asthma (248). In fact, in murine models, the age at exposure determines the severity of the eosinophilic infiltrate and the Th1/Th2 balance during RSV secondary infections (249).

Neonatal DC Functions and Vaccination

Major infectious diseases, such as tuberculosis, HIV, RSV and malaria, can be acquired very early in life. Protection against these pathogens requires the induction of strong Th1-type responses. It is therefore crucial to establish how this can be achieved in very young infants. Many existing as well as newly developed vaccines incorporate TLR ligands (250). The understanding of the neonatal DC response to TLR triggering will therefore be helpful for the rational development of effective adjuvants, which could convert weak responses into more intense and protective immune responses (131). For example, in newborn mice, CpG oligonucleotides or complete Freund's adjuvant are able to induce adult-like Th1 responses (251, 252). However, while animal studies are very useful models for the understanding of neonatal immune responses, vaccination strategies have to take into account the specificities of human immune responses. For example, CpG oligonucleotides strongly stimulate both mDC and pDC subsets in neonatal mice but they are unable to activate human mDC, since these cells do not express TLR9. Moreover, in vitro activation of neonatal pDC with CpG is strongly impaired as compared to adult cells. These observations indicate that such a strategy might not be as effective for human newborns.

Following World Health Organization recommendations, BCG, oral poliovirus and anti-hepatitis B vaccine are administered at birth in endemic regions. The cellular responses elicited by these vaccines have been studied. In response to hepatitis B or poliomyelitis vaccine, neonates display reduced IFN-γ production in comparison to adults, despite a strong humoral response (253, 254). In marked contrast, neonatal administration of BCG induces adult-like Th1 responses (200). Moreover, BCG modulates the response to co-administered unrelated vaccines, leading to increased cytokine and antibody production (255). It indicates that under adequate stimulation of the immune system, neonates are capable of developing protective Th1-type responses. The strong stimulatory potential of BCG on the neonatal immune system could be related to its direct effect on DC, as several components of BCG, such as peptidoglycan and cell wall skeleton were shown to activate TLR-2 and TLR-4 in a MyD88-dependent fashion (256, 257). In newborns, this could favor IL-23 production. Alternatively, "innate lymphocytes", such as $\gamma\delta$ T cells, NK or NK T cells could be involved as they could represent an IL-12-independent and early source of IFN-γ.

In adults, NK and $\gamma\delta$ T cells rapidly produce IFN-γ in response to mycobacteria (258, 259). Once activated, these cells interact with DC and promote IL-12 production (260–262). Not much is known about these cells early in life. Cytolytic activity and expression of adhesion molecules by cord blood NK cells is reduced as compared to adults (263). However, it remains to be determined whether neonatal NK cells have the capacity to induce DC maturation. $\gamma\delta$ T cells recognize microbial and tumor antigens, typically small pyrophosphomonoesters and alkylamines. It has been suggested that they could play a very important role early in life (264). Indeed, both V1 and V2 cells include a relatively high proportion of non-naive cells in cord blood. Within the first year of life, conversion to memory of the $\gamma\delta$ T cells is rapidly observed. $\gamma\delta$ T cells express perforin and are capable of producing IFN-γ after short-term in vitro stimulation (265). This represents the earliest described immunological maturation of any lymphocyte compartment in humans. In agreement with this observation, primary immune protection against an intestinal parasite was shown to require $\gamma\delta$ T cells in young mice but not in adults. It would be of interest to define $\gamma\delta$ T cell and DC interaction in early life (266).

NK T cells express a single Vα chain and recognize foreign and self glycolipids presented by the nonclassical MHC class I molecule CD1d. Administration of α-galactosylceramide (αGalCer), a synthetic glycolipid, induces in vivo maturation of splenic DCs and favors IL-12 synthesis (267). This adjuvant effect, mediated by NK T cells, strongly supports the development of Th1 responses. Of note, CD1d ligation alone is sufficient to induce bioactive IL-12 synthesis by DC (268). However, in the presence of αGalCer, cytokines or DC, cord blood NK T cells proliferate and preferentially produce IL-4 instead of IFN-γ (269). Therefore, the adjuvant potential of αGalCer should be studied in a neonatal context.

Because of the impaired responses of neonatal plasmacytoid and myeloid DC to purified TLR ligands, activation through TLR-independent pathways could represent a good strategy for early life vaccination. As discussed in this chapter, it remains to be determined whether "alternative" activation by innate lymphocytes or through intracytoplasmic receptors such as NOD or RIG-1 could lead to efficient stimulation of neonatal APCs. Moreover, synergy between different TLRs, for example between TLR-7/8 and TLR-3 or TLR-4 or between TLR and NOD, could also be useful for enhancing the Th1-driving potential of neonatal DC (270, 271). The short- and long-term safety of vaccines to be used in young infants will be the most important consideration for the development of such strategies.

Acknowledgments

We thank Arnaud Marchand for critical reading of this manuscript. SG is a research associate from the FRS-FNRS (Fonds National de la Recherche Scientifique, Belgium).

REFERENCES

1. Medzhitov R, Janeway C Jr. Innate immunity. N Engl J Med 343:338–344, 2000.
2. Reis e Sousa C. Toll-like receptors and dendritic cells: for whom the bug tolls. Semin Immunol 16:27–34, 2004.
3. Bell JK, Mullen GE, Leifer CA, et al. Leucine-rich repeats and pathogen recognition in Toll-like receptors. Trends Immunol 24:528–533, 2003.
4. Kobe B, Deisenhofer J. Proteins with leucine-rich repeats. Curr Opin Struct Biol 5:409–416, 1995.
5. Aravind L, Dixit VM, Koonin EV. Apoptotic molecular machinery: vastly increased complexity in vertebrates revealed by genome comparisons. Science 291:1279–1284, 2001.
6. Poltorak A, He X, Smirnova I, et al. Defective LPS signaling in C3H/HeJ, C57BL/10ScCr mice: mutations in Tlr4 gene. Science 282:2085–2088, 1998.
7. Qureshi ST, Lariviere L, Leveque G, et al. Endotoxin-tolerant mice have mutations in Toll-like receptor 4 (Tlr4). J Exp Med 189:615–625, 1999.
8. Hoshino K, Takeuchi O, Kawai T, et al. Cutting edge: Toll-like receptor 4 (TLR4)-deficient mice are hyporesponsive to lipopolysaccharide: evidence for TLR4 as the Lps gene product. J Immunol 162:3749–3752, 1999.
9. Takeuchi O, Hoshino K, Kawai T, et al. Differential roles of TLR2 and TLR4 in recognition of gram-negative and gram-positive bacterial cell wall components. Immunity 11:443–451, 1999.
10. Arbour NC, Lorenz E, Schutte BC, et al. TLR4 mutations are associated with endotoxin hyporesponsiveness in humans. Nat Genet 25:187–191, 2000.
11. Kiechl S, Lorenz E, Reindl M, et al. Toll-like receptor 4 polymorphisms and atherogenesis. N Engl J Med 347:185–192, 2002.
12. Schroder NW, Meister D, Wolff V, et al. Chronic periodontal disease is associated with single-nucleotide polymorphisms of the human TLR-4 gene. Genes Immun 6:448–451, 2005.
13. Wright SD. CD14 and innate recognition of bacteria. J Immunol 155:6–8, 1995.
14. Hailman E, Lichenstein HS, Wurfel MM, et al. Lipopolysaccharide (LPS)-binding protein accelerates the binding of LPS to CD14. J Exp Med 179:269–277, 1994.
15. Haziot A, Rong GW, Lin XY, et al. Recombinant soluble CD14 prevents mortality in mice treated with endotoxin (lipopolysaccharide). J Immunol 154:6529–6532, 1995.
16. Schromm AB, Lien E, Henneke P, et al. Molecular genetic analysis of an endotoxin nonresponder mutant cell line: a point mutation in a conserved region of MD-2 abolishes endotoxin-induced signaling. J Exp Med 194:79–88, 2001.
17. Shimazu R, Akashi S, Ogata H, et al. MD-2, a molecule that confers lipopolysaccharide responsiveness on Toll-like receptor 4. J Exp Med 189:1777–1782, 1999.
18. Beutler B. Tlr4: central component of the sole mammalian LPS sensor. Curr Opin Immunol 12:20–26, 2000.
19. Akira S, Takeda K. Toll-like receptor signalling. Nat Rev Immunol 4:499–511, 2004.
20. Iwaki D, Mitsuzawa H, Murakami S, et al. The extracellular toll-like receptor 2 domain directly binds peptidoglycan derived from Staphylococcus aureus. J Biol Chem 277:24315–24320, 2002.
21. Underhill DM, Ozinsky A, Smith KD, et al. Toll-like receptor-2 mediates mycobacteria-induced proinflammatory signaling in macrophages. Proc Natl Acad Sci USA 96:14459–14463, 1999.
22. Ozinsky A, Underhill DM, Fontenot JD, et al. The repertoire for pattern recognition of pathogens by the innate immune system is defined by cooperation between toll-like receptors. Proc Natl Acad Sci USA 97:13766–13771, 2000.
23. Takeuchi O, Hoshino K, Akira S. Cutting edge: TLR2-deficient and MyD88-deficient mice are highly susceptible to Staphylococcus aureus infection. J Immunol 165:5392–5396, 2000.

24. Takeuchi O, Sato S, Horiuchi T, et al. Cutting edge: role of Toll-like receptor 1 in mediating immune response to microbial lipoproteins. J Immunol 169:10–14, 2002.
25. Takeuchi O, Kawai T, Muhlradt PF, et al. Discrimination of bacterial lipoproteins by Toll-like receptor 6. Int Immunol 13:933–940, 2001.
26. Alexopoulou L, Holt AC, Medzhitov R, et al. Recognition of double-stranded RNA and activation of NF-kappaB by Toll-like receptor 3. Nature JID-0410462 413:732–738, 2001.
27. Kariko K, Bhuyan P, Capodici J, et al. Small interfering RNAs mediate sequence-independent gene suppression and induce immune activation by signaling through toll-like receptor 3. J Immunol 172:6545–6549, 2004.
28. Kariko K, Ni H, Capodici J, et al. mRNA is an endogenous ligand for Toll-like receptor 3. J Biol Chem 279:12542–12550, 2004.
29. Edelmann KH, Richardson-Burns S, Alexopoulou L, et al. Does Toll-like receptor 3 play a biological role in virus infections? Virology 322:231–238, 2004.
30. Tabeta K, Georgel P, Janssen E, Du X, et al. Toll-like receptors 9 and 3 as essential components of innate immune defense against mouse cytomegalovirus infection. Proc Natl Acad Sci USA 101:3516–3521, 2004.
31. Diebold SS, Montoya M, Unger H, et al. Viral infection switches non-plasmacytoid dendritic cells into high interferon producers. Nature 424:324–328, 2003.
32. Schulz O, Diebold SS, Chen M, et al. Toll-like receptor 3 promotes cross-priming to virus-infected cells. Nature 433:887–892, 2005.
33. Hayashi F, Smith KD, Ozinsky A, et al. The innate immune response to bacterial flagellin is mediated by Toll-like receptor 5. Nature JID-0410462 410:1099–1103, 2001.
34. Hawn TR, Verbon A, Lettinga KD, et al. A common dominant TLR5 stop codon polymorphism abolishes flagellin signaling and is associated with susceptibility to legionnaires' disease. J Exp Med 198:1563–1572, 2003.
35. Gewirtz AT, Navas TA, Lyons S, et al. Cutting edge: bacterial flagellin activates basolaterally expressed TLR5 to induce epithelial proinflammatory gene expression. J Immunol 167:1882–1885, 2001.
36. Diebold SS, Kaisho T, Hemmi H, et al. Innate antiviral responses by means of TLR7-mediated recognition of single-stranded RNA. Science 303:1529–1531, 2004.
37. Heil F, Hemmi H, Hochrein H, et al. Species-specific recognition of single-stranded RNA via toll-like receptor 7 and 8. Science 303:1526–1529, 2004.
38. Hornung V, Guenthner-Biller M, Bourquin C, et al. Sequence-specific potent induction of IFN-alpha by short interfering RNA in plasmacytoid dendritic cells through TLR7. Nat Med 11:263–270, 2005.
39. Hemmi H, Kaisho T, Takeuchi O, et al. Small anti-viral compounds activate immune cells via the TLR7 MyD88-dependent signaling pathway. Nat Immunol 3:196–200, 2002.
40. Jurk M, Heil F, Vollmer J, et al. Human TLR7 or TLR8 independently confer responsiveness to the antiviral compound R-848. Nat Immunol 3:499, 2002.
41. Lee J, Chuang TH, Redecke V, et al. Molecular basis for the immunostimulatory activity of guanine nucleoside analogs: activation of Toll-like receptor 7. Proc Natl Acad Sci USA 100:6646–6651, 2003.
42. Goodman MG, Reitz AB, Chen R, et al. Selective modulation of elements of the immune system by low molecular weight nucleosides. J Pharmacol Exp Ther 274:1552–1557, 1995.
43. Vasilakos JP, Smith RM, Gibson SJ, et al. Adjuvant activities of immune response modifier R-848: comparison with CpG ODN. Cell Immunol 204:64–74, 2000.
44. Kadowaki N, Ho S, Antonenko S, et al. Subsets of human dendritic cell precursors express different toll-like receptors and respond to different microbial antigens. J Exp Med 194:863–869, 2001.
45. Ito T, Amakawa R, Kaisho T, et al. Interferon-alpha and interleukin-12 are induced differentially by Toll-like receptor 7 ligands in human blood dendritic cell subsets. J Exp Med 195:1507–1512, 2002.
46. Gust TC, Diebold SS, Cotten M, et al. RNA-containing adenovirus/polyethylenimine transfer complexes effectively transduce dendritic cells and induce antigen-specific T cell responses. J Gene Med 6:464–470, 2004.
47. Lund JM, Alexopoulou L, Sato A, et al. Recognition of single-stranded RNA viruses by Toll-like receptor 7. Proc Natl Acad Sci USA 101:5598–5603, 2004.
48. Bauer S, Wagner H. Bacterial CpG-DNA licenses TLR9. Curr Top Microbiol Immunol 270:145–154, 2002.
49. Bauer S, Kirschning CJ, Hacker H, et al. Human TLR9 confers responsiveness to bacterial DNA via species-specific CpG motif recognition. Proc Natl Acad Sci USA 98:9237–9242, 2001.
50. Hemmi H, Kaisho T, Takeda K, et al. The roles of Toll-like receptor 9, MyD88, and DNA-dependent protein kinase catalytic subunit in the effects of two distinct CpG DNAs on dendritic cell subsets. J Immunol 170:3059–3064, 2003.
51. Krieg AM, Yi AK, Matson S, et al. CpG motifs in bacterial DNA trigger direct B-cell activation. Nature 374:546–549, 1995.
52. Heikenwalder M, Polymenidou M, Junt T, et al. Lymphoid follicle destruction and immunosuppression after repeated CpG oligodeoxynucleotide administration. Nat Med 10:187–192, 2004.
53. Sun CM, Deriaud E, Leclerc C, et al. Upon TLR9 signaling, CD5+ B cells control the IL-12-dependent Th1-priming capacity of neonatal DCs. Immunity 22:467–477, 2005.
54. Vollmer J, Weeratna R, Payette P, et al. Characterization of three CpG oligodeoxynucleotide classes with distinct immunostimulatory activities. Eur J Immunol 34:251–262, 2004.
55. Poeck H, Wagner M, Battiany J, et al. Plasmacytoid dendritic cells, antigen, and CpG-C license human B cells for plasma cell differentiation and immunoglobulin production in the absence of T-cell help. Blood 103:3058–3064, 2004.

56. Chu RS, Targoni OS, Krieg AM, et al. CpG oligodeoxynucleotides act as adjuvants that switch on T helper 1 (Th1) immunity. J Exp Med 186:1623–1631, 1997.

57. Brazolot Millan CL, Weeratna R, Krieg AM, et al. CpG DNA can induce strong Th1 humoral and cell-mediated immune responses against hepatitis B surface antigen in young mice. Proc Natl Acad Sci USA 95:15553–15558, 1998.

58. Sun S, Kishimoto H, Sprent J. DNA as an adjuvant: capacity of insect DNA and synthetic oligodeoxynucleotides to augment T cell responses to specific antigen. J Exp Med 187:1145–1150, 1998.

59. Sun S, Zhang X, Tough DF, et al. Type I interferon-mediated stimulation of T cells by CpG DNA. J Exp Med 188:2335–2342, 1998.

60. Krug A, French AR, Barchet W, et al. TLR9-dependent recognition of MCMV by IPC and DC generates coordinated cytokine responses that activate antiviral NK cell function. Immunity 21:107–119, 2004.

61. Lund J, Sato A, Akira S, et al. Toll-like receptor 9-mediated recognition of Herpes simplex virus-2 by plasmacytoid dendritic cells. J Exp Med 198:513–520, 2003.

62. Krug A, Luker GD, Barchet W, et al. Herpes simplex virus type 1 activates murine natural interferon-producing cells through toll-like receptor 9. Blood 103:1433–1437, 2004.

63. Coban C, Ishii KJ, Kawai T, et al. Toll-like receptor 9 mediates innate immune activation by the malaria pigment hemozoin. J Exp Med 201:19–25, 2005.

64. Zhang D, Zhang G, Hayden MS, et al. A toll-like receptor that prevents infection by uropathogenic bacteria. Science 303:1522–1526, 2004.

65. Yarovinsky F, Zhang D, Andersen JF, et al. TLR11 activation of dendritic cells by a protozoan profilin-like protein. Science, 2005.

66. Yang YL, Reis LF, Pavlovic J, et al. Deficient signaling in mice devoid of double-stranded RNA-dependent protein kinase. EMBO J 14:6095–6106, 1995.

67. Zheng X, Bevilacqua PC. Activation of the protein kinase PKR by short double-stranded RNAs with single-stranded tails. RNA 10:1934–1945, 2004.

68. Balachandran S, Roberts PC, Brown LE, et al. Essential role for the dsRNA-dependent protein kinase PKR in innate immunity to viral infection. Immunity 13:129–141, 2000.

69. Williams BR. PKR; a sentinel kinase for cellular stress. Oncogene 18:6112–6120, 1999.

70. Goh KC, deVeer MJ, Williams BR. The protein kinase PKR is required for p38 MAPK activation and the innate immune response to bacterial endotoxin. EMBO J 19:4292–4297, 2000.

71. Kumar A, Yang YL, Flati V, et al. Deficient cytokine signaling in mouse embryo fibroblasts with a targeted deletion in the PKR gene: role of IRF-1 and NF-kappaB. EMBO J 16:406–416, 1997.

72. Levy DE, Marie IJ. RIGging an antiviral defense—it's in the CARDs. Nat Immunol 5:699–701, 2004.

73. Tanner NK, Linder P. DExD/H box RNA helicases: from generic motors to specific dissociation functions. Mol Cell 8:251–262, 2001.

74. Yoneyama M, Kikuchi M, Natsukawa T, et al. The RNA helicase RIG-I has an essential function in double-stranded RNA-induced innate antiviral responses. Nat Immunol 5:730–737, 2004.

75. Inohara N, Nunez G. NODs: intracellular proteins involved in inflammation and apoptosis. Nat Rev Immunol 3:371–382, 2003.

76. Inohara N, Chamaillard M, McDonald C, et al. NOD-LRR proteins: role in host-microbial interactions and inflammatory disease. Annu Rev Biochem 74:355–383, 2004.

77. Chamaillard M, Hashimoto M, Horie Y, et al. An essential role for NOD1 in host recognition of bacterial peptidoglycan containing diaminopimelic acid. Nat Immunol 4:702–707, 2003.

78. Girardin SE, Boneca IG, Carneiro LA, et al. Nod1 detects a unique muropeptide from Gram-negative bacterial peptidoglycan. Science 300:1584–1587, 2003.

79. Watanabe T, Kitani A, Murray PJ, et al. NOD2 is a negative regulator of Toll-like receptor 2-mediated T helper type 1 responses. Nat Immunol 5:800–808, 2004.

80. O'Neill LA. The interleukin-1 receptor/Toll-like receptor superfamily: signal transduction during inflammation and host defense. Sci STKE 2003 (171):re3, 2003.

81. Takeda K, Kaisho T, Akira S. Toll-like receptors. Annu Rev Immunol 21:335–376, 2003.

82. Adachi O, Kawai T, Takeda K, et al. Targeted disruption of the MyD88 gene results in loss of IL-1- and IL-18-mediated function. Immunity 9:143–150, 1998.

83. Kawai T, Adachi O, Ogawa T, et al. Unresponsiveness of MyD88-deficient mice to endotoxin. Immunity 11:115–122, 1999.

84. Hoebe K, Du X, Georgel P, et al. Identification of Lps2 as a key transducer of MyD88-independent TIR signalling. Nature 424:743–748, 2003.

85. Hoebe K, Janssen EM, Kim SO, et al. Upregulation of costimulatory molecules induced by lipopolysaccharide and double-stranded RNA occurs by Trif-dependent and Trif-independent pathways. Nat Immunol 4:1223–1229, 2003.

86. Kaisho T, Takeuchi O, Kawai T, et al. Endotoxin-induced maturation of MyD88-deficient dendritic cells. J Immunol 166:5688–5694, 2001.

87. Yamamoto M, Sato S, Hemmi H, et al. Role of adaptor TRIF in the MyD88-independent toll-like receptor signaling pathway. Science 301:640–643, 2003.

88. Yamamoto M, Takeda K, Akira S. TIR domain-containing adaptors define the specificity of TLR signaling. Mol Immunol 40:861–868, 2004.

89. Kaisho T, Hoshino K, Iwabe T, et al. Endotoxin can induce MyD88-deficient dendritic cells to support T(h)2 cell differentiation. Int Immunol 14:695–700, 2002.

90. Iwasaki A, Medzhitov R. Toll-like receptor control of the adaptive immune responses. Nat Immunol 5:987–995, 2004.

91. Pasare C, Medzhitov R. Toll-dependent control mechanisms of CD4 T cell activation. Immunity 21:733–741, 2004.

92. Jankovic D, Kullberg MC, Hieny S, et al. In the absence of IL-12, CD4(+) T cell responses to intracellular pathogens fail to default to a Th2 pattern and are host protective in an IL-10(-/-) setting. Immunity 16:429–439, 2002.

93. Feng CG, Scanga CA, Collazo-Custodio CM, et al. Mice lacking myeloid differentiation factor 88 display profound defects in host resistance and immune responses to Mycobacterium avium infection not exhibited by Toll-like receptor 2 (TLR2)- and TLR4-deficient animals. J Immunol 171:4758–4764, 2003.

94. Fitzgerald KA, Palsson-McDermott EM, Bowie AG, et al. Mal (MyD88-adapter-like) is required for Toll-like receptor-4 signal transduction. Nature 413:78–83, 2001.

95. Horng T, Barton GM, Medzhitov R. TIRAP: an adapter molecule in the Toll signaling pathway. Nat Immunol 2:835–841, 2001.

96. Horng T, Barton GM, Flavell RA, et al. The adaptor molecule TIRAP provides signalling specificity for Toll-like receptors. Nature 420:329–333, 2002.

97. Yamamoto M, Sato S, Hemmi H, et al. Essential role for TIRAP in activation of the signalling cascade shared by TLR2 and TLR4. Nature 420:324–329, 2002.

98. Fitzgerald KA, Rowe DC, Barnes BJ, et al. LPS-TLR4 signaling to IRF-3/7 and NF-κB involves the Toll adapters TRAM and TRIF. J Exp Med 198:1043–1055, 2003.

99. Hoebe K, Du X, Goode J, et al. Lps2: a new locus required for responses to lipopolysaccharide, revealed by germline mutagenesis and phenotypic screening. J Endotoxin Res 9:250–255, 2003.

100. Yamamoto M, Sato S, Hemmi H, et al. TRAM is specifically involved in the Toll-like receptor 4-mediated MyD88-independent signaling pathway. Nat Immunol 4:1144–1150, 2003.

101. Marie I, Durbin JE, Levy DE. Differential viral induction of distinct interferon-alpha genes by positive feedback through interferon regulatory factor-7. EMBO J 17:6660–6669, 1998.

102. Prakash A, Smith E, Lee CK, et al. Tissue-specific positive feedback requirements for production of type I interferon following virus infection. J Biol Chem 280:18651–18657, 2005.

103. Honda K, Yanai H, Negishi H, et al. IRF-7 is the master regulator of type-I interferon-dependent immune responses. Nature 434:772–777, 2005.

104. Kawai T, Sato S, Ishii KJ, et al. Interferon-alpha induction through Toll-like receptors involves a direct interaction of IRF7 with MyD88 and TRAF6. Nat Immunol 5:1061–1068, 2004.

105. Honda K, Yanai H, Mizutani T, et al. Role of a transductional-transcriptional processor complex involving MyD88 and IRF-7 in Toll-like receptor signaling. Proc Natl Acad Sci USA 101:15416–15421, 2004.

106. Uematsu S, Sato S, Yamamoto M, et al. Interleukin-1 receptor-associated kinase-1 plays an essential role for Toll-like receptor (TLR)7- and TLR9-mediated interferon-alpha induction. J Exp Med 201:915–923, 2005.

107. Takaoka A, Yanai H, Kondo S, et al. Integral role of IRF-5 in the gene induction programme activated by Toll-like receptors. Nature 434:243–249, 2005.

108. Schoenemeyer A, Barnes BJ, Mancl ME, et al. The interferon regulatory factor, IRF5, is a central mediator of toll-like receptor 7 signaling. J Biol Chem 280:17005–17012, 2005.

109. Banchereau J, Briere F, Caux C, et al. Immunobiology of dendritic cells. Annu Rev Immunol 18:767–811, 2000.

110. O'Doherty U, Peng M, Gezelter S, et al. Human blood contains two subsets of dendritic cells, one immunologically mature and the other immature. Immunology 82:487–493, 1994.

111. Romani N, Gruner S, Brang D, et al. Proliferating dendritic cell progenitors in human blood. J Exp Med 180:83–93, 1994.

112. Sallusto F, Lanzavecchia A. Efficient presentation of soluble antigen by cultured human dendritic cells is maintained by granulocyte/macrophage colony-stimulating factor plus interleukin 4 and downregulated by tumor necrosis factor alpha. J Exp Med 179:1109–1118, 1994.

113. Randolph GJ, Beaulieu S, Lebecque S, et al. Differentiation of monocytes into dendritic cells in a model of transendothelial trafficking. Science 282:480–483, 1998.

114. Randolph GJ, Inaba K, Robbiani DF, et al. Differentiation of phagocytic monocytes into lymph node dendritic cells in vivo. Immunity 11:753–761, 1999.

115. Banchereau J, Briere F, Caux C, et al. Immunobiology of dendritic cells. Annu Rev Immunol 18:767–811, 2000.

116. Pulendran B. Modulating TH1/TH2 responses with microbes, dendritic cells, and pathogen recognition receptors. Immunol Res 29:187–196, 2004.

117. Olweus J, BitMansour A, Warnke R, et al. Dendritic cell ontogeny: a human dendritic cell lineage of myeloid origin. Proc Natl Acad Sci USA 94:12551–12556, 1997.

118. Perussia B, Fanning V, Trinchieri G. A leukocyte subset bearing HLA-DR antigens is responsible for in vitro alpha interferon production in response to viruses. Nat Immun Cell Growth Regul 4:120–137, 1985.

119. Siegal FP, Kadowaki N, Shodell M, et al. The nature of the principal type 1 interferon-producing cells in human blood. Science 284:1835–1837, 1999.

120. Jarrossay D, Napolitani G, Colonna M, et al. Specialization and complementarity in microbial molecule recognition by human myeloid and plasmacytoid dendritic cells. Eur J Immunol 31:3388–3393, 2001.

121. Kadowaki N, Ho S, Antonenko S, et al. Subsets of human dendritic cell precursors express different toll-like receptors and respond to different microbial antigens. J Exp Med 194:863–869, 2001.

122. Krug A, Towarowski A, Britsch S, et al. Toll-like receptor expression reveals CpG DNA as a unique microbial stimulus for plasmacytoid dendritic cells which synergizes with CD40 ligand to induce high amounts of IL-12. Eur J Immunol 31:3026–3037, 2001.

123. Hornung V, Rothenfusser S, Britsch S, et al. Quantitative expression of toll-like receptor 1–10 mRNA in cellular subsets of human peripheral blood mononuclear cells and sensitivity to CpG oligodeoxynucleotides. J Immunol 168:4531–4537, 2002.

124. Ito T, Amakawa R, Fukuhara S. Roles of toll-like receptors in natural interferon-producing cells as sensors in immune surveillance. Hum Immunol 63:1120–1125, 2002.

125. Gorden KB, Gorski KS, Gibson SJ, et al. Synthetic TLR agonists reveal functional differences between human TLR7 and TLR8. J Immunol 174:1259–1268, 2005.

126. Brown MA, Rad PY, Halonen MJ. Method of birth alters interferon-gamma and interleukin-12 production by cord blood mononuclear cells. Pediatr Allergy Immunol 14:106–111, 2003.

127. Buonocore G, De Filippo M, Gioia D, et al. Maternal and neonatal plasma cytokine levels in relation to mode of delivery. Biol Neonate 68:104–110, 1995.

128. De Jongh RF, Bosmans EP, Puylaert MJ, et al. The influence of anaesthetic techniques and type of delivery on peripartum serum interleukin-6 concentrations. Acta Anaesthesiol Scand 41:853–860, 1997.

129. Malamitsi-Puchner A, Protonotariou E, et al. The influence of the mode of delivery on circulating cytokine concentrations in the perinatal period. Early Hum Dev 81:387–392, 2005.

130. Romani N, Reider D, Heuer M, et al. Generation of mature dendritic cells from human blood. An improved method with special regard to clinical applicability. J Immunol Methods 196:137–151, 1996.

131. Siegrist CA. Vaccination in the neonatal period and early infancy. Int Rev Immunol 19:195–219, 2000.

132. Dakic A, Shao QX, D'Amico A, et al. Development of the dendritic cell system during mouse ontogeny. J Immunol 172:1018–1027, 2004.

133. Muthukkumar S, Goldstein J, Stein KE. The ability of B cells and dendritic cells to present antigen increases during ontogeny. J Immunol 165:4803–4813, 2000.

134. Sun CM, Fiette L, Tanguy M, et al. Ontogeny and innate properties of neonatal dendritic cells. Blood 102:585–591, 2003.

135. Chang MD, Pollard JW, Khalili H, et al. Mouse placental macrophages have a decreased ability to present antigen. Proc Natl Acad Sci USA 90:462–466, 1993.

136. Simpson CC, Woods GM, Muller HK. Impaired CD40-signalling in Langerhans' cells from murine neonatal draining lymph nodes: implications for neonatally induced cutaneous tolerance. Clin Exp Immunol 132:201–208, 2003.

137. Dadaglio G, Sun CM, Lo-Man R, et al. Efficient in vivo priming of specific cytotoxic T cell responses by neonatal dendritic cells. J Immunol 168:2219–2224, 2002.

138. Nelson DJ, Holt PG. Defective regional immunity in the respiratory tract of neonates is attributable to hyporesponsiveness of local dendritic cells to activation signals. J Immunol 155:3517–3524, 1995.

139. Kampalath B, Cleveland RP, Kass L. Reduced CD4 and HLA-DR expression in neonatal monocytes. Clin Immunol Immunopathol 87:93–100, 1998.

140. Marodi L, Kaposzta R, Campbell DE, et al. Candidacidal mechanisms in the human neonate. Impaired IFN-gamma activation of macrophages in newborn infants. J Immunol 153:5643–5649, 1994.

141. Hunt DW, Huppertz HI, Jiang HJ, et al. Studies of human cord blood dendritic cells: evidence for functional immaturity. Blood 84:4333–4343, 1994.

142. Sorg RV, Kogler G, Wernet P. Identification of cord blood dendritic cells as an immature CD11c-population. Blood 93:2302–2307, 1999.

143. Borras FE, Matthews NC, Lowdell MW, et al. Identification of both myeloid CD11c+ and lymphoid CD11c- dendritic cell subsets in cord blood. Br J Haematol 113:925–931, 2001.

144. De Wit D, Tonon S, Olislagers V, et al. "FOCIS": impaired responses to toll-like receptor 4 and toll-like receptor 3 ligands in human cord blood. J Autoimmun 3:277–281, 2003.

145. De Wit D, Olislagers V, Goriely S, et al. Blood plasmacytoid dendritic cell responses to CpG oligodeoxynucleotides are impaired in human newborns. Blood 103:1030–1032, 2004.

146. Goriely S, Demonte D, Nizet S, et al. Human IL-12(p35) gene activation involves selective remodeling of a single nucleosome within a region of the promoter containing critical Sp1-binding sites. Blood 101:4894–4902, 2003.

147. Langrish CL, Buddle JC, Thrasher AJ, et al. Neonatal dendritic cells are intrinsically biased against Th-1 immune responses. Clin Exp Immunol 128:118–123, 2002.

148. Salio M, Dulphy N, Renneson J, et al. Efficient priming of antigen-specific cytotoxic T lymphocytes by human cord blood dendritic cells. Int Immunol 15:1265–1273, 2003.

149. Weatherstone KB, Rich EA. Tumor necrosis factor/cachectin and interleukin-1 secretion by cord blood monocytes from premature and term neonates. Pediatr Res 25:342–346, 1989.

150. Cohen L, Haziot A, Shen DR, et al. CD14-independent responses to LPS require a serum factor that is absent from neonates. J Immunol 155:5337–5342, 1995.

151. Levy O, Zarember KA, Roy RM, et al. Selective impairment of TLR-mediated innate immunity in human newborns: neonatal blood plasma reduces monocyte TNF-alpha induction by bacterial lipopeptides, lipopolysaccharide, and imiquimod, but preserves the response to R-848. J Immunol 173:4627–4634, 2004.

152. Yan SR, Qing G, Byers DM, et al. Role of MyD88 in diminished tumor necrosis factor alpha production by newborn mononuclear cells in response to lipopolysaccharide. Infect Immun 72:1223–1229, 2004.

153. Trinchieri G. Interleukin-12 and the regulation of innate resistance and adaptive immunity. Nat Rev Immunol 3:133–146, 2003.

154. Lee SM, Suen Y, Chang L, et al. Decreased interleukin-12 (IL-12) from activated cord versus adult peripheral blood mononuclear cells and upregulation of interferon-gamma, natural killer, and lymphokine-activated killer activity by IL-12 in cord blood mononuclear cells. Blood 88:945–954, 1996.

155. Joyner JL, Augustine NH, Taylor KA, et al. Effects of group B streptococci on cord and adult mononuclear cell interleukin-12 and interferon-gamma mRNA accumulation and protein secretion. J Infect Dis 182:974–977, 2000.

156. Upham JW, Lee PT, Holt BJ, et al. Development of interleukin-12-producing capacity throughout childhood. Infect Immun 70:6583–6588, 2002.

157. Tonon S, Goriely S, Aksoy E, et al. Bordetella pertussis toxin induces the release of inflammatory cytokines and dendritic cell activation in whole blood: impaired responses in human newborns. Eur J Immunol 32:3118–3125, 2002.

158. Karlsson H, Hessle C, Rudin A. Innate immune responses of human neonatal cells to bacteria from the normal gastrointestinal flora. Infect Immun 70:6688–6696, 2002.

159. Goriely S, Vincart B, Stordeur P, et al. Deficient IL-12(p35) gene expression by dendritic cells derived from neonatal monocytes. J Immunol 166:2141–2146, 2001.

160. Wong OH, Huang FP, Chiang AK. Differential responses of cord and adult blood-derived dendritic cells to dying cells. Immunology 116:13–20, 2005.

161. Upham JW, Rate A, Rowe J, et al. Dendritic cell immaturity during infancy restricts the capacity to express vaccine-specific T-cell memory. Infect Immun 74:1106–1112, 2006.

162. Marodi L, Goda K, Palicz A, et al. Cytokine receptor signalling in neonatal macrophages: defective STAT-1 phosphorylation in response to stimulation with IFN-gamma. Clin Exp Immunol 126:456–460, 2001.

163. Sun CM, Deriaud E, Leclerc C, et al. Upon TLR9 signaling, CD5+ B cells control the IL-12-dependent Th1-priming capacity of neonatal DCs. Immunity 22:467–477, 2005.

164. Hunter CA. New IL-12-family members: IL-23 and IL-27, cytokines with divergent functions. Nat Rev Immunol 5:521–531, 2005.

165. Vanden Eijnden S, Goriely S, De Wit D, et al. Preferential production of the IL-12(p40)/IL-23(p19) heterodimer by dendritic cells from human newborns. Eur J Immunol 36:21–26, 2006.

166. D'Andrea A, Rengaraju M, Valiante NM, et al. Production of natural killer cell stimulatory factor (interleukin 12) by peripheral blood mononuclear cells. J Exp Med 176:1387–1398, 1992.

167. Buzby JS, Lee SM, Van Winkle P, et al. Increased granulocyte-macrophage colony-stimulating factor mRNA instability in cord versus adult mononuclear cells is translation-dependent and associated with increased levels of A+U-rich element binding factor. Blood 88:2889–2897, 1996.

168. Qian JX, Lee SM, Suen Y, et al. Decreased interleukin-15 from activated cord versus adult peripheral blood mononuclear cells and the effect of interleukin-15 in upregulating antitumor immune activity and cytokine production in cord blood. Blood 90:3106–3117, 1997.

169. Suen Y, Lee SM, Qian J, et al. Dysregulation of lymphokine production in the neonate and its impact on neonatal cell mediated immunity. Vaccine 16:1369–1377, 1998.

170. Grumont R, Hochrein H, O'Keeffe M, et al. c-Rel regulates interleukin 12 p70 expression in CD8(+) dendritic cells by specifically inducing p35 gene transcription. J Exp Med 194:1021–1032, 2001.

171. Liu J, Cao S, Herman LM, et al. Differential regulation of interleukin (IL)-12 p35 and p40 gene expression and interferon (IFN)-gamma-primed IL-12 production by IFN regulatory factor 1. J Exp Med 198:1265–1276, 2003.

172. Liu J, Guan X, Tamura T, et al. Synergistic activation of interleukin-12 p35 gene transcription by interferon regulatory factor-1 and interferon consensus sequence-binding protein. J Biol Chem 279:55609–55617, 2004.

173. Goriely S, Molle C, Nguyen M, et al. Interferon regulatory factor 3 is involved in Toll-like receptor 4 (TLR4)- and TLR3-induced IL-12p35 gene activation. Blood 107:1078–1084, 2006.

174. Smale ST, Fisher AG. Chromatin structure and gene regulation in the immune system. Annu Rev Immunol 20:427–462, 2002.

175. Goriely S, Van Lint C, Dadkhah R, et al. A defect in nucleosome remodeling prevents IL-12(p35) gene transcription in neonatal dendritic cells. J Exp Med 199:1011–1016, 2004.

176. Suhara W, Yoneyama M, Kitabayashi I, et al. Direct involvement of CREB-binding protein/p300 in sequence-specific DNA binding of virus-activated interferon regulatory factor-3 holocomplex. J Biol Chem 277:22304–22313, 2002.

177. Yang K, Puel A, Zhang S, et al. Human TLR-7-, -8-, and -9-mediated induction of IFN-alpha/beta and -lambda Is IRAK-4 dependent and redundant for protective immunity to viruses. Immunity 23:465–478, 2005.

178. Honda K, Yanai H, Takaoka A, et al. Regulation of the type I IFN induction: a current view. Int Immunol 17:1367–1378, 2005.

179. Colonna M, Trinchieri G, Liu YJ. Plasmacytoid dendritic cells in immunity. Nat Immunol 5:1219–1226, 2004.

180. Ito T, Wang YH, Liu YJ. Plasmacytoid dendritic cell precursors/type I interferon-producing cells sense viral infection by Toll-like receptor (TLR) 7 and TLR9. Springer Semin Immunopathol 26:221–229, 2005.

181. Bauer S, Kirschning CJ, Hacker H, et al. Human TLR9 confers responsiveness to bacterial DNA via species-specific CpG motif recognition. Proc Natl Acad Sci USA 98:9237–9242, 2001.

182. Lund JM, Alexopoulou L, Sato A, et al. Recognition of single-stranded RNA viruses by Toll-like receptor 7. Proc Natl Acad Sci USA 101:5598–5603, 2004.

183. Gibson SJ, Lindh JM, Riter TR, et al. Plasmacytoid dendritic cells produce cytokines and mature in response to the TLR7 agonists, imiquimod and resiquimod. Cell Immunol 218:74–86, 2002.

184. Hemmi H, Kaisho T, Takeuchi O, et al. Small anti-viral compounds activate immune cells via the TLR7 MyD88-dependent signaling pathway. Nat Immunol 3:196–200, 2002.

185. Dai J, Megjugorac NJ, Amrute SB, et al. Regulation of IFN regulatory factor-7 and IFN-alpha production by enveloped virus and lipopolysaccharide in human plasmacytoid dendritic cells. J Immunol 173:1535–1548, 2004.

186. Honda K, Yanai H, Negishi H, et al. IRF-7 is the master regulator of type-I interferon-dependent immune responses. Nature 434:772–777, 2005.

187. Honda K, Ohba Y, Yanai H, et al. Spatiotemporal regulation of MyD88-IRF-7 signalling for robust type-I interferon induction. Nature 434:1035–1040, 2005.

188. Fitzgerald KA, McWhirter SM, Faia KL, et al. IKKepsilon and TBK1 are essential components of the IRF3 signaling pathway. Nat Immunol.2003.May.;4(5):491.-6. 4:491–496, 2003.

189. Kadowaki N, Ho S, Antonenko S, et al. Subsets of human dendritic cell precursors express different toll-like receptors and respond to different microbial antigens. J Exp Med 194:863–869, 2001.

190. Toshchakov V, Jones BW, Perera PY, et al. TLR4, but not TLR2, mediates IFN-beta-induced STAT1alpha/beta-dependent gene expression in macrophages. Nat Immunol 3:392–398, 2002.

191. Honda K, Sakaguchi S, Nakajima C, et al. Selective contribution of IFN-alpha/beta signaling to the maturation of dendritic cells induced by double-stranded RNA or viral infection. Proc Natl Acad Sci USA 100:10872–10877, 2003.

192. Wilson CB. Immunologic basis for increased susceptibility of the neonate to infection. J Pediatr 108:1–12, 1986.

193. Whitley RJ. Herpes simplex virus in children. Curr Treat Options Neurol 4:231–237, 2002.

194. Shearer WT, Quinn TC, LaRussa P, et al. Viral load and disease progression in infants infected with human immunodeficiency virus type 1. Women and Infants Transmission Study Group. N Engl J Med 336:1337–1342, 1997.

195. Smith S, Jacobs RF, Wilson CB. Immunobiology of childhood tuberculosis: a window on the ontogeny of cellular immunity. J Pediatr 131:16–26, 1997.

196. Edmunds WJ, Medley GF, Nokes DJ, et al. The influence of age on the development of the hepatitis B carrier state. Proc R Soc Lond B Biol Sci 253:197–201, 1993.

197. Marchant A, Goldman M. T cell-mediated immune responses in human newborns: ready to learn? Clin Exp Immunol 141:10–18, 2005.

198. Hermann E, Truyens C, Alonso-Vega C, et al. Human fetuses are able to mount an adultlike CD8 T-cell response. Blood 100:2153–2158, 2002.

199. Marchant A, Appay V, Van Der SM, et al. Mature CD8(+) T lymphocyte response to viral infection during fetal life. J Clin Invest 111:1747–1755, 2003.

200. Marchant A, Goetghebuer T, Ota MO, et al. Newborns develop a Th1-type immune response to Mycobacterium bovis bacillus Calmette-Guerin vaccination. J Immunol 163:2249–2255, 1999.

201. Mascart F, Verscheure V, Malfroot A, et al. Bordetella pertussis infection in 2-month-old infants promotes type 1 T cell responses. J Immunol 170:1504–1509, 2003.

202. Vollstedt S, O'Keeffe M, Odermatt B, et al. Treatment of neonatal mice with Flt3 ligand leads to changes in dendritic cell subpopulations associated with enhanced IL-12 and IFN-alpha production. Eur J Immunol 34:1849–1860, 2004.

203. Vollstedt S, Franchini M, Hefti HP, et al. Flt3 ligand-treated neonatal mice have increased innate immunity against intracellular pathogens and efficiently control virus infections. J Exp Med 197:575–584, 2003.

204. Mattner F, Magram J, Ferrante J, et al. Genetically resistant mice lacking interleukin-12 are susceptible to infection with Leishmania major and mount a polarized Th2 cell response. Eur J Immunol 26:1553–1559, 1996.

205. Elkins KL, Cooper A, Colombini SM, et al. In vivo clearance of an intracellular bacterium, Francisella tularensis LVS, is dependent on the p40 subunit of interleukin-12 (IL-12) but not on IL-12 p70. Infect Immun 70:1936–1948, 2002.

206. Decken K, Kohler G, Palmer-Lehmann K, et al. Interleukin-12 is essential for a protective Th1 response in mice infected with Cryptococcus neoformans. Infect Immun 66:4994–5000, 1998.

207. Lehmann J, Bellmann S, Werner C, et al. IL-12p40-dependent agonistic effects on the development of protective innate and adaptive immunity against Salmonella enteritidis. J Immunol 167:5304–5315, 2001.

208. Holscher C, Atkinson RA, Arendse B, et al. A protective and agonistic function of IL-12p40 in mycobacterial infection. J Immunol 167:6957–6966, 2001.

209. Lankford CS, Frucht DM. A unique role for IL-23 in promoting cellular immunity. J Leukoc Biol 73:49–56, 2003.

210. Happel KI, Dubin PJ, Zheng M, et al. Divergent roles of IL-23 and IL-12 in host defense against Klebsiella pneumoniae. J Exp Med 202:761–769, 2005.

211. Khader SA, Pearl JE, Sakamoto K, et al. IL-23 compensates for the absence of IL-12p70 and is essential for the IL-17 response during tuberculosis but is dispensable for protection and antigen-specific IFN-gamma responses if IL-12p70 is available. J Immunol 175:788–795, 2005.

212. Fieschi C, Casanova JL. The role of interleukin-12 in human infectious diseases: only a faint signature. Eur J Immunol 33:1461–1464, 2003.
213. Dupuis S, Jouanguy E, Al Hajjar S, et al. Impaired response to interferon-alpha/beta and lethal viral disease in human STAT1 deficiency. Nat Genet 33:388–391, 2003.
214. Pikora CA, Sullivan JL, Panicali D, et al. Early HIV-1 envelope-specific cytotoxic T lymphocyte responses in vertically infected infants. J Exp Med 185:1153–1161, 1997.
215. Luzuriaga K, Holmes D, Hereema A, et al. HIV-1-specific cytotoxic T lymphocyte responses in the first year of life. J Immunol 154:433–443, 1995.
216. Wasik TJ, Jagodzinski PP, Hyjek EM, et al. Diminished HIV-specific CTL activity is associated with lower type 1 and enhanced type 2 responses to HIV-specific peptides during perinatal HIV infection. J Immunol 158:6029–6036, 1997.
217. Tu W, Chen S, Sharp M, et al. Persistent and selective deficiency of CD4+ T cell immunity to cytomegalovirus in immunocompetent young children. J Immunol 172:3260–3267, 2004.
218. Pass RF, Stagno S, Britt WJ, et al. Specific cell-mediated immunity and the natural history of congenital infection with cytomegalovirus. J Infect Dis 148:953–961, 1983.
219. Janssen EM, Lemmens EE, Wolfe T, et al. CD4+ T cells are required for secondary expansion and memory in CD8+ lymphocytes. Nature 421:852–856, 2003.
220. Shedlock DJ, Shen H. Requirement for CD4 T cell help in generating functional CD8 T cell memory. Science 300:337–339, 2003.
221. Sun JC, Bevan MJ. Defective CD8 T cell memory following acute infection without CD4 T cell help. Science 300:339–342, 2003.
222. Carter LL, Murphy KM. Lineage-specific requirement for signal transducer and activator of transcription (Stat)4 in interferon gamma production from CD4(+) versus CD8(+) T cells. J Exp Med 189:1355–1360, 1999.
223. White GP, Watt PM, Holt BJ, et al. Differential patterns of methylation of the IFN-gamma promoter at CpG, non-CpG sites underlie differences in IFN-gamma gene expression between human neonatal and adult CD. J Immunol 168:2820–2827, 2002.
224. Lund J, Sato A, Akira S, et al. Toll-like receptor 9-mediated recognition of Herpes simplex virus-2 by plasmacytoid dendritic cells. J Exp Med 198:513–520, 2003.
225. Beignon AS, McKenna K, Skoberne M, et al. Endocytosis of HIV-1 activates plasmacytoid dendritic cells via Toll-like receptor-viral RNA interactions. J Clin Invest 115:3265–3275, 2005.
226. Hornung V, Schlender J, Guenthner-Biller M, et al. Replication-dependent potent IFN-alpha induction in human plasmacytoid dendritic cells by a single-stranded RNA virus. J Immunol 173:5935–5943, 2004.
227. Kato H, Sato S, Yoneyama M, et al. Cell type-specific involvement of RIG-I in antiviral response. Immunity 23:19–28, 2005.
228. Yoneyama M, Kikuchi M, Natsukawa T, et al. The RNA helicase RIG-I has an essential function in double-stranded RNA-induced innate antiviral responses. Nat Immunol 5:730–737, 2004.
229. Levy DE, Marie IJ. RIGging an antiviral defense—it's in the CARDs. Nat Immunol 5:699–701, 2004.
230. Holt PG, Thomas WR. Sensitization to airborne environmental allergens: unresolved issues. Nat Immunol 6:957–960, 2005.
231. Holt PG. Postnatal maturation of immune competence during infancy and childhood. Pediatr Allergy Immunol 6:59–70, 1995.
232. Prescott SL, Macaubas C, Holt BJ, et al. Transplacental priming of the human immune system to environmental allergens: universal skewing of initial T cell responses toward the Th2 cytokine profile. J Immunol 160:4730–4737, 1998.
233. Miyawaki T, Seki H, Taga K, et al. Dissociated production of interleukin-2 and immune (gamma) interferon by phytohaemagglutinin stimulated lymphocytes in healthy infants. Clin Exp Immunol 59:505–511, 1985.
234. Rowe J, Macaubas C, Monger TM, et al. Antigen-specific responses to diphtheria-tetanus-acellular pertussis vaccine in human infants are initially Th2 polarized. Infect Immun 68:3873–3877, 2000.
235. Holt PG, Clough JB, Holt BJ, et al. Genetic 'risk' for atopy is associated with delayed postnatal maturation of T-cell competence. Clin Exp Allergy 22:1093–1099, 1992.
236. Kondo N, Kobayashi Y, Shinoda S, et al. Reduced interferon gamma production by antigen-stimulated cord blood mononuclear cells is a risk factor of allergic disorders—6-year follow-up study. Clin Exp Allergy 28:1340–1344, 1998.
237. Tang ML, Kemp AS, Thorburn J, et al. Reduced interferon-gamma secretion in neonates and subsequent atopy. Lancet 344:983–985, 1994.
238. Prescott SL, Taylor A, King B, et al. Neonatal interleukin-12 capacity is associated with variations in allergen-specific immune responses in the neonatal and postnatal periods. Clin Exp Allergy 33:566–572, 2003.
239. Morahan G, Huang D, Wu M, et al. Association of IL12B promoter polymorphism with severity of atopic and non-atopic asthma in children. Lancet 360:455–459, 2002.
240. Wold AE. The hygiene hypothesis revised: is the rising frequency of allergy due to changes in the intestinal flora? Allergy 53:20–25, 1998.
241. Mazmanian SK, Liu CH, Tzianabos AO, et al. An immunomodulatory molecule of symbiotic bacteria directs maturation of the host immune system. Cell 122:107–118, 2005.
242. Lauener RP, Birchler T, Adamski J, et al. Expression of CD14 and Toll-like receptor 2 in farmers' and non-farmers' children. Lancet 360:465–466, 2002.
243. Braun-Fahrlander C, Riedler J, Herz U, et al. Environmental exposure to endotoxin and its relation to asthma in school-age children. N Engl J Med 347:869–877, 2002.

244. Baldini M, Lohman IC, Halonen M, et al. A polymorphism* in the 5′ flanking region of the CD14 gene is associated with circulating soluble CD14 levels and with total serum immunoglobulin E. Am J Respir Cell Mol Biol 20:976–983, 1999.

245. Sigurs N, Bjarnason R, Sigurbergsson F, et al. Respiratory syncytial virus bronchiolitis in infancy is an important risk factor for asthma and allergy at age 7. Am J Respir Crit Care Med 161:1501–1507, 2000.

246. Openshaw P, Murphy EE, Hosken NA, et al. Heterogeneity of intracellular cytokine synthesis at the single-cell level in polarized T helper 1 and T helper 2 populations. J Exp Med 182:1357–1367, 1995.

247. Varga SM, Wang X, Welsh RM, et al. Immunopathology in RSV infection is mediated by a discrete oligoclonal subset of antigen-specific CD4(+) T cells. Immunity 15:637–646, 2001.

248. Stein RT, Sherrill D, Morgan WJ, et al. Respiratory syncytial virus in early life and risk of wheeze and allergy by age 13 years. Lancet 354:541–545, 1999.

249. Culley FJ, Pollott J, Openshaw PJ. Age at first viral infection determines the pattern of T cell-mediated disease during reinfection in adulthood. J Exp Med 196:1381–1386, 2002.

250. van Duin D, Medzhitov R, Shaw AC. Triggering TLR signaling in vaccination. Trends Immunol 27:49–55, 2006.

251. Barrios C, Brandt C, Berney M, et al. Partial correction of the TH2/TH1 imbalance in neonatal murine responses to vaccine antigens through selective adjuvant effects. Eur J Immunol 26:2666–2670, 1996.

252. Kovarik J, Bozzotti P, Love-Homan L, et al. CpG oligodeoxynucleotides can circumvent the Th2 polarization of neonatal responses to vaccines but may fail to fully redirect Th2 responses established by neonatal priming. J Immunol 162:1611–1617, 1999.

253. Vekemans J, Ota MO, Wang EC, et al. T cell responses to vaccines in infants: defective IFNgamma production after oral polio vaccination. Clin Exp Immunol 127:495–498, 2002.

254. Ota MO, Vekemans J, Schlegel-Haueter SE, et al. Hepatitis B immunisation induces higher antibody and memory Th2 responses in new-borns than in adults. Vaccine 22:511–519, 2004.

255. Ota MO, Vekemans J, Schlegel-Haueter SE, et al. Influence of Mycobacterium bovis bacillus Calmette-Guerin on antibody and cytokine responses to human neonatal vaccination. J Immunol 168:919–925, 2002.

256. Means TK, Wang S, Lien E, et al. Human toll-like receptors mediate cellular activation by Mycobacterium tuberculosis. J Immunol 163:3920–3927, 1999.

257. Tsuji S, Matsumoto M, Takeuchi O, et al. Maturation of human dendritic cells by cell wall skeleton of Mycobacterium bovis bacillus Calmette-Guerin: involvement of toll-like receptors. Infect Immun 68:6883–6890, 2000.

258. Hoft DF, Brown RM, Roodman ST. Bacille Calmette-Guerin vaccination enhances human gamma delta T cell responsiveness to mycobacteria suggestive of a memory-like phenotype. J Immunol 161:1045–1054, 1998.

259. Kemp K, Hviid L, Kharazmi A, Kemp M. Interferon-gamma production by human T cells and natural killer cells in vitro in response to antigens from the two intracellular pathogens Mycobacterium tuberculosis and Leishmania major. Scand J Immunol 46:495–499, 1997.

260. Gerosa F, Baldani-Guerra B, Nisii C, et al. Reciprocal activating interaction between natural killer cells and dendritic cells. J Exp Med 195:327–333, 2002.

261. Mailliard RB, Son YI, Redlinger R, et al. Dendritic cells mediate NK cell help for Th1 and CTL responses: two-signal requirement for the induction of NK cell helper function. J Immunol 171:2366–2373, 2003.

262. Ismaili J, Olislagers V, Poupot R, et al. Human gamma delta T cells induce dendritic cell maturation. Clin Immunol 103:296–302, 2002.

263. Tanaka H, Kai S, Yamaguchi M, et al. Analysis of natural killer (NK) cell activity and adhesion molecules on NK cells from umbilical cord blood. Eur J Haematol 71:29–38, 2003.

264. Hayday AC. [gamma][delta] cells: a right time and a right place for a conserved third way of protection. Annu Rev Immunol 18:975–1026, 2000.

265. De Rosa SC, Andrus JP, Perfetto SP, et al. Ontogeny of gamma delta T cells in humans. J Immunol 172:1637–1645, 2004.

266. Ramsburg E, Tigelaar R, Craft J, et al. Age-dependent requirement for gammadelta T cells in the primary but not secondary protective immune response against an intestinal parasite. J Exp Med 198:1403–1414, 2003.

267. Fujii S, Shimizu K, Smith C, et al. Activation of natural killer T cells by alpha-galactosylceramide rapidly induces the full maturation of dendritic cells in vivo and thereby acts as an adjuvant for combined CD4 and CD8 T cell immunity to a coadministered protein. J Exp Med 198:267–279, 2003.

268. Yue SC, Shaulov A, Wang R, et al. CD1d ligation on human monocytes directly signals rapid NF-kappaB activation and production of bioactive IL-12. Proc Natl Acad Sci USA 102:11811–11816, 2005.

269. Kadowaki N, Antonenko S, Ho S, et al. Distinct cytokine profiles of neonatal natural killer T cells after expansion with subsets of dendritic cells. J Exp Med 193:1221–1226, 2001.

270. van Heel DA, Ghosh S, Butler M, et al. Synergistic enhancement of Toll-like receptor responses by NOD1 activation. Eur J Immunol 35:2471–2476, 2005.

271. Napolitani G, Rinaldi A, Bertoni F, et al. Selected Toll-like receptor agonist combinations synergistically trigger a T helper type 1-polarizing program in dendritic cells. Nat Immunol 6:769–776, 2005.

Chapter 9

Maternally Mediated Neonatal Autoimmunity

Neelufar Mozaffarian, MD, PhD •
Anne M. Stevens, MD, PhD

Maternal Antibodies and Neonatal Autoimmunity

Maternal Microchimerism (MMc) and Neonatal Autoimmunity

Role of T Regulatory Cells in Neonatal Autoimmunity

Conclusions

Transplacental passage of maternal antibodies was first described in 1895 with the finding of anti-diphtheria toxin antibodies in fetal blood by Fischl and Von Wundscheim (reviewed in ref. 1). Over the past century, the role of maternally derived antibodies in passive neonatal immunity has been extensively studied, but this protection against infection comes with a price: self-reactive antibodies transferred to the fetus may result in neonatal autoimmunity. The resultant antibody-mediated disease phenotype depends not only on the antigen-specificity, titer, and affinity of the antibody transferred, but on the gestational age and underlying health of the newborn, as these factors can influence the transplacental and gastrointestinal acquisition of immunoglobulins from the mother (2–4).

In addition to maternal–fetal antibody transfer, several investigators have demonstrated transplacental acquisition and retention of whole maternal cells by the human fetus (5–7), a phenomenon not previously believed to be possible. These maternal cells persist and are detectable in healthy individuals for years after birth (8), signifying a chronic chimeric state termed maternal microchimerism (MMc).

In the first half of this chapter, we will review examples of maternal antibody-mediated autoimmunity in the neonate (Table 9-1), and speculate on hypothetical roles for maternal antibodies in modulating the risk of autoimmune disease. In the second half, we will outline the latest findings with respect to the relationship between MMc and neonatal autoimmune disease, and summarize what is known regarding the role of T regulatory cells in these types of neonatal autoimmunity.

MATERNAL ANTIBODIES AND NEONATAL AUTOIMMUNITY

Normal Physiology

Humans begin to receive immunoglobulins (Ig) from their mothers during fetal development. Transfer of maternal IgG to the fetus involves initiation of antibody transport shortly after the first trimester through term, with the majority of antibody acquisition occurring in the third trimester (9). Transplacental transfer of maternal antibodies is effected by the interaction of Annexin II with neonatal Fc

Table 9-1 Some of the Transplacentally Acquired Maternal Autoantibodies and the Associated Disease in the Fetus/infant

Maternal antibodies	Associated disease
	Collagen vascular diseases
Anti-SSA/Ro, anti-SSB/La, and anti-RNP antibodies	Neonatal lupus syndrome/heart block
Anti-neutrophil cytoplasmic antibodies (ANCA)	Neonatal vasculitis
Monoclonal IgG	Type I cryoglobulinemia
Monoclonal IgG	Glomerulonephritis
	Hematologic diseases
Anti-erythrocyte	Neonatal anemia
Anti-platelet	Neonatal thrombocytopenia
Anti-neutrophil	Neonatal neutropenia
Anti-lymphocyte	Neonatal lymphopenia
	Endocrine diseases
Anti-thyroid antibodies	Neonatal hyper/hypothyroidism
Diabetes-related antibodies	Unknown
Anti-adrenal antibodies	Unknown
	Neuromuscular junction diseases
Anti-acetylcholine receptor (ACh R) antibodies	Neonatal myasthenia gravis
Unknown	Neonatal Guillain-Barre
Anti-ganglioside GM-1 antibodies	Neonatal lower motor neuron disease
	Cardiac diseases
Anti-beta-adrenoceptor/cholinergic receptor antibodies	Neonatal cardiac disease
Anti-myolemmal antibodies	Fetal arrhythmias
	Skin diseases
Anti-desmoglein antibodies	Neonatal pemphigus
	Nutritional deficiencies
Anti-folate receptor antibodies	Neural tube defects
Anti-intrinsic factor antibodies	Neonatal B12 deficiency
	Complications of pregnancy
Anti-angiotensin II receptor antibodies	Preeclampsia
Anti-phospholipid antibodies	Preeclampsia, IUGR, fetal loss
Anti-laminin-1 antibodies	Spontaneous abortion
Anti-tissue transglutaminase antibodies	Spontaneous abortion, IUGR
Anti-AChR antibodies	Complications of labor
	Liver diseases
Anti-nuclear antibodies (ANA)	Neonatal liver diseases
Antibodies to unknown target(s)	Neonatal hemochromatosis

receptors (FcRn) on placental syncytiotrophoblasts (10, 11). These FcRn actively transport IgG in a subclass-specific fashion; for example, IgG_1 and IgG4 are more efficiently transferred to the fetus than IgG_2 or IgG_3 (9, 12, 13). Although placental cells regulate the isotype, amount, and timing of antibody transfer, transfer is inherently dependent on the circulating antibody levels in the pregnant mother. Alterations in maternal immunoglobulin titers or infusion of exogenous immunoglobulins to the pregnant woman will directly affect fetal antibody acquisition. These are important considerations as maternally derived antibodies do not merely play a passive role in neonatal immunity but can direct the development of the newborn's immune system (14, 15). At birth, the infant's IgG levels are similar to or higher than those of his mother (13), providing early protection against infection, as the half-life of maternal IgG in the infant is approximately 30–50 days (16). Postnatally, the levels of maternal IgG in the infant steadily decline, until over half of the maternal IgG load is lost after 3 months, and virtually all of it is catabolized by 6–9 months of age.

In addition to IgG, there is evidence for prenatal IgE uptake. Fetal gut lymphoid follicles express IgE receptors after week 16 of gestation, and human amniotic fluid samples from 16–18 week gestations contain intact IgE, probably derived from the maternal circulation (17). Therefore, maternal IgE may be acquired by the fetus via ingestion of amniotic fluid, possibly to protect from parasitic infections in endemic areas. Additionally, interaction of maternal IgG and IgE may modulate neonatal autoimmunity. IgE levels at birth correlate with the infant's risk of developing atopic disease, but protection from atopy is seen in newborns with high titers of IgG anti-IgE, acquired from the maternal circulation (18).

To further enhance the immunoglobulin repertoire, the newborn receives additional maternal antibodies via ingestion of breast milk, which provides substantial amounts of IgA (mostly dimeric), some IgM, and some subtypes of IgG (19). The initial colostrum contains the highest titers of IgA, putatively to coat the newborn's unprotected mucosal surfaces. Gastrointestinal passage of breast milk does not result in proteolysis of the immunoglobulins. For example, protective anti-enteropathogenic *E. coli* IgA antibodies acquired via colostrum can be found intact in the feces of breast-fed neonates (20). In addition to providing mucosal protection, breast milk immunoglobulins may be transferred to the neonatal circulation. Human intestinal cells have been found to express the neonatal Fc receptor, suggesting a mechanism for IgG acquisition from gastrointestinal sources (21).

The importance of acquired antibody in protection against infection and its effects on infant vaccination have been previously described (reviewed in refs 22–24). But antibody acquisition can also lead to fetal or neonatal disease. Potential pathogenic mechanisms for maternal antibodies in neonatal disease include antibody-mediated depletion of specific cell types (via complement- or cell-mediated lysis, reticuloendothelial clearance, or initiation of apoptosis), interference with normal cellular/metabolic processes, immune complex (IC) formation and deposition, and/or initiation of a T cell-mediated immune response. Although some disease-related maternal autoantibodies can be routinely screened for in the neonate, it is likely that there are other, as yet unknown antibodies which remain to be identified.

Developmental Differences between the Fetus and Newborn

As discussed above, maternal antibody transfer to the fetus takes place throughout gestation, with postnatal ingestion of colostrum and breast milk providing additional antibody sources for the infant. We are only beginning to understand the normal and pathogenic roles of the various components provided via maternal blood, colostrum, and breast milk, and how these factors interact with the fetal and neonatal immune systems.

With respect to antibody-mediated diseases, there are several developmentally regulated proteins expressed only in the fetal or neonatal period, or expressed in a "fetal" or "neonatal" form which later transitions to the "adult" form (e.g., fetal acetylcholinesterase receptor, fetal hemoglobin), suggesting that some of the disorders we currently know as "congenital" or "idiopathic" are actually a result of maternally derived antibodies which bind fetal/neonatal antigens, and cause little or no disease in the mother. If the mother is asymptomatic, an underlying antibody disorder is not suspected, and the infant would not be tested. Therefore, the true prevalence of maternal antibody-mediated disease in neonates may be underestimated. Conversely, neonates may be protected from antibody-mediated diseases due to differences in antigen expression or presentation. For example, infants are resistant to the development of anti-glomerular basement membrane (anti-GBM)-mediated glomerulonephritis due to decreased antigen accessibility in fetal and neonatal renal tissues (25, 26), and to antibody-mediated pemphigus folaceous due to redundant expression of cell adhesion proteins (27).

Special Physiologic Aspects of Preterm Infants

As most of the transplacental antibody transfer occurs in the third trimester, preterm birth can result in diminished antibody acquisition. However, full gestation does not necessarily ensure normal antibody levels in the neonate. Umbilical cord serum samples from low birth weight infants born at term revealed reduced IgG levels, similar to those seen in preterm infants of adequate weight (28). Both the low birth weight and preterm infants were also found to have qualitative differences in maternal IgG acqustion, with disproportionately reduced concentrations of IgG1 and IgG2 subclasses. After birth, immune development may be further altered in preterm or low birth weight infants, due to decreased intake of breast milk (29). It is not known whether gastrointestinal antibody uptake in these neonates is also qualitatively different. What role altered antibody transfer then plays in the development of neonatal autoimmunity is not known.

The Role of Breast Milk in Neonatal Autoimmunity

The ability of breast milk to provide species-specific immunity to infants was first demonstrated by Paul Erlich in 1892 (reviewed in ref. 1). However, the influence of breast milk on the progeny's risk of autoimmunity is only beginning to be understood. For example, lupus-associated autoantibodies may cause fetal or neonatal lupus syndrome when acquired transplacentally, but breast-fed infants of women with these autoantibodies were not found to have an increased risk of disease, although breast milk samples contain these autoantibodies in both IgA and IgG isotypes (30). Ingestion of breast milk from asthmatic women has been linked to increased allergy risk in human infants (31), but this was not confirmed in other studies (32–34). To test whether substances transferred in breast milk could promote atopy, an experimental mouse model was created. Pups born to asthmatic and non-asthmatic mice were switched at birth and adoptively nursed (35). After ingestion of breast milk from asthmatic mothers, the healthy pups also developed airway hyper-reactivity. Whether this is related to transfer of IgE, IgG anti-IgE, or other breast milk components is not known. Further studies are needed to determine the specific mechanisms which mediate atopy transfer in this model, and whether they hold true in humans.

Relevance of Physiologic Differences to the Disease Process

The fetus and preterm, term, and breast-fed infant exhibit significant differences in maternal antibody acquisition, function of the endogenous immune system, and expression of target antigens due to developmental, nutritional, and environmental factors. These factors play a role in neonatal autoimmunity as transfer of maternal autoantibody alone is not sufficient to cause disease. For example, lupus-associated autoantibodies can cause significant cutaneous inflammation in neonates exposed to sunlight, while the fetus is usually protected from antibody-mediated skin disease due to lack of this environmental factor. Further evidence that maternal antibodies are necessary but not sufficient for neonatal autoimmunity is demonstrated by sets of twins and triplets discordant for autoimmune diseases.

Potential Mechanisms of Antibody-Mediated Autoimmune Disease

Acquired maternal antibodies can cause fetal or neonatal disease via multiple pathogenic mechanisms. Some autoantibodies cause disease by binding to antigen targets normally sequestered within the plasma and/or nuclear membranes of individual cells. Exposure of these antigens to the immune system may occur during apoptosis – a type of programmed cell death initiated by cellular insults such as infection, and also invoked in regulated waves during developmental remodeling (36). The apoptotic program results in the processing of several intracellular and intranuclear proteins and their presentation at the cell surface. Antibodies to these antigens have been implicated in the pathogenesis of systemic lupus erythematosus and other autoimmune diseases. Examples of maternally derived antibodies to intracellular targets include: anti-SSA/Ro, anti-SSB/La and anti-nuclear antibodies (ANA).

Other maternally derived antibodies cause neonatal disease by binding cell surface molecules, resulting in loss of the targeted cell from the circulation or tissues (via complement-mediated lysis, antibody-mediated cellular cytotoxicity, reticulo-endothelial clearance, or induction of apoptosis). Neonatal cytopenias are often caused by these types of antibodies. Rarely, these antibodies are true maternal autoantibodies, causing disease in the mother as well as the fetus, but more typically, they are *allo*antibodies, reacting against paternal antigens expressed by the fetus. Alloantibodies do not cause symptoms in the mother, as her cells do not express the antigenic targets. Antibody-mediated neonatal cytopenias can be quite severe, and may lead to death of the affected neonate if not aggressively treated. Examples of these antibodies include: anti-erythrocyte, anti-platelet, anti-neutrophil, and anti-lymphocyte antibodies.

Maternal anti-receptor antibodies bind endogenous cell surface molecules and act as receptor agonists or antagonists. Anti-receptor antibodies can bind their targets at the normal ligand binding site or at another location, and may alter receptor interaction with endogenous ligand, depending on whether or not the antibody causes steric hindrance or a conformational change in the receptor. These autoantibodies may also alter receptor turnover or expression at the cell surface, or bind to and clear a soluble receptor from the circulation or tissues. As noted above, cell surface-bound antibodies may also lead to destruction of the targeted cell. In general, agonistic anti-receptor antibodies cause active cell signaling, with the problem that the antibodies are not cleared, degraded, or regulated as endogenous ligand would be by the normal feedback pathways, resulting in signaling that can be tonic, mistimed, in aberrant locations, and/or at abnormal levels. These antibodies may act as partial agonists, full agonists, or supraphysiologic agonists at the targeted receptor. An example of this type of antibody is the agonistic anti-thyroid-stimulating hormone receptor (TSH-R) antibody. In contrast, antagonistic anti-receptor antibodies typically reduce normal cell signaling. Examples of antagonistic anti-receptor antibodies include the anti-beta-1-adrenoceptor and anti-acetylcholine receptor antibodies.

Antibodies to cell adhesion molecules are similar to the anti-receptor antibodies in that their targets are endogenous surface proteins, but in this case they disrupt cell–cell interactions important in signaling and/or maintaining tissue integrity; for example: anti-desmoglein antibodies.

Another type of anti-receptor antibody is the anti-nutrient antibody. These maternal autoantibodies bind to endogenous receptors and interfere with fetal or neonatal nutrient acquisition. Antibody-mediated nutritional deficiency can result in a neonatal phenotype indistinguishable from true nutritional deficiency or congenital absence of the relevant receptor. However, it is important to make the distinction between these types of neonatal disease, in order to initiate the appropriate treatment and/or preventative measures. Examples of these types of antibody include the anti-folate receptor and anti-intrinsic factor receptor antibodies.

Anti-ligand antibodies bind to and limit the amount of endogenous ligand available for signaling. The affected individual must then increase production of the targeted protein or suffer the consequences of diminished signaling, or both. Like other autoantibodies, these may cross-react with more than one target, causing pleiotropic effects in the fetus or neonate. An example is the anti-insulin antibody.

Some maternal antibodies cause disease by binding target antigens to form immune complexes. These immune complexes can be acquired by the fetus and may circulate at very high titers. In addition to altering blood viscosity, immune complexes may deposit in organs or vessel walls. Alternatively, transplacentally transferred maternal antibodies may form immune complexes directly in situ, in fetal tissues which contain their target antigen. In either case, these antibody–antigen complexes cause disease by inciting an intense, localized inflammatory response. Cryoglobulinemia is one example of maternal immune complex-mediated neonatal disease.

Interaction of Maternally Derived Antibodies with the Neonatal Immune System

Transplacental transfer of maternal autoantibodies alone does not necessarily lead to disease in the fetus or infant. Autoimmune disease initiated by maternally derived antibodies may depend on the presence of other factors, including an intact adaptive immune system. In murine studies, acquisition of maternal autoantibodies against a specific ovarian protein resulted in neonatal autoimmune ovarian disease (AOD) and premature ovarian failure, but only if T cells were also present (37). Passive transfer of T cells from mice with AOD resulted in disease in the recipients, demonstrating that once the process was initiated by autoantibodies, antigen-specific effector T cells could mediate disease independently. These findings have important implications for the human neonate, as maternal antibodies could prime an autoimmune T cell response which would continue even after the loss of the transiently acquired maternal antibodies.

Maternal Alloimmunization due to Genetic Mutation

Although maternal antibodies against specific targets such as blood group antigens often develop because the woman lacks these alleles as a result of normal variation, there have been descriptions of maternal alloimmunization related to idiosyncratic genetic mutations. Absence of a normal gene may cause the encoded protein to appear foreign to the mother's immune system, leading to antibody production. For example, the gene for CD36 encodes a protein normally expressed on platelets, monocytes, and endothelial cells; a woman lacking CD36 expression due to genetic mutation developed anti-CD36 IgG, and normal transplacental antibody transfer resulted in hydrops fetalis in her infants (38). In another case, neonatal disease was caused by maternal antibodies to neutral endopeptidase (NEP), a protein normally expressed on renal podocytes (39). Women with mutations in the gene for NEP become alloimmunized to this protein during pregnancy, when it is produced by placental syncytiotrophoblasts. Transplacental transfer of anti-NEP IgG antibodies results in antenatal membranous glomerulonephritis.

These examples raise the possibility that other neonatal diseases may be a result of alloimmunization in women with unusual genetic mutations. Typically, women with these types of genetic mutations have no antibody-related symptoms, as they lack the target antigens. Since these maternal antibodies are not suspected, the first pregnancies are at greatest risk for complications. Subsequent fetuses have an improved prognosis as they are more likely to be closely monitored. To protect the fetus from maternal antibody-mediated disease, pregnant women with known genetic mutations should be monitored for antibody titer and isotype, and possibly treated with intravenous immunoglobulin (IVIG) and/or plasma exchange, although there have been no clinical trials for these types of syndromes. Whether neutralizing agents, such as anti-D antibodies used in women at risk for alloimmunization to erythrocyte antigens, will be developed and/or useful for these diseases remains to be seen.

Specific Maternal Antibody-Mediated Neonatal Autoimmune Diseases

For each antibody-mediated syndrome, we will summarize pathogenesis, clinical manifestations, and diagnostic considerations, followed by what is currently known regarding the prevention, treatment, and management of these rare diseases.

Neonatal Cardiac Diseases

The presence of any of several known anti-cardiac autoantibodies and/or immune complexes may lead to neonatal cardiac disease, resulting in a myriad of inflammatory pathologies in the heart, including myositis, fibrosis, and even myocyte apoptosis (40). The best-studied are the lupus-associated anti-Ro/SSA and anti-La/SSB autoantibodies, which can lead to severe congenital heart block CHB. However, CHB and cardiac arrhythmias have also been associated with antibodies to cardiac adrenoceptors, muscarinic cholinergic receptors, and myolemmal antigens (41).

In most cases, autoantibodies implicated in cardiac conduction disorders may actually play a protective role, as they also bind antigens derived from infectious agents: antibodies to the bundle of His, SSB/La, cardiac myosin heavy chain, or the laminin B1 chain crossreact with antigens from *Streptococcus pyogenes*; and antibodies to sarcolemmal epitopes crossreact with antigens from Coxsackie viruses (42). It is not clear which factors are required to turn a protective antibody into a pathogenic one, but the affinity, isotype, and titer of each particular antibody, characteristics of the target antigens themselves, major histocompatibility complex (MHC) alleles, and cellular immune system of the host all probably play a role.

NEONATAL LUPUS SYNDROME AND CONGENITAL HEART BLOCK

Neonatal lupus syndrome (NLS), not to be confused with systemic lupus erythematosus (SLE), is an autoimmune disease initiated during gestation by transplacental passage of maternal autoantibodies to intranuclear antigens, typically anti-SSA/Ro, anti-SSB/La, and/or anti-U1-ribonuclear protein (anti-RNP). Mothers with these autoantibodies classically have Sjogren's syndrome or SLE, but can be clinically asymptomatic – although this latter group often develops autoimmune disease in the years following delivery (43). NLS has also been associated with maternal leukocytoclastic vasculitis (44, 45). Fetal acquisition of these lupus-related autoantibodies may lead to systemic or limited syndromes which include cardiac disease, cutaneous lesions, nephritis, cytopenias, pneumonitis, central nervous system disorders, and/or hepatobiliary disease (46). Infants with NLS do not appear to have an increased risk of developing SLE (47), but may be at risk for developing other connective tissue disorders (48, 49). However, siblings of neonates with NLS have been reported to have an elevated risk of developing SLE, even if healthy at birth, supporting the idea that there is an underlying genetic susceptibility for lupus in these families. Like SLE, NLS has a gender predilection. Females are more likely to be affected than males, with a 2:1 ratio for cardiac disease, and

3:1 ratio for skin lesions (50). However, in contrast to SLE, NLS does not appear to preferentially affect a particular racial group.

NLS occurs in approximately 1 in 12 500–20 000 live births, and is felt to represent the combination of both pathogenic antibody acquisition and genetic/environmental factors (50). Only 2–5% of infants who acquire these maternal autoantibodies manifest signs and symptoms of NLS, supporting the idea that other factors are required for disease pathogenesis (reviewed in refs 51 and 52). In fact, discordant clinical expression of NLS has been reported in sets of twins where both infants were positive for maternally derived autoantibodies (53–55). Discordant expression of NLS has also been reported in a set of triplets carried by a mother with anti-SSA/Ro and anti-SSB/La autoantibodies (56). Certain major histocompatibility complex (MHC) class I and II alleles in the mothers have been associated with development of NLS in their infants (57). However, there appears to be no correlation between the development of NLS and the HLA alleles of the infants themselves (58), suggesting that maternal *cells* acquired by the fetus may play a role in the pathogenesis of NLS. Although there are many potential clinical manifestations of NLS, nearly half of the infants with NLS develop cutaneous lesions in sun-exposed areas in the first few weeks after birth, while the other half are born with complete or incomplete heart block; 10% suffer from concurrent skin and cardiac disease (50). Like SLE, NLS can cause life-threatening nephritis; however, unlike SLE, this manifestation is extremely rare.

The skin lesions of NLS typically consist of scaly, annular erythematous plaques at sun-exposed areas (often the head and neck), but other variations have been described (59). Exposure to sunlight causes ultraviolet radiation (UV)-induced apoptosis of skin cells, with presentation of normally sequestered intranuclear antigens. This process becomes problematic in the context of acquired maternal autoantibodies, which bind the apoptotic targets and incite a perivascular inflammatory infiltrate. Of note, sunlight is not absolutely required for the development of skin disease, as some antibody-positive infants exhibit cutaneous NLS at birth (59). Infants with NLS-related skin inflammation can be treated with topical corticosteroids and prevention of sun exposure. The skin lesions generally resolve over several months without residual effects, although they can result in permanent scarring in severe cases. In general, neonates with only skin, hematologic, or hepatic involvement have a better prognosis than those with cardiac disease, as these types of NLS typically remit with decline of the maternal autoantibodies in the infant's circulation (60).

The most significant problem in NLS is the development of congenital heart block (CHB), which carries a high morbidity and mortality (61). CHB was reported as early as 1901, but was not linked to maternal autoantibodies until the 1980s (62, 63). We now know that antibody-mediated NLS is responsible for most cases of CHB (50). More than 85% of fetuses who have conduction defects in the setting of a structurally normal heart have mothers with these autoantibodies (64, 65), but only 2% of women who have these pathogenic autoantibodies will have a child with CHB (66, 67). Unlike other manifestations of NLS, CHB is irreversible, even after loss of the maternal autoantibodies from the infant's circulation. This may be due to the fact that the antibody-mediated cardiac damage occurs in utero, as evidenced by detectable conduction abnormalities before the third trimester of gestation.

NLS-related CHB is associated with inflammatory fibrosis of the cardiac conducting system, endocardial fibroelastosis, endocardial hyperplasia, and other cardiomyopathies(68–70). Infants with CHB who survive often require pacemaker insertion, and can develop left ventricular cardiomyopathy even with adequate treatment (71). Cardiomyocyte apoptosis is required for the development of NLS, to allow exposure of target antigens at the lipid membrane of dying cells (72). Injection of human anti-SSB/La antibodies into pregnant mice resulted in antibody binding to apoptotic cells in selected organs, including the fetal heart, skin, liver, and bone (73), supporting the role of these autoantibodies in the pathogenesis of NLS. Antibody-coated apoptotic blebs may promote tissue scarring by stimulating local macrophages to produce transforming growth factor-beta (TGF-beta), a pro-fibrotic cytokine (74). Genetic polymorphisms linked to high TGF-beta production have been associated with increased risk for CHB (75).

In fetuses at risk for acquiring lupus-related autoantibodies, careful prenatal monitoring is warranted, including measurement of maternal autoantibody titers and Doppler evaluation to detect cardiac conduction defects in utero, as fetal CHB carries a 50% death rate (61, 68, 76). Women with these antibodies and a history of an affected fetus have a 2–3-fold higher risk of fetal CHB in subsequent pregnancies (61). Maternal plasmapheresis or immunoabsorption with and without dexamethasone may be beneficial during pregnancy (77–80), and in some cases dexamethasone has been associated with reversal of fetal conduction abnormalities, and increased survival at 1 year (68, 81). However, in cases that respond to corticosteroid administration, heart block may progress over time, even after the maternal antibodies have been degraded (47, 82). Treatment of affected neonates is largely symptomatic. Most infants with CHB will require pacemaker insertion and long-term monitoring, as CHB-related morbidity is high, and neonatal mortality approximates 10%.

CONGENITAL HEART BLOCK AND ANTI-ADRENOCEPTOR/CHOLINERGIC RECEPTOR ANTIBODIES

An antibody that binds both the cardiac beta-1-adrenoceptor and muscarinic acetylcholine receptor has been found in patients with "idiopathic" dilated cardiomyopathy (DCM) (83), DCM-associated atrial fibrillation (84), and congestive heart failure (85). Binding of this antibody to a ribosomal protein of *Trypanosoma cruzi* has also suggested a role for it in Chagas disease-associated cardiomyopathy, and implies an infectious etiology for its existence (86–89). Although it does not cause DCM in neonates, this autoantibody has been identified in infants with congential heart block (CHB) (41, 90). Using rat heart tissue samples, anti-adrenoceptor and anti-muscarinic cholinergic receptor IgG were found in infants with CHB and in their mothers, but not in controls. These autoantibodies could bind to and activate cardiac receptors, block ligand binding, and alter myocardial contractility, but only in neonatal rat tissues, suggesting a fetal antigen as the pathogenic target.

Although normally receptor agonists, these IgG antibodies act as receptor inhibitors when enzymatically cleaved to form monovalent antigen-binding fragments (Fab) by removal of the antibody constant region (91). In laboratory studies, monovalent Fab fragments derived from a stimulatory anti-beta-2-adrenoceptor IgG antibody acted as receptor antagonists, inducing conformational changes in the adrenoceptor and preventing ligand binding. The Fab fragments reacquired agonist activity when they were cross-linked to form divalent antibody. These findings are potentially relevant to neonatal disease as high-affinity IgG-derived Fab fragments comprise the major form of immunoglobulin in the meconium, even in babies who have not been breast-fed, suggesting a transplacental source (92). Thus, the effect of maternal autoantibodies in the neonate may depend not only on the antigen specificity, affinity, and antibody isotype, but also on whether or not the antibody is in a dimeric state. As the role of these anti-neurotransmitter antibodies in CHB is not yet well-understood, affected neonates should receive standard cardiac care. Comparison of fetal outcomes with measurement of antibody titers in women with previously affected infants or with a history of Chagas disease may provide a rationale for prenatal treatment in the future.

Fetal Arrhythmias and Anti-Myolemmal Antibodies

Anti-myolemmal antibodies (AMLA) cause lysis of cardiomyocytes in vitro, and have been implicated in adult cardiac diseases, including DCM and viral myocarditis. Transplacental transfer of AMLA from women with myocarditis may be responsible for fetal cardiac arrhythmia (93). Cord blood of infants born to mothers with and without myocarditis revealed that in 18 cases of fetal arrhythmia of unknown etiology, 13 mothers were positive for AMLA, as were five infants. In 19 healthy women, only three were found to have AMLA, and unaffected infants did not have these autoantibodies. Management of fetal arrhythmias has been previously discussed (94), but there are currently no guidelines for prenatal treatment of AMLA-exposed fetuses.

Hematopoietic Cell Diseases

Hemolytic Disease of the Newborn/Neonatal Anemia

Hemolytic disease of the newborn (HDN) has been well-described (95), and will only be briefly summarized here. Nearly all autoimmune HDN is caused by antibodies to Rhesus group antigen D (RhD), produced by women who lack the gene for this protein and thus do not express RhD on their own erythrocytes. The incidence of anti-RhD-related HDN is currently 1–6 per 1000 live births (95). First pregnancies are usually not affected. Women typically develop anti-RhD antibodies after delivery or loss of an RhD-positive infant, placing their subsequent pregnancies at risk for transplacental antibody transfer and disease. The anti-RhD antibodies are usually of IgG1 or IgG3 isotypes, and IgG1 is more pathogenic to the fetus than IgG3 (96).

For prevention of anti-RhD disease, infusion of anti-D antibodies to RhD-negative women has greatly improved neonatal outcomes by inhibiting maternal alloimmunization (reviewed in ref. 97). Fortunately, administration of anti-D immunoglobulin to pregnant women at risk for developing anti-RhD antibodies has not been found to result in fetal or neonatal hemolysis (98). For women who already have anti-RhD antibodies, anti-D infusion is not useful, and various maneuvers have been attempted to reduce fetal morbidity and mortality, including maternal plasmapheresis, high dose IVIG, and neonatal exchange transfusion, with variable success (99–102). In infants at risk of HDN, the occurence of hydrops fetalis and other complications has been greatly reduced by fetal blood sampling and in utero erythrocyte transfusions (103). In affected neonates, early serum bilirubin measurements are helpful in predicting whether an infant will develop severe hemolysis and significant hyperbilirubinemia (104, 105). The use of exchange transfusion in infants with ABO-incompatible HDN was found to have significant risks, including mortality (106). One randomized clinical trial of single versus double volume exchange transfusion for HDN showed that single volume exchange transfusion was as effective as double volume, and with less risk (107).

Although antibodies to RhD are the most common, transplacental transfer of maternal antibodies to other erythrocyte antigens may also lead to fetal anemia, including: anti-other Rh antigens (c, C, e, E), anti-ABO, anti-MNS, anti-Kell (K, k), anti-Duffy (Fya, Fyb), anti-Kidd (Jka, Jkb), anti-Lewis, anti-Lutheran, anti-Diego, and others (108–110). Moreover, the mechanism of action of these antibodies may involve more than just hemolysis. For example, the anti-Kell antibodies have been found to cause fetal anemia in part by inhibiting bone marrow erythropoesis (111). In these cases, measurement of maternal antibody titers or amniotic bilirubin levels are less useful for monitoring, and direct fetal blood sampling is required (112). Postnatal injections of erythropoietin have been successfully used to treat infants with anti-Kell-related anemia (113).

Neonatal thrombocytopenia can be caused by the transplacental transfer of anti-platelet antibodies from the mother to the fetus. Rarely, these antibodies are auto-reactive, and cause thrombocytopenia in the mother as well as the fetus, such as in cases of maternal idiopathic thrombocytopenic purpura (ITP). More commonly, however, the maternal antibodies are a result of feto-maternal incompatibility for human platelet-specific antigens (HPA) (114) and cause neonatal alloimmune thrombocytopenia (NAIT). NAIT is the primary cause of severe neonatal thrombocytopenia, occurring in approximately 1 in 1500–5000 live births (115).

Unlike maternal antibody-related hemolytic anemia, which requires sensitization to erythrocyte antigens in a prior pregnancy, most cases of NAIT occur in the first pregnancy, as the woman is sensitized to fetally expressed paternal antigens during gestation. Although many maternal antibody-mediated cytopenias resolve over time with loss of the offending maternal antibody, fetal thrombocytopenias can be severe enough in utero to cause life-threatening intracranial hemorrhage. Even if the fetus survives, intracranial hemorrhage may result in significant sequelae, including neonatal spasticity/hypotonia, seizures, developmental delay, or cortical blindness (116). In NAIT, the incidence of intracranial hemorrhage has been estimated at 20–30%, and neonatal death at approximately 10% (115, 117). In reality, the overall complication rate is even higher, as these numbers included closely monitored second pregnancies in women with a history of NAIT. When taking only the firstborn infants into account, the incidence and fatality rates increase to 47% and 24% respectively (117).

Management of NAIT has been recently reviewed (116). Prevention of NAIT-related complications includes fetal blood sampling to measure platelet counts as early as the 20th week of gestation. Women with currently affected fetuses or with a history of severely affected fetuses may benefit from weekly IVIG, with the addition of corticosteroids if the fetal platelet count does not respond. In fetuses with significant thrombocytopenia just prior to delivery, intrauterine platelet transfusions or delivery by cesarian section has been beneficial (117). Postnatally, infants may require IVIG or platelet transfusions. Platelet levels should be followed for at least 1 month after birth, until maternal antibodies have diminished (116).

NEONATAL NEUTROPENIA

Anti-neutrophil IgG transmitted to the fetus across the placenta may result in profound neutropenia. Neutropenia becomes a significant problem shortly after birth, as these neonates are susceptible to severe bacterial infections which can lead to death or permanent disability (118). As with neonatal thrombocytopenia, neonatal neutropenia may be caused by maternal autoantibodies which also cause neutropenia in the mother, or, more commonly, by maternal alloantibodies which only cause disease in the fetus (119). The incidence of neonatal alloimmune neutropenia is approximately 1 in 2000 live births (120), and true autoimmune neutropenia is rare.

Most of the maternal anti-neutrophil antibodies target the human neutrophil-specific antigens (HNA) (121, 122), but there are several reports of antibodies against neutrophil targets other than HNA (118, 123–125), and neonatal lupus syndrome may also cause neutropenia (126, 127). Prenatal management of IgG-mediated neutropenia involves monitoring of maternal anti-neutrophil antibody titers (and maternal neutrophil counts, in cases of autoimmune neutropenia). After delivery the infant's neutrophil count can be followed, and neonates treated with antibiotics as needed. Prenatal and postnatal administration of recombinant human granulocyte colony-stimulating factor has also been shown to be beneficial in the treatment of both auto- and alloimmune neonatal neutropenia (121, 128).

NEONATAL LYMPHOCYTOPENIA

Maternal antibody-mediated neonatal lymphocytopenia is rare. Two infants with severe antibody-mediated lymphocytopenia and thrombocytopenia were born to a woman who had been sensitized to fetally expressed paternal antigens during her five previous pregnancies (129). Antibody transfer resulted in congenital immuno-deficiency in both infants. One of the affected neonates died 16 days after birth due to severe graft-versus-host disease (GVHD), caused by transplacental acquisition of maternal lymphocytes. The other infant was diagnosed with sepsis and treated with exchange transfusion, which resulted in reversal of the antibody-mediated cytope-nias and recovery. IgG from the mother was found to react with non-HLA paternal antigens expressed on neonatal leukocytes, and serial testing after her last pregnancy revealed a steady decline in her anti-paternal IgG titers.

Neonatal Endocrine Diseases

NEONATAL HYPOTHYROIDISM AND ANTAGONISTIC ANTI-THYROID ANTIBODIES

Circulating autoantibodies in pregnant women with autoimmune thyroid disease may cross the placenta and cause aberrant thyroid function in the fetus and neonate (130). In a series of infants with transient congenital hypothyroidism, maternal autoimmune thyroid disease was found in every case, suggesting that the infants had acquired maternal autoantibodies (131). Autoantibodies associated with auto-immune hypothyroidism include anti-thyroid-stimulating hormone (anti-TSH) antibodies, antagonistic TSH receptor (TSH-R) antibodies, or anti-thyroid perox-idase antibodies. As with other maternal antibody-mediated diseases, neonatal manifestations usually resolve with catabolism of the relevant autoantibodies. However, severe cases of maternal antibody-mediated gestational hypothyroidism can lead to permanent damage, including abnormal brain development or fetal loss (132). The long-term effects of transient exposure to maternal anti-thryoid auto-antibodies is not known, but the presence of anti-thyroid peroxidase antibodies in cord blood has been associated with an increased risk of future autoimmune thy-roiditis (133) and with lower scores on cognitive testing, even in offspring of mothers who were euthyroid (134).

Fetuses of women with autoimmune thyroiditis are at risk for acquiring other maternal autoantibodies as well, due to the association of autoimmune thyroid disease with other connective tissue disorders such as Sjogren syndrome or SLE (135–137). In addition, fetal disease caused by other maternally derived autoanti-bodies can be exacerbated in the context of maternal hypothyroidism. Infants of women with lupus-associated anti-SSA/La or anti-SSB/Ro antibodies had a 9-fold increased risk of developing complete CHB if the mother was also hypothyroid (138). However, the mechanism of this synergy is not clear.

Management of neonatal hypothyroidism involves laboratory monitoring of the mother throughout pregnancy, with exogenous thyroxine administration as needed, taking into account her gestational requirements (139). After birth, the neonate can be followed with serial evaluations of thyroid function and maternal autoantibody titers, and treated with thyroxine until thyroid function has normalized.

NEONATAL HYPERTHYROIDISM AND AGONISTIC ANTI-TSH RECEPTOR ANTIBODIES

Neonatal hyperthyroidism is less common than neonatal hypothyroidism. The prevalence of Graves disease among pregnant women is estimated to be 0.2%, and clinically apparent hyperthyroidism due to transplacental transmission of stim-ulatory anti-TSH-R antibodies occurs in less than 1% of these pregnancies (140). As with other maternal antibody-mediated diseases, neonatal hyperthyroidism typically resolves with loss of maternal antibodies in the first 4 months of life (141). However, if untreated, fetal and neonatal thyrotoxicosis may lead to death.

Although the anti-TSH R antibodies produced in Graves disease are typically agonistic, antagonistic antibodies are often produced as well. In a study of pregnant women over time, the ratio of these antibody types was found to change during pregnancy, such that the antibody specificity became predominantly one of TSH-R blockade (142). Although maternal autoantibody-mediated effects on the developing fetus were not evaluated in this particular study, it is clear that there are potential dangers for induction of both neonatal hyper- and hypothyroidism during pregnancies complicated by Graves disease.

Management of neonatal thyroid disease involves laboratory evaluation of the mother throughout pregnancy, as well as monitoring of fetal growth and heart rate. Prenatal thyroid status can be followed using ultrasonography to measure fetal thyroid gland size and progression of skeletal maturation (143). In selected cases, umbilical cord blood sampling can be used to directly measure thyroid hormone levels (144). Fetal hyperthyroidism can be treated by administration of medications to the pregnant woman. After birth, the infant should have serial laboratory evaluations of thyroid function, and pharmacotherapy until thyroid function has normalized (141, 145).

Neonatal Exposure to Diabetes-Related Autoantibodies

Type I diabetes mellitus (DM I) is caused by the autoimmune destruction of pancreatic beta cells, and is associated with the presence of specific autoantibodies against insulin, the insulin receptor, and various islet cell antigens. These diabetes-associated autoantibodies can be transferred to the fetus.

Anti-insulin Autoantibodies. Transplacental acquisition of anti-insulin autoantibodies (AIA) or insulin-AIA complexes has been documented in infants of women with these IgG (146–149). Individuals with AIA also often produce its anti-idiotypic antibody (150). The anti-idiotypes bind not only AIA, but can block the insulin receptor, leading to neonatal fatality in some cases. However, if both AIA and anti-idiotype are present at high levels, they will bind to and neutralize each other, preventing interference with insulin signaling (see Fig. 9-1). Recent work has demonstrated that approximately one-third of polyclonal AIA from diabetic patients also cross-reacts with nerve growth factor (NGF) (150). Transplacental transfer of these antibodies could potentially lead to NGF-depletion during fetal development, suggesting a mechanism for the neuropathy seen in children born to mothers with AIA.

In genetically susceptible non-obese diabetic (NOD) mice, the risk of neonatal diabetes did not seem to correlate with the presence or absence of maternally

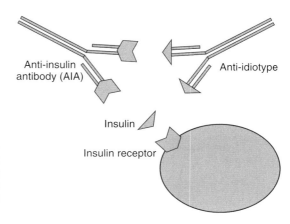

Figure 9-1 Anti-insulin and anti-idiotype autoantibodies. Anti-insulin antibody (AIA) can bind either insulin or anti-idiotype antibodies. The anti-idiotype antibody can bind AIA or the insulin receptor. If both antibodies are present in adequate concentrations, they can bind and neutralize each other.

derived AIA (151), while under other experimental conditions, maternal AIA appeared to play a central role in neonatal disease (152, 153). In human neonates, the transient presence of AIA has not been associated with the future development of diabetes (154, 155); however, the presence of autoantibodies after 9 months of age, by which time the maternally derived antibodies should have cleared, is associated with increased risk (154). As it has not been shown whether diabetes-related maternal autoantibodies cause neonatal disease, there are no known preventive measures or specific treatments recommended at this time. Infants who manifest signs of hyperglycemia should receive standard diabetes management.

Anti-islet Cell, Anti-glutamic Acid Decarboxylase, and Anti-IA-2 Protein Autoantibodies. Other maternal autoantibodies associated with DM I include anti-islet cell antibodies (ICA), anti-glutamic acid decarboxylase (anti-GAD) antibodies, and anti-protein tyrosine phosphatase IA-2 (anti-IA-2) antibodies, all of which have been found to be transplacentally transferred. Levels of these autoantibodies in the serum of pregnant women were compared to those in their infant's cord blood after birth (156). Of the women with DM I, almost 40% had ICA, 55% had anti-GAD, and 54% had anti-IA-2. Of the infants born to diabetic mothers, 33% had ICA, 50% had anti-GAD, and 51% had anti-IA-2. In non-diabetic mothers, 5.2% had ICA, 5.2% had anti-GAD, and 3% had anti-IA-2. Of the infants born to non-diabetic mothers, 6% had ICA, 2.2% had anti-GAD, and none had anti-IA-2. Infants of mothers lacking these autoantibodies had no autoantibodies in their cord blood. It is not clear whether exposure to these autoantibodies in utero increases the risk of developing DM I, but infants with anti-GAD, anti-IA-2, or AIA in their cord blood were not found to have significantly altered birth weights or insulin concentrations when compared to controls (157, 158).

Anti-adrenal Autoantibodies. Little is known regarding the fetal effects of maternal autoantibodies related to other autoimmune endocrine diseases. Transplacental transfer of anti-adrenal autoantibodies has been reported in rare cases. One infant born to a mother with Addison disease and gestational DM was found to have anti-adrenal cortex and anti-islet cells antibodies at birth, but no signs or symptoms of disease (159). Another infant born to a woman with autoimmune polyendocrine syndrome type II (Addison disease, DM I, and autoimmune thyroiditis) had anti-adrenal cortex and anti-steroid-21-hydroxylase autoantibodies at birth, but also remained clinically asymptomatic (160). Although these cases suggest that anti-adrenal autoantibodies do not cause fetal pathology, establishing treatment recommendations will require screening a larger number of selected infants for subclinical adrenal disease.

Neuromuscular Diseases

NEONATAL MYASTHENIA GRAVIS AND ANTI-ACETYLCHOLINE RECEPTOR ANTIBODIES

Neonatal myasthenia gravis (NMG) is an uncommon autoimmune disease resulting from transplacental acquisition of maternal anti-AChR antibodies (161). These antibodies result in pathologic muscle weakness which typically presents within the first 72 h of life. As in other types of maternal antibody-mediated syndromes, the severity of disease does not necessarily correlate with the antibody titer in the mother or infant. There are reports of neonates with acquired anti-AChR antibodies who remain clinically asymptomatic (162), and cases of NMG in which only one fetus of a twin gestation is affected (163, 164), suggesting that antibody acquisition alone may not be enough to cause clinical manifestations (165).

Some maternal anti-AChR antibodies are specific for the *fetal* form of AChR, and cause NMG only in the fetus, while the mother remains asymptomatic (166, 167).

Examination of human skeletal muscle revealed that the fetal form of AChR is present until 31 weeks of gestation (168), suggesting that antibody-mediated damage may take place early in development. Clinical disease is generally more severe in cases with anti-fetal AChR antibodies, and the risk of NMG in the subsequent pregnancies of these women is estimated to be 100%. Although the absolute autoantibody levels in women vary greatly, the ratio of anti-fetal/anti-adult AChR remains fairly constant in individual mothers over time, and is a much better predictor of the development of NMG (169). NMG usually resolves as maternal antibody is lost from the neonatal circulation between 1 and 6 months of age (170). However, if the disease is severe enough during gestation, there may be long-term, irreversible sequelae. For example, anti-AChR antibody-mediated major fetal akinesia may lead to arthrogryposis multiplex congenita (congenital polyarticular contractures), abnormal pulmonary development, velopharyngeal incompetence, and even death (166, 167, 171, 172).

There are no known preventive measures for NMG. Maternal myasthenia gravis is not an absolute contraindication to pregnancy, and successful pregnancy can be achieved with the appropriate pre- and postnatal care (164, 173). Prevention of NMG involves identifying women with myasthenia gravis, but this is complicated by the fact that some women with anti-AChR antibodies are completely asymptomatic (174). If the fetus is affected by NMG, ultrasonography may reveal reduced fetal movement or polyhydramnios due to decreased swallowing, and the pregnant woman may note a change in fetal activity. An oxytocin challenge can be used to evaluate fetal health, and continuous fetal monitoring may be beneficial in selected cases. After delivery, infants suspected of having NMG can be tested using neostigmine or other cholinesterase inhibitors.

Management of NMG consists of supportive treatment. Neonatal autoantibody levels can be monitored with the expectation that clinical manifestations of NMG will regress within the first 2 months as antibody levels decline. Some have tried using neonatal plasmapheresis or IVIG to speed the recovery process (175, 176). However, unlike in adults, treatment with IVIG has not been proven to be effective in NMG (176), and IVIG use in any patient is associated with serious risks, including anaphylactic reactions, aseptic meningitis, acute renal failure, cardiovascular thromboses, transmission of viral pathogens, and other complications (reviewed in refs 177 and 178).

NEONATAL GUILLAIN-BARRE

Campylobacter jejuni enteritis is associated with the development of Guillain-Barre syndrome in one in 1000 cases (179, 180). In susceptible individuals, production of an anti-*Campylobacter* antibody cross-reactive with a human peripheral nerve antigen may lead to Guillain-Barre syndrome. Infants of women with Guillain-Barre syndrome can develop a transient version of this neuromuscular disease, called neonatal Guillain-Barre (NGB). Cases of NGB have also been described in infants born to women with active ulcerative colitis during pregnancy (181, 182). This is interesting as inflammatory bowel disease has also been linked to a history of bacterial enteritis. However, the responsible antibody and antigenic target(s) have not been identified.

One infant born to a woman with active Guillain-Barre syndrome developed NGB 12 days after birth, characterized by flaccid paralysis and respiratory distress (183). As he had not been breast-fed, his disease was attributed to transplacental transfer of maternal autoantibodies. In laboratory testing, IgG from the mother or infant blocked neuromuscular transmission in murine diaphragmatic muscle explants. However, IgG-mediated neuromuscular blockade did not require interaction with complement components or leukocyte Fc receptors, as monovalent antigen-binding fragments (Fab) of this antibody had the same effect.

Diaphragmatic muscles from mice younger than 5 days of age were not affected by this antibody, and there were no clinical signs in the infant until nearly 2 weeks after birth, suggesting that the target antigen is not expressed, active, or accessible in fetal tissues. Thus, acquisition of maternal autoantibody against a developmentally regulated protein spared the fetus from disease, but caused neuromuscular pathology in the neonate.

As with many of the rare maternal antibody-mediated neonatal diseases, prevention and treatment of NGB has not been systematically studied. In the case of maternally derived NGB described above, the infant was treated with IVIG and recovered quickly. He had no further sequelae, and subsequent laboratory testing showed loss of the pathogenic IgG from his circulation by 3 months of age (183).

NEONATAL LOWER MOTOR NEUROPATHY AND ANTI-GANGLIOSIDE ANTIBODY

Maternal autoantibodies associated with other neuropathies can also be transferred during gestation. For example, anti-ganglioside GM-1 antibodies were transplacentally acquired by the fetus of a woman with multifocal motor neuropathy, although she had been treated with monthly IVIG throughout pregnancy (184). Monoclonal IgG was detectable in neonatal serum for 4 months after birth, and distal muscle atrophy and weakness were present both pre- and post-natally. Although the infant's distal motor function improved over time, he suffered long-term sequelae, revealed by abnormal nerve conduction studies in childhood.

Collagen-Vascular Diseases

ANTI-NEUTROPHIL CYTOPLASMIC ANTIBODY

Anti-neutrophil cytoplasmic antibodies (ANCA) directed at neutrophil-derived myeloperoxidase (MPO) are associated with systemic small vessel vasculitides. Transmission of maternal MPO-ANCA to the fetus can result in neonatal vasculitis. A pregnant woman with MPO-ANCA gave birth at 33 weeks of gestation to an infant who developed life-threatening pulmonary hemorrhage and renal disease on day 2 of life (185). Anti-MPO antibody was present in the infant's cord blood at birth. The neonate was treated with high-dose corticosteroids on day 2 and with exchange transfusion on day 5, resulting in undetectable antibody by day 25, and no further recurrence of the disease.

Women with ANCA-associated diseases should be carefully monitored and the antibody levels well-controlled at the time of pregnancy. It is unknown whether corticosteroid treatment during pregnancy would improve neonatal outcome, but extrapolation from other maternal antibody-mediated diseases suggests that this may be beneficial. However, the benefits of prenatal and postnatal corticosteroid administration must be weighed against its potential adverse effects, which include perinatal death, cardiovascular disease, neurologic abnormalities (186–188), and possibly, an increased risk of future autoimmunity (189).

MONOCLONAL GAMMOPATHIES

Neonatal connective tissue diseases may result from the transfer of monoclonal maternal antibodies or immune complexes. A neonate born to a woman with monoclonal IgG-lambda developed glomerulonephritis and acute renal failure within the first week after delivery (190). This infant was found to have an antibody which was elecrophoretically identical to that found in her mother. Treatment with neonatal exchange transfusion was successful in resolving her clinical symptoms. In another case, a woman with a diagnosis of essential type I cryoglobulinemia gave birth to a set of twins who developed cyanotic macules when exposed to cold (191). They both had the same monoclonal IgG as their mother, and their clinical manifestations resolved after 6 months, supporting a direct role for maternal antibodies as the cause of this neonatal disease. In another case, a preterm infant was incidentally found to have a monoclonal gammopathy identical to that of his mother (192), suggesting that the incidence of neonatal monoclonal gammopathies may be higher than expected, as these antibodies do not always cause clinically apparent disease. Due to the heterogeneity of this rare syndrome, infants with monoclonal gammopathies can only be managed on a case-by-case basis.

Nutritional Deficiencies

NEURAL TUBE DEFECTS AND ANTI-FOLATE RECEPTOR ANTIBODIES

Folate deficiency during gestation results in neural tube defects, fetal loss, preterm birth, and intrauterine growth restriction (IUGR) (193). Although folate supplementation in pregnant women greatly reduces the risk of neural tube defects, the majority of women with affected fetuses do not have clinical folate deficiency during pregnancy, suggesting that the additional folate is needed to overcome a block to folate uptake by the developing fetus (194). In support of this hypothesis, autoantibodies to the folate receptor were found in nine of 12 women with a pregnancy complicated by neural tube defects and in two of 20 controls (although these antibodies were of lower affinity) (194). These maternal autoantibodies were found to bind folate receptors isolated from human placenta, suggesting a mechanism of action for fetal pathogenesis.

Of note, a majority of the affected fetuses in this study were the result of a first pregnancy, making it difficult to ascertain whether the maternal autoantibodies had been generated as a result of alloimmunization during pregnancy or in response to an unrelated antigen. Due to the high rate of disease in first-born infants, and lack of clinical signs in their mothers, screening for anti-folate receptor autoantibodies is not feasible or cost-effective. Rather, all women should receive folate supplementation throughout conception, gestation, and breast-feeding, as supplementation appears to be able to overcome the effect of these maternal autoantibodies (194).

NEONATAL PERNICIOUS ANEMIA AND ANTI-INTRINSIC FACTOR ANTIBODIES

Transplacental transfer of maternal autoantibodies which bind intrinsic factor may lead to cobalamin (vitamin B12) deficiency. In adults, these autoantibodies interfere with intrinsic factor-mediated uptake of cobalamin from the gut, leading to pernicious anemia, neuropathy, and atrophic gastritis in severely affected cases (reviewed in ref. 195). Anti-intrinsic factor autoantibodies acquired during gestation can cause fetal cobalamin deficiency with cytopenias, failure to thrive, and neurologic deficits (196).

Like many autoantibodies, the presence of anti-intrinsic factor antibodies indicates an increased risk of other maternal autoimmune diseases, including autoimmune thyroiditis, DM I, and SLE, as these syndromes often coexist (197–199). Therefore, the finding of anti-intrinsic factor antibodies in the neonate should prompt consideration for other maternal autoantibody-mediated diseases, and vice-versa. To prevent fetal pathology, pregnant women with anti-intrinsic factor autoantibodies should receive cobalamin supplementation to ensure adequate serum levels. Neonates can be supplemented with cobalamin until loss of maternal autoantibody has been verified.

Skin Disease

NEONATAL PEMPHIGUS AND ANTI-DESMOGLEIN ANTIBODIES

Desmogleins (Dsg) are cadherin-like adhesion molecules which function to maintain tissue integrity and facilitate cell-cell communication. These proteins are the target antigens in epidermal blistering diseases such as pemphigus, caused by

Table 9-2 Correlation of Autoantibodies with Adult and Neonatal Skin Disease

	Anti-Dsg-1 antibodies	Anti-Dsg-3 antibodies
Adult disease	Pemphigus folaceous	Pemphigus vulgaris
Neonatal disease	Rare effects	Pemphigus vulgaris

autoantibody-mediated acantholysis (disruption of keratinocyte adhesion) (200). To date, four isoforms of desmogleins (Dsg1–4) have been identified in humans (201). These isoforms are differentially expressed in various epithelial tissues, so that antibody specificity plays a significant role in determining the clinical outcome. For example, autoantibodies to Dsg-1 cause pemphigus foliaceus (PF) in adults, with prominent skin blistering in the upper layers of the epidermis, while anti-Dsg-3 antibodies cause pemphigus vulgaris (PV), with blistering in the suprabasal layer of the skin and in the mucous membranes (200). Transplacental transfer of auto-antibodies from women with PF only rarely causes clinical symptoms in infants (27), as the Dsg target isoforms have a different distribution (Table 9-2). The neonatal epidermal Dsg pattern more closely resembles that of adult mucous membranes, suggesting that the high levels of Dsg-3 can compensate for antibody-mediated loss of Dsg-1 (202). Functional studies using transgenic mice engineered to express human Dsg-3 in their epidermis confirmed protection from human anti-Dsg-1 antibodies. The importance of Dsg-3 in neonatal disease is further exemplified by case reports of infants with extensive PV following acquisition of maternal anti-Dsg-3 (203, 204), including one case where the mother's PV was in remission (205).

Adult PV is endemic in Brazil, and there is a correlation between individuals with anti-Dsg-1 and a history of infectious disease, notably onchocerciasis and Chagas disease (206). It is interesting to speculate that transplacental transfer of anti-Dsg-1 in endemic areas may be meant to protect the offspring from infection without causing pemphigus, due to the skewed fetal expression of desmogleial isoforms as outlined above. The heterogeneity of the anti-epidermal anti-bodies makes prediction of neonatal disease difficult; investigators found that a subset of antibodies to Dsg-1 could cross-react with the Dsg-4 isoform (207), revealing that the pathogenic profile of anti-Dsg antibodies varies not only based on the distribution of Dsg isoforms in the affected individual, but on antigen-specificity of the autoantibody. The autoantibody production in these diseases is typically polyclonal, with IgG4 produced early in disease, and IgG1 later; both of these IgG isotypes may cross the placenta (200). There may be other important factors involved in mediating pemphigus as well. Anti-Dsg serum antibody titers were found to correlate with dermal dendritic cell numbers in lesioned skin, suggesting that cellular immune factors may play a role (208), but there are currently no data regarding dermal dendritic cells in neonatal pemphigus.

Clinical disease is not only painful, but subjects the neoate to risk of infection, fluid loss, and weight loss due to diminished feeding (200). There are no known preventive measures. In women with active or historical blistering skin disease, serial measurements of autoantibody titers can guide treatment, which may include plasma exchange and/or corticosteroids (209, 210). Infants of these women are monitored for disease and treated symptomatically. In animal models, cholinergic agonists block antibody-induced acantholysis (211), and application of wheat germ agglutinin can interfere with autoantibody binding to Dsg-1 (212), but these approaches have not yet been tried in humans.

Neonatal Liver Diseases

Neonatal Liver Disease and Antinuclear Antibody

Mothers of infants with idiopathic neonatal cholestasis, biliary atresia, or other liver diseases were found to have a higher than expected frequency of serum antinuclear antibodies (ANA), suggesting a link between maternal autoimmunity and neonatal liver disease (213). However, no specific role for ANA has been elucidated, and it is unclear whether the ANA are directly pathogenic or merely markers of disease.

Neonatal Hemochromatosis

Neonatal hemochromatosis (NH) is a rare disease manifested by cirrhosis, liver fibrosis, and intra- and extrahepatic siderosis (214). Fetuses with NH often suffer from IUGR, and can die during gestation. Those surviving until delivery may have oligohydramnios or renal dysgenesis, and may develop fulminant hepatic failure necessitating transplantation. Although twins and triplets discordant for NH have been described, their apparently healthy siblings also have abnormal measures of hepatic function on laboratory testing, suggesting an underestimation of the true incidence of NH (215, 216).

Transmission of NH is unusual; no genetic mutation for this disease has been identified, and after a woman has one infant with NH, her chance of having a subsequently affected pregnancy is approximately 80% (217). In light of these facts, investigators hypothesized that NH is caused by transplacental transfer of maternal antibodies to a fetal liver antigen not expressed in the mother. Studies to identify this antigen are currently underway.

There is no specific prenatal testing for NH. However, in a clinical trial, 15 women with previously affected pregnancies received weekly IVIG starting in week 18 of gestation until delivery (218). All 16 babies born to these women survived without surgical treatment, although 12 had signs of NH. In contrast to prior pregnancies, there were no cases of IUGR, fetal distress, or oligohydramnios, suggesting that this treatment was highly beneficial. Postnatal management of NH includes the use of MRI for detection of siderosis in neonatal tissues, and measurement of serum AFP and ferritin as sensitive markers of disease (216). Chelation therapies and antioxidant cocktails administered to newborns with NH have only had limited success, with a high morbidity and mortality (219, 220).

Complications of Pregnancy

Several maternal autoantibodies have been linked to decreased fertility and/or pregnancy complications (221). Although some of these antibodies cause maternal autoimmune disease which can be directly associated with decreased fertility, these autoantibodies may also bind fetal-placental antigens and cause gestational disease in a manner unrelated to their primary mode of action.

Anti-Angiotensin II Receptor Antibody

Anti-angiotensin II receptor (anti-AT-1) autoantibodies in the serum of pregnant women have been associated with preeclampsia. Antibody-mediated receptor stimulation upregulates production of tissue factor by vascular smooth muscle cells, expression of plasminogen activator inhibitor-1 and interleukin-6 by trophoblasts and mesangial cells, and increases the rate of cardiomyocyte contraction (222–224). In an experimental animal model, rats with anti-AT-1 autoantibodies also develop a preeclampsia-like syndrome (225), supporting a pathogenic role for these antibodies in vivo.

Although these autoantibodies have been linked to preeclampsia, it is not known whether transplacental transfer of these antibodies causes autoimmune disease in the neonate. Recent studies reveal the presence of these autoantibodies in patients with renal-allograft rejection and malignant hypertension (226), suggesting that transfer of these antibodies to the fetus may cause renovascular disease.

ANTI-PHOSPHOLIPID ANTIBODY

Antiphospholipid antibodies (APLA) are found in nearly 40% of women with SLE, and approximately 5% of the child-bearing population (227). The presence of maternal APLA has been associated with spontaneous abortion, fetal death, IUGR, and preeclampsia (reviewed in ref. 228). APLA mediate their negative perinatal effects via pleiotropic mechanisms. These include interference with normal trophoblast function in early and late gestation, and creation of a hypercoagulable state (by inhibition of endogenous anticoagulants, activation of platelets and endothelial cells, and disruption of vascular endothelium), leading to spontaneous abortion and/or placental thrombosis and infarction (229).

APLA can be transplacentally acquired–neonatal APLA antibody titers, isotypes, and specificities correlate with the maternal levels (230, 231). These autoantibodies are not generally associated with disease in the neonate (230), but there are reports of fetal stroke in pregnant women with high APLA titers (232). In the neonate, APLA levels decline over time, becoming undetectable at 6 months, consistent with transplacental acquisition of maternal autoantibodies. It is not known whether perinatal exposure to APLA has any effect on future development of SLE.

Many interventions have been attempted for the prevention of fetal disease in women with symptomatic APLA syndrome; however, the most promising treatment involves the use of heparin (228). Many APLA effects are related to excessive antibody-mediated complement activation, which is blocked by heparin (233, 234). Current recommendations for pregnant women include treatment with heparin or heparin-derived compounds in conjunction with low-dose aspirin (reviewed in refs 228 and 229). Cases refractory to pharmacotherapy can be treated with high-dose IVIG.

ANTI-LAMININ-1 ANTIBODY

The laminin-1 glycoproteins in uterine and fetal tissues play an integral role in normal implantation and are required for maintenance of placental integrity (235–237). Maternal anti-laminin-1 autoantibodies have been linked to recurrent spontaneous abortion (237, 238), and pathogenicity of these antibodies was demonstrated in an animal model which revealed increased fetal resorption rates in mice immunized with laminin-1 (235). Pregnant mice with anti-laminin-1 autoantibodies also had underweight fetuses and placentas compared to controls. There are no data regarding the effect of transplacental acquisition of anti-laminin-1 autoantibodies on infants who survive to term.

ANTI-TISSUE TRANSGLUTAMINASE ANTIBODY

Autoantibodies to tissue transglutaminase (anti-tTg) are classically associated with celiac disease and dermatitis herpetiformis, as its target protein is expressed in both the gastrointestinal tract and skin (239). However, women with celiac disease also have decreased fertility, higher rates of spontaneous abortion, IUGR, and low birth weight infants, all of which vastly improve with adherence to a gluten-free diet (240). These observations have led to the hypothesis that anti-tTg antibodies are directly detrimental to the fetus. In support of this idea, human tissue transglutaminase has been found to be temporally and compartmentally expressed in placental stromal cells, trophoblasts, and decidual cells, and was shown to be functionally active in fibroblast extracellular matrix and syncytial microvillous membranes (241, 242). These data suggest an important role for tissue transglutaminase in normal placental development and function. It is not known whether the maternal autoantibodies traverse the placenta and cause disease in the fetus itself, but maternal anti-tTg antibodies are detectable in cord blood (239). Anti-tTg antibodies in the neonate do not appear to increase the risk of developing future celiac disease.

Anti-AChR Antibody

Women with myasthenia gravis have an increased rate of premature rupture of membranes, major congenital anomalies, necessity for cesarean section, and other complications, all of which significantly increase fetal morbidity and mortality (243). These effects are not merely due to maternal disease, as women with asymptomatic myasthenia gravis – either in remission or prior to initial diagnosis – also have a higher rate of protracted labor, induced labor, and perinatal mortality (244).

Anti-Thyroid Antibody

Anti-thyroid autoantibodies may cause gestational complications such as preterm birth and spontaneous abortion, even if the mother is euthyroid (245, 246). Maternal *hypo*thyroidism-related autoantibodies have been linked to spontaneous abortion, preterm delivery, and neuropsychiatric abnormalities. Maternal *hyper*thyroidism-related autoantibodies have been linked to spontaneous abortion, preterm delivery, placenta abruptio, congestive heart failure, preeclampsia, and fetal thyrotoxicosis (247). The mechanisms of autoantibody action in some of the above complications are not known.

Maternally Derived Antibodies and the Development of Future Autoimmunity

Although autoantibody-mediated diseases in the newborn often resolve upon the loss of maternal antibodies, autoimmunity that develops later in life may have its origins in the perinatal period, making even the transient presence of maternally derived antibodies a critical factor. In fact, rather than autoantigens, most maternal antibodies are directed against infectious agents. However, these anti-pathogen antibodies could also play a role in promotion or prevention of autoimmunity. For example, transfer of maternal antibodies against a virus or bacterium may alter the fetal or neonatal immune response and/or level of infection, thereby changing the role of this pathogen in the development of autoimmunity. Conversely, the antibody may promote transplacental transfer of a virus or other pathogen which could infect the fetus and influence future autoimmunity. Maternal antibodies may transfer non-infectious proteins which could trigger a cross-reactive autoimmune response in the fetus, or alter cytokine and chemokine expression via interaction with fetal/neonatal leukocyte Fc receptors. Theoretically, environmental toxins could also cross the placenta via binding to maternal antibodies, resulting in vertical transmission of mutagens which may play a role in autoimmunity. Food or other environmental antigens/allergens in the fetus may also be targets of maternal antibodies, with the resultant immune complexes playing a role in the development of autoimmunity.

One example of the link between early antibody transfer and future autoimmunity is seen in relation to the development of type I diabetes mellitus (DM I). The prevalence of DM I in a population is inversely correlated with maternal anti-enterovirus antibody levels, suggesting that maternal anti-pathogen antibodies may protect against the development of DM I (248). Moreover, the production of diabetes-associated autoantibodies (anti-insulin, anti-ICA, anti-GAD, or anti-IA-2) in susceptible children has been associated with antecedent enteroviral infection, with 13% of the infections in this study occurring prior to 6 months of age (249). In another study, enterovirus infections led to the production of antibodies which were crossreactive with IA-2 in 7% of patients, supporting the idea that these infections lead to production of antibodies against DM I-associated antigens (250). Whether maternal anti-enterovirus antibodies mediate protection from autoimmunity by preventing viral propagation and immune stimulation, by blocking pathogenic antigens crossreactive with host proteins, or by interacting with other antibodies or viruses unrelated to the primary infection is unknown.

MATERNAL MICROCHIMERISM (MMc) AND NEONATAL AUTOIMMUNITY

Normal Physiology

Fetal–maternal two-way cell traffic during pregnancy had been described as early as 1960 (251, 252). The small number of maternal cells living within a child is termed maternal microchimerism (MMc) (8), to signify the origin of the allogeneic cells in the chimeric offspring, and it has been hypothesized that increased maternal–fetal blood exchange in complicated pregnancies or traumatic deliveries leads to increased MMc in the fetus. Maternal DNA can be detected in the healthy human fetus as early as the 13th week of gestation (253), while in the mouse, maternal cell transfer begins between 9 and 12 days of gestation, when the placental circulation develops and fetal hematopoieisis begins (254). In contrast to maternal antibody titer, which is low in preterm infants and increases with gestational age, the level of MMc in the blood does not seem to be affected by gestational age (253, 255). However, the levels of MMc in developing organs have yet to be quantitated.

One major challenge in this field has been the accurate quantification of MMc. Previous methods used semi-quantitative PCR or tedious cell counting of female cells identified in male subjects. To quantitate low levels of MMc in patients and controls, a panel of real-time Q-PCR assays to target non-shared maternal HLA genes has been developed (256). With 14 specific HLA sequences, the assay panel is informative for 90% of patient-mother pairs, with a sensitivity of one in 100 000. Importantly, these assays have been validated in 47 cell lines expressing different HLA alleles to demonstrate that there is no cross-reactivity. In an initial study of MMc, maternal DNA was detected in genomic DNA isolated from peripheral blood mononuclear cells in 22% of healthy adults, with levels ranging from 0 to 68.6 genome equivalents per million host cells, suggesting that MMc is a normal and not infrequent occurrence in the general population (256).

MMc is commonly found in cord blood. Early studies used labeled maternal blood re-transfused into the mother shortly before delivery to track transfer of maternal cells into the cord blood during parturition (252, 257). More recently, the presence of maternal DNA in 40–100% of human umbilical cord blood samples was revealed using the high-sensitivity quantitative polymerase chain reaction (Q-PCR) (255, 258–260). However, it is known that cell-free DNA may circulate between the mother and fetus, and thus detection of DNA alone does not prove cell trafficking. In fact, when examining mother-to-fetus cell transfer, the fractional concentration of maternal DNA in cord plasma samples was more than 10-fold greater than maternal nucleated cells detected (261). Using fluorescence in situ hybridization (FISH) for X- and Y-chromosome sequences in whole cells, 20% of male cord blood samples were found to contain female cells, presumably maternal (5).

It is not known how maternal cells transfer to the fetus, or what regulates the transfer. After birth, maternal cells may also be acquired by infants during breast-feeding. MMc has been found in multiple peripheral blood cell types, including macrophages, B cells, natural killer cells, and natural killer T cells (262), and maternal T lymphocytes have been identified in cases of childhood disease (263, 264). That maternal T lymphocytes are active after transfer is evidenced by the finding of cells retaining their original antigen specificity. For example, approximately 15% of neonates born to women with anti-tuberculin immunity had lymphocytes reactive to purified protein derivative (PPD) 4–6 weeks after birth, while none of the infants born to non-immune women did (265). These data support the idea that not only had the infants acquired maternal T lymphocytes, but that these cells were functional after transfer. Of note, the anti-PPD response waned by 3 months of age, suggesting death of the maternal cells, and/or activation of infant regulatory cells to control the maternal anti-PPD response postnatally.

MMc in the newborn may also transmit malignancy. Hodgkin disease was hypothesized to be derived from unregulated maternal cells in children almost 50 years ago (251), and since then there have been case reports of infants with monocytic leukemia, natural killer cell lymphoma, and malignant melanomas derived from maternal blood (266–269).

Maternally derived cells have been found not only as circulating leukocytes in the offspring (5), but as differentiated tissue cells in every human organ examined to date, including: skin, thymus, heart, lung, pancreas, liver, spleen, kidney, muscle, and bone marrow (6, 7, 270, 271). These findings support the idea that an undifferentiated maternal stem cell engrafts into the fetal bone marrow and provides a continuous source of allogeneic precursors. These maternal stem cells may normally be recruited into the fetal tissues during early development to participate in organogenesis along with the fetal cells, and may provide a source of cells for tissue repair and regeneration in areas of injury. Although the role of MMc in these processes remains speculative, recent data from a mouse model of renal disease demonstrated that bone marrow transplant-derived stem cells were recruited to damaged glomeruli, where they participated in healing (272). Alternatively, maternal cells expressing antigens not inherited by the fetus could act as targets for the fetal/neonatal immune system, or even for neonatally acquired maternal autoantibodies.

Regulation of MMc Levels in Infants

Assuming that the PCR-based DNA detection and FISH methods are reproducible and sensitive enough to omit large variation by chance, it is not clear why MMc is found in the circulation of some healthy persons, but not others. One explanation is that MMc is transferred with higher frequency in some pregnancies or deliveries. Factors regulating the transplacental transfer of maternal cells to the fetus are not fully understood, but high-risk deliveries with antepartum problems such as fetal anomalies, preeclampsia, placental insufficiency and chorioamnionitis have been associated with increased maternal–fetal cell transfer (273–277). However, a direct comparison of MMc levels in normal vaginal delivery, complicated delivery with excess bleeding, and cesarian section has not been performed. After birth, breastfeeding may affect the levels of MMc. Some breast milk may contain a higher number of maternal cells, or have cell subsets with different survival advantages in the neonate. Maternal alloantigens may induce antigen-specific tolerance in the neonatal immune system; this may be dependent on the genes of both the mother and the fetus. In a mouse study, levels of MMc were influenced by maternal–fetal histocompatibility, where MHC homozygous progeny had slightly higher levels of MMc than heterozygous progeny (278). MHC alleles may also affect the transfer, survival or expansion of chimeric cells in humans. Data reveal that the level of MMc in human peripheral blood correlates with maternal–fetal compatibility at MHC class II molecules DRB1 and DQB1, and with specific DQA1*0501 and DQB1*0301 alleles (255, 263, 279). It is not known how specific HLA molecules contribute to higher levels of microchimerism in the blood.

The fact that any "foreign" maternal cells are tolerated by the neonatal immune system suggests that maternally derived cells and/or antigens may play a role in thymic education. In support of this hypothesis, studies reveal the presence of maternal DNA in human and murine thymuses (278, 280). Regulatory T cells educated in the thymus may also play a role in mediating tolerance to MMc, but this has not yet been demonstrated.

Although a role for maternal cells in autoimmunity has been suggested, they probably play a beneficial role in most individuals. MMc may assist with protection against infection, autoimmunity, and even cancer, and may play a role in normal pregnancy and fetal/neonatal development. Maternal cells expressing allogeneic antigens may also provide a source of constant stimulation to host T lymphocytes to maintain the T cell receptor repertoire (281).

Other Sources of Microchimerism

In addition to maternal and fetal microchimerism, there are other potential sources of foreign cells derived during pregnancy, including from a twin, an unrecognized vanished twin, (estimated to occur in 5% of pregnancies), or siblings in a multiplex pregnancy (282–285). One case report describes a fertile, healthy woman, who was found to have near-complete replacement of her hematopoietic system with male cells (99% of cells examined), although her somatic karyotype was female. She had a twin brother who died shortly after birth, suggesting that successful, naturally occurring feto–fetal transfusion had occurred during gestation (286).

Fetal cells can be detected for decades in a woman after delivery, or even after an early spontaneous abortion (287–289), suggesting that a subsequent fetus could theoretically receive not only his mother's cells, but also cells from any prior pregnancies carried by his mother. As his mother may also be carrying cells acquired during her own gestation, the fetus could receive cells from his maternal grandmother and maternal aunts, uncles, and so on. In this sense, each infant is potentially a multi-chimeric organism composed of cells from not just multiple individuals, but multiple generations. In samples from females too young to have been pregnant, male microchimerism has been detected in five of six girls and seven of eleven fetuses, supporting the idea that cells from older siblings may also be transferred via the transplacental route (290).

Developmental Differences between Fetus and Newborn

The stage of development at which a foreign (i.e., maternal or transfused) cell is transferred to the fetus may influence the outcome. MMc has been detected as early as 13 weeks gestation, and NLS-related heart block is usually detected at 17 weeks gestation, supporting the idea that maternal cells may play a role in the pathogenesis of atrioventricular (AV) node inflammation (7, 253). MMc may also alter the effect of transplacentally acquired maternal antibodies, depending on whether or not maternal cells carry the target antigens and/or are integrated into host tissues.

The fate of allogeneic maternal cells transferred to the fetus may be hypothesized to parallel the fate of donor cells transplanted during gestation. In some cases, in utero transplantation leads to long-lasting tolerance in the recipient (291–295). In immunocompetent mice, in utero hematopoietic stem cell transplantation with MHC-mismatched bone marrow cells resulted in durable low-level engraftment beyond 20 weeks of age (well into adulthood) (293). However, in other cases, cells acquired during gestation do not induce tolerance, and may even be pathogenic. Transfusion of spleen cell subsets to mice in utero was found to result in persistent microchimerism, but did not improve acceptance of skin grafts placed

6 months after birth (296). Rather, accelerated rejection of donor tissues was observed in the previously transfused mice. In some murine studies, early postnatal infusion of homozygous parental cells to heterozygous offspring caused GVHD with many features of SLE (297). GVHD has also been observed in immunocompetent human infants following intrauterine and exchange transfusions for hemolytic disease (298). Thus, the outcome of maternal cell acquisition by the neonate depends upon the route of transfer, recipient's age, developmental stage, genetic profiles of the donor and recipient, and cell type transferred (296, 299, 300).

The Role of Breast Milk in Acquisition and Function of MMc

Studies in mice have suggested that persistence of maternal cells in blood and tissues derived in utero is dependent on oral tolerance induced by breast milk antigens ingested by the neonate (301). Maternal HLA molecules may play a role in this process, as they are found as both soluble and cell-membrane-associated proteins in breast milk (302). The protective effect of breast feeding on the future development of autoimmune disease suggests that maternal cells, antibodies, or antigens contained in breast milk may interact with the neonatal immune system in a beneficial way (303).

Maternal cells in breast milk are believed to pass into the infant's circulation, although evidence for this is indirect. Cell types in breast milk are varied, but the vast majority are granulocytes, macrophages, and other antigen-presenting cells, along with 1–7% lymphocytes (304–307). The majority of T lymphocytes in human milk are activated or memory cells, thus the infant may benefit from his mother's immunological experience (305, 306). The role of maternal immune cells in the infant is not well-understood, but maternal B cells appear to become antibody-secreting mucosal plasma cells which can protect the newborn against gastrointestinal and respiratory pathogens, while the infant's intrinsic immune system is still developing (308). Immunocompetent mouse pups who were nursed by lymphopenic mothers were found to have reduced antibody production, suggesting that maternal lymphocytes and/or immunoglobulins in breast milk normally contribute to the neonatal immune response (309).

Exposure to maternal antigens during gestation may regulate neonatal B cell development. Female mice expressing specific MHC I antigens were bred to male mice with high or moderate-affinity germline B cell receptors against these proteins (310). Pups who did not inherit the genes for these antigens, but were presumed to have been exposed to the maternal antigens during gestation and breast-feeding, showed changes in their antigen-specific B cell populations. Their high-affinity antigen-specific B cells were deleted, while their moderate-affinity B cells showed an activated phenotype. These results demonstrate that B cell development may be affected by neonatal exposure to maternal antigens as well as by the affinity of the B cell receptor for its antigen.

Exposure to maternal milk may alter the host T lymphocyte response to MMc and other antigens. Newborn calves fed whole colostrum exhibited increased T cell responses in a mixed leukocyte reaction within 24 h of feeding, but this did not occur in calves fed cell-free colostrum until 2 or more weeks after birth (311). Moreover, calves who ingested whole colostrum developed reduced reactivity to maternal alloantigens, which may lead to tolerance and persistence of MMc, preventing a chronic inflammatory response against HLA-mismatched maternal cells.

Whole maternal cells in bovine colostrum are not digested in the gut, but traceable in the circulation between 12 and 36 h after ingestion (312). Of note, ingestion of maternal cells without colostrum resulted in diminished entry into the circulation. Although normal maternal lymphoid cells in colostrum are absorbed from the gastrointestinal tract, heat-treated lymphoid cells or those isolated from peripheral blood are not (313), suggesting that a heat-labile surface molecule is required for survival and/or transfer of maternal cells across the epithelial barrier.

Relevance of Physiologic Differences to the Disease Process

MMc in Immunodeficient Infants

Observations in infants with severe combined immunodeficiency (SCID) have provided evidence that host immune tolerance plays a role in the level of maternal cell acquisition. Infants with immunodeficiencies have long been known to harbor high levels of maternal hematopoietic cells (314, 315), suggesting that the immunocompetent host limits the amount of MMc normally accepted. However, MMc does not reconstitute a functional immune system in these infants, although engrafted infants may have a survival advantage over those without maternal cells. Maternal T cells that are transferred do not respond normally to in vitro stimulation and express a limited T cell receptor repertoire (316, 317), suggesting that a few T cells may be transferred to immunocompromised offspring and expand in response to specific antigenic stimuli, or that only small T cell subsets are allowed to transfer or persist in allogeneic individuals.

In immunodeficient infants, engraftment with maternal cells leads to GVHD in 60% of cases (318). The T cells transferred may already be expanded in the mother, as evidenced by the case of a 5-month-old male with SCID and chronic GVHD with skin and hepatic manifestations (319). He had aberrant peripheral T cell subsets which included rare $CD4^+$ T cells and a $CD8^+$ gamma/delta$^+$ population of which more than 50% were maternally derived clonal T cells. The clonal $CD8^+$ gamma/delta$^+$ T cell population comprised 10% of the mother's peripheral blood mononuclear cells, which decreased over time after delivery. These cells may have been stimulated by paternal antigens carried by the fetus, with transplacental transfer of these maternal anti-paternal T cells to the immunodeficient fetus. In support of this hypothesis, studies in transgenic mice reveal a 3-fold increase in anti-fetal $CD8^+$ T cells specific for inherited paternal MHC class I antigens, especially in lymph nodes draining the uterus (320). The fact that major immunodeficiency can lead to high levels of MMc raises the question of whether more subtle immune defects, such as those seen in common variable immunodeficiency, chronic granulomatous disease, and hyperIgM syndrome, could also lead to increased maternal engraftment. Whether the autoimmune diseases that occur in these patients are related to MMc also remains to be examined.

MMc in Neonatal Autoimmunity

Just as maternal cells in immunodeficient infants can cause GVHD, maternal cells in immunocompetent individuals may sometimes be involved in the initiation or perpetuation of autoimmune disease (256).

NEONATAL SCLERODERMA

Systemic sclerosis is a rare autoimmune disease resembling GVHD. MMc has been detected in adult scleroderma patients (321), and a role for MMc (and/or maternal autoantibodies) in neonatal scleroderma is suggested by rare case reports of affected infants born to mothers with connective tissue disease (322–325). Infants affected by systemic sclerosis can present with diffuse cutaneous involvement (tight, shiny skin) at birth, with or without visceral involvement. In one reported case, the neonate's condition gradually improved over time (323), consistent with the idea that a large initial load of MMc may have played a role in disease pathogenis. Neonates with autoimmune disease are currently treated with immunosuppression as needed for skin, vascular, and musculoskeletal manifestations. With the recent findings of MMc in affected infants, it is hoped that more targeted therapy will be developed.

NEONATAL LUPUS SYNDROME

MMc has been investigated in the context of neonatal lupus syndrome (NLS), an autoimmune disease that develops in utero. Infants born to mothers with lupus-associated autoantibodies are at risk for developing NLS, with rash, cytopenias, hepatitis, and the life-threatening complication of AV node inflammation and congenital heart block (47). Although maternally derived autoantibodies are necessary for the development of NLS congenital heart block (CHB), they are not sufficient. Over 95% of infants born to women with anti-SSA and/or anti-SSB antibodies are healthy (47, 326). One factor implicated in the pathogenesis of CHB has been the presence of allogeneic cells in the child that may interact with the host immune system. Using Q-PCR, both maternal and sibling microchimerism have been detected in the peripheral blood of twins and triplets discordant for CHB (285). In one set of triplets, microchimerism was present in the blood of two infants affected with CHB, but not in their sibling, who only had a transient hepatitis. Moreover, evolution of the disease in these two siblings correlated with measurements of microchimerism in serial peripheral blood samples. In contrast, in a pair of discordantly affected twins, microchimerism was detected in the healthy infant, and not in the twin with CHB.

To further investigate the role of MMc in CHB, heart tissues from male infants with and without NLS were analyzed for female (maternal) cells using FISH to identify X- and Y-chromosome-specific sequences (7). Maternal cells were found in all 15 sections of heart tissue from four NLS patients, comprising 0.025–2.2% of the myocardial cells. Maternal cells were also found in two of eight control cardiac sections, but at lower levels (0.05–0.1%). A minority of maternal cells expressed CD45, suggesting that these were maternally derived leukocytes, but a majority expressed sarcomeric alpha-actin, a marker specific for cardiac myocytes. The finding of maternal cardiomyocytes at the site of disease has important implications for autoimmunity, as maternal cells may be the pathogenic target of transplacentally acquired maternal autoantibodies, or may be beneficial to the neonate, by contributing to the process of tissue repair.

MMc and the Risk of Future Autoimmune Disease

Although many autoimmune diseases only become apparent years after birth, their origins may be inherently dependent on the acquisition of MMc during the fetal and neonatal periods. MMc has been implicated in the pathogenesis of several autoimmune diseases affecting children and adults, including systemic sclerosis (256), myositis (263, 264, 327), pityriasis lichenoides (271), rheumatoid arthritis (328), and a case of chronic idiopathic GVHD-type syndrome (329). Using FISH to identify X- and Y-chromosomes, MMc was found in ten of ten skin and muscle biopsies from boys with juvenile idiopathic inflammatory myopathy (264). Only two of ten biopsies from children with non-inflammatory muscle disorders were positive for MMc. In eight of nine children with autoimmune myositis, MMc was also noted in peripheral blood T cells (264). Rare cases of inflammatory myopathy have also been described in neonates (330, 331), suggesting that MMc may be involved in myositis early in life.

Inherited and Non-Inherited Maternal Genes in the Risk for Neonatal Disease

Human leukocyte antigen (HLA) alleles have been associated with many autoimmune diseases, although the mechanisms for how they contribute to disease are not known (332). It has been shown that HLA compatibility of the mother and fetus at MHC class II loci increases the risk for both neonatal and future autoimmunity (58). Males who develop lupus are more likely to be HLA-identical with their mothers at the HLA DRB1 locus (333), suggesting a mechanism whereby they could tolerate greater MMc acquisition during gestation and breast-feeding. Other studies have shown that *non-inherited* maternal alleles can also be associated with an increased risk of developing autoimmune disease, although this is controversial (328, 334–337). For example, in humans, several studies have demonstrated correlation between the mother's HLA alleles and the neonate's development of CHB, but no correlation between fetal HLA alleles and CHB (338–342), suggesting that maternal cells are transferred to the fetus and play a direct role in the pathogenesis of heart block. Therefore, immunologic studies in neonates should include the contribution of antigens inherited via microchimerism as well as those inherited genetically.

The mechanisms whereby non-inherited maternal alleles affect the offspring's immune system are not known. One possibility is that MMc can tolerize the neonatal immune system to maternal cells. For example, in experimental murine studies, bone marrow transplants from offspring to half-matched adults resulted in lower GVHD if the donor's mother matched the recipient, suggesting that the donor had been exposed to the non-inherited allele perinatally (343). The reduced GVHD in this study was found to be dependent on the presence of donor T regulatory cells, possibly generated as a result of exposure to maternal cells in utero. Support for the idea of perinatal tolerization in humans comes from studies of RhD-negative women, who are typically susceptible to alloimmunization following pregnancy with an RhD-positive fetus. These women were found to be less likely to develop an anti-RhD antibody response if their own mothers were RhD positive, suggesting they had become tolerant of this antigen during exposure in utero (344). Another example of tolerance to non-inherited maternal antigens involves the anti-HLA response generated in recipients of multiple blood transfusions. Fifty percent of these transfusion recipients were found to lack antibodies to non-inherited maternal HLA, suggesting that they had been tolerized to these antigens perinatally (345). More evidence comes from retrospective evaluation of renal and hematopoietic stem cell transplants, which has revealed better outcomes in cases where a donor–recipient HLA-mismatch was compensated for by HLA alleles of the donor's mother (reviewed in ref. 346). However, in contrast, a review of 5000 renal transplants did not find that offspring were more tolerant of maternal antigens, as there was no apparent advantage of maternal-to-child over paternal-to-child renal donations (347). It should be noted, however, that findings in humans are confounded by the issue of compliance to immunosuppressive regimens, and whether or not the patient was breast-fed as an infant, as this may be a necessary factor for full tolerization to maternal cells acquired in utero (301). Overall, the evidence for perinatal tolerization to non-inherited maternal alleles is strong, and implies that MMc acquired early in life may play a significant role in immune development.

ROLE OF T REGULATORY CELLS IN NEONATAL AUTOIMMUNITY

Much has been recently learned regarding the role of T regulatory cells (Treg) in human autoimmunity, but less is known with respect to their function in fetal/neonatal disease. Several types of Treg have been described to date, but we will use the term Treg here to mean the "classic" CD4$^+$, CD25$^+$ Foxp3$^+$ T regulatory cells, found to be pivotal in the prevention and amelioration of multiple forms of human and animal autoimmunity (348–350). After positive selection in the thymus, Treg enter the circulation to monitor ongoing immune responses and to mediate their suppressive effects. In mice, Treg do not appear in the circulation until approximately 3 days after birth, so thymectomy prior to this time leads to widespread autoimmune disease. However, in humans, Treg enter the circulation before birth, so that neonatal thymectomy does not usually result in overt autoimmunity (351). In both mice and humans, not only are circulating Treg found very early in life, but they are also functional at these stages (352, 353). For example, in an animal model of neonatal autoimmune ovarian disease (AOD), mice were susceptible to autoantibody-initiated, T cell-dependent AOD, but only before 7 days of age (37). Resistance to disease gained after 7 days of life correlated with the presence of and response to CD4+/CD25+ Treg.

Although human maternal Treg increase in the circulation during pregnancy, are found in the early decidua, and contribute to maternal tolerance of the fetus (354, 355), it is not clear whether maternal Treg can be acquired transplacentally. It is known that Treg are present and functional in human cord blood (356), and a recent study demonstrated that cord blood Treg were more potent inhibitors of an in vitro anti-myelin oligodendrocyte glycoprotein (MOG) thymocyte response than Treg derived from neonatal thymus (357). The cord blood Treg inhibited both T effector interferon-gamma production and cell proliferation, while Treg derived from thymic tissue only suppressed cytokine production. This discordance in Treg function may be a result of further Treg development after thymic egress, but it would be interesting to determine whether any of the cord blood Treg were maternally derived.

Treg may be a major factor mediating the offspring's tolerance of maternal cells. To evaluate the role of Treg in tolerance to non-inherited maternal antigens, an experimental mouse model was created by breeding a female mouse heterozygous for class I histocompatibility alleles with a male mouse homozygous at this locus. Pups who lacked the maternal antigen were examined for their immune response to the non-inherited allele. Testing of CD4+ splenic T cells from these offspring revealed a reduced in vitro immune response to maternal cells compared to control mice, and injection of their splenic CD4+ T cells into lethally irradiated recipients with the same non-inherited allele resulted in less T cell expansion and GVHD compared to donors whose mothers lacked this allele (343). Of note, the donor's tolerance of non-inherited maternal alleles was lost if CD4+CD25+ T cells were depleted prior to infusion, supporting the idea that in utero exposure to non-inherited maternal alleles had resulted in induction of antigen-specific T reg. However, this study did not examine the level of MMc in these offspring or whether there were any maternal Treg among the CD4+CD25+ Treg population which may have played a role in tolerance to non-inherited maternal alleles.

The effects of MMc (and maternal antibody acquisition) on the development and function of Treg in the human fetus and neonate are not known. Cord blood-derived mononuclear cells from babies born to atopic mothers have decreased expression of Treg-related genes upon stimulation with peptidoglycans in vitro (354). However, it is not clear whether these differences are intrinsic to the newborn or are maternally mediated, and the implications of these findings are not yet fully understood. Thus, the importance of Treg in maternally derived neonatal autoimmunity is an exciting area that remains to be explored.

CONCLUSIONS

We are just beginning to understand the complex short- and long-term immune interactions between the maternal and fetal immune systems. These signals are composed not only of transplacentally and nutritionally acquired immunoglobulins, lymphocytes, antigen-presenting cells, and immature precursor cells, but also numerous protein- and nucleic acid-based signaling molecules, such as growth factors, cytokines, chemokines, and free-floating DNA. Fetal–maternal interaction can result in protection of the neonate from infection, but can also promote autoimmune disease, depending on the antigen specificity of the antibodies or leukocytes involved, variations in maternal–fetal HLA composition, genetic and environmental factors, and physiologic maturity of the host. Studies in these areas may lead to improved diagnostic and therapeutic maneuvers not only in neonatal autoimmunity, but also in infection, pregnancy, and transplantation biology.

Acknowledgments

The authors would like to thank Dr. Kristina Adams for her critical review of the manuscript and Ms. Debra George IBCLC for her input regarding the role of breast milk.

Abbreviations

AChR	acetylcholine receptor
AIA	anti-insulin antibodies
AMLA	anti-myolemmal antibodies
ANCA	anti-neutrophil cytoplasmic antibodies
ANA	anti-nuclear antibodies
AOD	autoimmune ovarian disease
APLA	antiphospholipid antibodies
AT-1	antiogensin II receptor
AV	atrioventricular
CHB	congenital heart block
DCM	dilated cardiomyopathy
DM	diabetes mellitus
DNA	deoxyribonucleic acid
Dsg	desmoglein
Fab	fragment, antigen binding (monovalent antibody)
FISH	fluorescence in situ hybridization
GAD	glutamic acid decarboxylase
GVHD	graft-versus-host disease
HLA	human leukocyte antigen
HDN	hemolytic disease of the newborn
IA-2	protein tyrosine phosphatase IA-2
ICA	islet cell antibodies
Ig	immunoglobulins
IVIG	intravenous immunoglobulins
IUGR	intrauterine growth restriction
MHC	major histocompatibility complex
MMc	maternal microchimerism
MPO	myeloperoxidase
NAIT	neonatal alloimmune thrombocytopenia
NEP	neutral endopeptidase
NGB	neonatal Guillain-Barre
NH	neonatal hemochromatosis
NLS	neonatal lupus syndrome
NMG	neonatal myasthenia gravis
NOD	non-obese-diabetic (mouse strain)
PF	pemphigus folaceous
PPD	purified protein derivative
PV	pemphigus vulgaris
Q-PCR	quantitative PCR
Rh	Rhesus group antigen
RNP	ribonuclear protein

SCID   severe combined immunodeficiency
SLE   systemic lupus erythematosus
Treg   T regulatory cells
TSH   thyroid-stimulating hormone
TSH-R   thyroid-stimulating hormone receptor
tTg   tissue transglutaminase

REFERENCES

1. Kaul A, Smith GF. Immunobiology of the fetus and newborn – historical perspectives and recent advances. 1980.
2. Linder N, et al. Placental transfer and decay of varicella-zoster virus antibodies in preterm infants. J Pediatr 137 (1):85–89, 2000.
3. Wesumperuma HL, et al. The influence of prematurity and low birthweight on transplacental antibody transfer in Sri Lanka. Ann Trop Med Parasitol 93 (2):169–177, 1999.
4. Hanson LA, et al. The transfer of immunity from mother to child. Ann N Y Acad Sci 987:199–206, 2003.
5. Hall JM, et al. Detection of maternal cells in human umbilical cord blood using fluorescence in situ hybridization. Blood 86 (7):2829–2832, 1995.
6. Srivatsa B, et al. Maternal cell microchimerism in newborn tissues. J Pediatr 142 (1):31–35, 2003.
7. Stevens AM, et al. Myocardial-tissue-specific phenotype of maternal microchimerism in neonatal lupus congenital heart block. Lancet 362 (9396):1617–1623, 2003.
8. Maloney S, et al. Microchimerism of maternal origin persists into adult life. J Clin Invest 104 (1):41–47, 1999.
9. Simister NE. Placental transport of immunoglobulin G. Vaccine 21 (24):3365–3369, 2003.
10. Saji F, et al. Dynamics of immunoglobulins at the feto-maternal interface. Rev Reprod 4 (2):81–89, 1999.
11. Kristoffersen EK, Matre R. Co-localization of the neonatal Fc gamma receptor and IgG in human placental term syncytiotrophoblasts. Eur J Immunol 26 (7):1668–1671, 1996.
12. Baril L, et al. Natural materno-fetal transfer of antibodies to PspA and to PsaA. Clin Exp Immunol 135 (3):474–477, 2004.
13. Garty BZ, et al. Placental transfer of immunoglobulin G subclasses. Clin Diagn Lab Immunol 1 (6):667–669, 1994.
14. Hanson LA, et al. Immune system modulation by human milk. Adv Exp Med Biol 503:99–106, 2002.
15. Bednar-Tantscher E, Mudde GC, Rot A. Maternal antigen stimulation downregulates via mother's milk the specific immune responses in young mice. Int Arch Allergy Immunol 126 (4):300–308, 2001.
16. Watanaveeradej V, et al. Transplacentally transferred maternal-infant antibodies to dengue virus. Am J Trop Med Hyg 69 (2):123–128, 2003.
17. Thornton CA, et al. Fetal exposure to intact immunoglobulin E occurs via the gastrointestinal tract. Clin Exp Allergy 33 (3):306–311, 2003.
18. Vassella CC, et al. High anti-IgE levels at birth are associated with a reduced allergy prevalence in infants at risk: a prospective study. Clin Exp Allergy 24 (8):771–777, 1994.
19. Van de Perre P. Transfer of antibody via mother's milk. Vaccine 21 (24):3374–3376, 2003.
20. de Souza Campos Fernandes RC, Quintana Flores VM, Medina-Acosta E. Prevalent transfer of human colostral IgA antibody activity for the enteropathogenic Escherichia coli bundle-forming pilus structural repeating subunit A in neonates. Diagn Microbiol Infect Dis 44 (4):331–336, 2002.
21. Israel EJ, et al. Expression of the neonatal Fc receptor, FcRn, on human intestinal epithelial cells. Immunology 92 (1):69–74, 1997.
22. Hanson LA, Korotkova M. The role of breastfeeding in prevention of neonatal infection. Semin Neonatol 7 (4):275–281, 2002.
23. Pabst HF, Spady DW. Effect of breast-feeding on antibody response to conjugate vaccine. Lancet 336 (8710):269–270, 1990.
24. Kelleher SL, Lonnerdal B. Immunological activities associated with milk. Adv Nutr Res 10:39–65, 2001.
25. Wingen AM, et al. Evidence for developmental changes of type IV collagen in glomerular basement membrane. Nephron 45 (4):302–305, 1987.
26. Jeraj K, et al. Development and heterogeneity of antigens in the immature nephron. Reactivity with human antiglomerular basement membrane autoantibodies. Am J Pathol 117 (2):180–183, 1984.
27. Hirsch R, et al. Neonatal pemphigus foliaceus. J Am Acad Dermatol 49 (2 Suppl Case Reports):S187–189, 2003.
28. Okoko BJ, et al. The transplacental transfer of IgG subclasses: influence of prematurity and low birthweight in the Gambian population. Ann Trop Paediatr 22 (4):325–332, 2002.
29. Lemons PK, Lemons JA. Transition to breast/bottle feedings: the premature infant. J Am Coll Nutr 15 (2):126–135, 1996.

30. Askanase AD, et al. The presence of IgG antibodies reactive with components of the SSA/Ro-SSB/La complex in human breast milk: implications in neonatal lupus. Arthritis Rheum 46 (1):269–271, 2002.

31. Wright AL, et al. Factors influencing the relation of infant feeding to asthma and recurrent wheeze in childhood. Thorax 56 (3):192–197, 2001.

32. Oddy WH, Peat JK, de Klerk NH. Maternal asthma, infant feeding, and the risk of asthma in childhood. J Allergy Clin Immunol 110 (1):65–67, 2002.

33. Friedman NJ, Zeiger RS. The role of breast-feeding in the development of allergies and asthma. J Allergy Clin Immunol 115 (6):1238–1248, 2005.

34. Rothenbacher D, et al. Breastfeeding, soluble CD14 concentration in breast milk and risk of atopic dermatitis and asthma in early childhood: birth cohort study. Clin Exp Allergy 35 (8):1014–1021, 2005.

35. Leme AS, et al. Role of breast milk in a mouse model of maternal transmission of asthma susceptibility. J Immunol 176 (2):762–769, 2006.

36. Martin DA, Elkon KB. Mechanisms of apoptosis. Rheum Dis Clin North Am 30 (3):441–454, vii, 2004.

37. Setiady YY, Samy ET, Tung KS. Maternal autoantibody triggers de novo T cell-mediated neonatal autoimmune disease. J Immunol 170 (9):4656–4664, 2003.

38. Okajima S, et al. Two sibling cases of hydrops fetalis due to alloimmune anti-CD36 (Nak a) antibody. Thromb Haemost 95 (2):267–271, 2006.

39. Debiec H, et al. Role of truncating mutations in MME gene in fetomaternal alloimmunisation and antenatal glomerulopathies. Lancet 364 (9441):1252–1259, 2004.

40. Ristic AD, Maisch B. Cardiac rhythm and conduction disturbances: what is the role of autoimmune mechanisms? Herz 25 (3):181–188, 2000.

41. Camusso JJ, et al. Antibodies against beta adrenoceptors in mothers of children with congenital heart block. Acta Physiol Pharmacol Ther Latinoam 44 (3):94–99, 1994.

42. Maisch B, Ristic AD. Immunological basis of the cardiac conduction and rhythm disorders. Eur Heart J 22 (10):813–824, 2001.

43. Julkunen H, et al. Autoimmune response in mothers of children with congenital and postnatally diagnosed isolated heart block: a population based study. J Rheumatol 31 (1):183–189, 2004.

44. Borrego L, et al. Neonatal lupus erythematosus related to maternal leukocytoclastic vasculitis. Pediatr Dermatol 14 (3):221–225, 1997.

45. Penate Y, et al. [Neonatal lupus erythematosus: 4 cases and clinical review]. Actas Dermosifiliogr 96 (10):690–696, 2005.

46. Brucato A, Cimaz R, Stramba-Badiale M. Neonatal lupus. Clin Rev Allergy Immunol 23 (3):279–299, 2002.

47. Buyon JP, Clancy RM. Neonatal lupus syndromes. Curr Opin Rheumatol 15 (5):535–541, 2003.

48. Martin V, et al. Long-term followup of children with neonatal lupus and their unaffected siblings. Arthritis Rheum 46 (9):2377–2383, 2002.

49. Burch JM, Lee LA, Weston WL. Neonatal lupus erythematosus. Dermatol Nurs 14 (3):157–160, 2002.

50. Boh EE, Neonatal lupus erythematosus. Clin Dermatol 22 (2):125–128, 2004.

51. Cimaz R, et al. Incidence and spectrum of neonatal lupus erythematosus: a prospective study of infants born to mothers with anti-Ro autoantibodies. J Pediatr 142 (6):678–683, 2003.

52. Lee LA. Transient autoimmunity related to maternal autoantibodies: neonatal lupus. Autoimmun Rev 4 (4):207–213, 2005.

53. Watson RM, et al. Neonatal lupus erythematosus. Report of serological and immunogenetic studies in twins discordant for congenital heart block. Br J Dermatol 130 (3):342–348, 1994.

54. Batard ML, et al. Cutaneous neonatal lupus erythematosus: discordant expression in identical twins. Ann Dermatol Venereol 127 (10):814–817, 2000.

55. Solomon BA, Laude TA, Shalita AR. Neonatal lupus erythematosus: discordant disease expression of U1RNP-positive antibodies in fraternal twins–is this a subset of neonatal lupus erythematosus or a new distinct syndrome? J Am Acad Dermatol 32 (5 Pt 2):858–862, 1995.

56. Fesslova V, et al. Neonatal lupus: fetal myocarditis progressing to atrioventricular block in triplets. Lupus 12 (10):775–778, 2003.

57. Siren MK, et al. Role of HLA in congenital heart block: susceptibility alleles in children. Lupus 8 (1):60–67, 1999.

58. Miyagawa S, et al. Neonatal lupus erythematosus: haplotypic analysis of HLA class II alleles in child/mother pairs. Arthritis Rheum 40 (5):982–983, 1997.

59. Cimaz R, et al. Ultraviolet light exposure is not a requirement for the development of cutaneous neonatal lupus. Lupus 11 (4):257–260, 2002.

60. Selander B, Cedergren S, Domanski H. A case of severe neonatal lupus erythematosus without cardiac or cutaneous involvement. Acta Paediatr 87 (1):105–107, 1998.

61. Buyon JP, et al. Autoimmune-associated congenital heart block: demographics, mortality, morbidity and recurrence rates obtained from a national neonatal lupus registry. J Am Coll Cardiol 31 (7):1658–1666, 1998.

62. Scott JS, et al. Connective-tissue disease, antibodies to ribonucleoprotein, and congenital heart block. N Engl J Med 309 (4):209–212, 1983.

63. Buyon J, Szer I. Passively acquired autoimmunity and the maternal fetal dyad in systemic lupus erythematosus. Springer Semin Immunopathol 9 (2–3):283–304, 1986.

64. Buyon JP, Rupel A, Clancy RM. Neonatal lupus syndromes. Lupus 13 (9):705–712, 2004.

65. Lee LA, Neonatal lupus erythematosus. J Invest Dermatol 100 (1):9S–13S, 1993.

66. Cimaz R, Duquesne A. Neonatal lupus syndromes. Arch Pediatr 13 (5):473–478, 2006.

67. Brucato A, et al. Risk of congenital complete heart block in newborns of mothers with anti-Ro/SSA antibodies detected by counterimmunoelectrophoresis: a prospective study of 100 women. Arthritis Rheum 44 (8):1832–1835, 2001.

68. Raboisson MJ, et al. Fetal Doppler echocardiographic diagnosis and successful steroid therapy of Luciani-Wenckebach phenomenon and endocardial fibroelastosis related to maternal anti-Ro and anti-La antibodies. J Am Soc Echocardiogr 18 (4):375–380, 2005.

69. Costedoat-Chalumeau N, et al. Anti-SSA/Ro antibodies and the heart: more than complete congenital heart block? A review of electrocardiographic and myocardial abnormalities and of treatment options. Arthritis Res Ther 7 (2):69–73, 2005.

70. Nield LE, et al. Maternal anti-Ro and anti-La antibody-associated endocardial fibroelastosis. Circulation 105 (7):843–848, 2002.

71. Moak JP, et al. Congenital heart block: development of late-onset cardiomyopathy, a previously underappreciated sequela. J Am Coll Cardiol 37 (1):238–242, 2001.

72. Neufing PJ, et al. Exposure and binding of selected immunodominant La/SSB epitopes on human apoptotic cells. Arthritis Rheum 52 (12):3934–3942, 2005.

73. Tran HB, et al. Anti-La/SSB antibodies transported across the placenta bind apoptotic cells in fetal organs targeted in neonatal lupus. Arthritis Rheum 46 (6):1572–1579, 2002.

74. Clancy RM, et al. Transdifferentiation of cardiac fibroblasts, a fetal factor in anti-SSA/Ro-SSB/La antibody-mediated congenital heart block. J Immunol 169 (4):2156–2163, 2002.

75. Clancy RM, Buyon JP. Autoimmune-associated congenital heart block: dissecting the cascade from immunologic insult to relentless fibrosis. Anat Rec A Discov Mol Cell Evol Biol 280 (2):1027–1035, 2004.

76. Nii M, et al. Assessment of fetal atrioventricular time intervals by tissue Doppler and pulse Doppler echo cardiography: normal values and correlation with fetal electrocardiography. Heart 92 (12):1831–1837, 2006.

77. Claus R, et al. Identification and management of fetuses at risk for, or affected by, congenital heart block associated with autoantibodies to SSA (Ro), SSB (La), or an HsEg5-like autoantigen. Rheumatol Int, 2006:1–10.

78. Hickstein H, et al. Autoimmune-associated congenital heart block: treatment of the mother with immunoadsorption. Ther Apher Dial 9 (2):148–153, 2005.

79. Buyon JP, et al. Intrauterine therapy for presumptive fetal myocarditis with acquired heart block due to systemic lupus erythematosus. Experience in a mother with a predominance of SS-B (La) antibodies. Arthritis Rheum 30 (1):44–49, 1987.

80. Jaeggi ET, et al. Is immune-mediated complete fetal atrioventricular block reversible by transplacental dexamethasone therapy? Ultrasound Obstet Gynecol 23 (6):602–605, 2004.

81. Jaeggi ET, et al. Transplacental fetal treatment improves the outcome of prenatally diagnosed complete atrioventricular block without structural heart disease. Circulation 110 (12):1542–1548, 2004.

82. Buyon JP. Neonatal lupus: bedside to bench and back. Scand J Rheumatol 25 (5):271–276, 1996.

83. Matsui S, et al. Dilated cardiomyopathy defines serum autoantibodies against G-protein-coupled cardiovascular receptors. Autoimmunity 21 (2):85–88, 1995.

84. Baba A, et al. Autoantibodies against M2-muscarinic acetylcholine receptors: new upstream targets in atrial fibrillation in patients with dilated cardiomyopathy. Eur Heart J 25 (13):1108–1115, 2004.

85. Zhang L, et al. Autoantibodies against the myocardial beta1-adrenergic and M2-muscarinic receptors in patients with congestive heart failure. Chin Med J (Engl) 115 (8):1127–1131, 2002.

86. Wallukat G, et al. Autoantibodies against the beta- and muscarinic receptors in cardiomyopathy. Herz 25 (3):261–266, 2000.

87. Matsui S, Fu ML. Myocardial injury due to G-protein coupled receptor-autoimmunity. Jpn Heart J 39 (3):261–274, 1998.

88. Ferrari I, et al. Molecular mimicry between the immunodominant ribosomal protein P0 of Trypanosoma cruzi and a functional epitope on the human beta 1-adrenergic receptor. J Exp Med 182 (1):59–65, 1995.

89. Elies R, et al. Structural and functional analysis of the B cell epitopes recognized by anti-receptor autoantibodies in patients with Chagas' disease. J Immunol 157 (9):4203–4211, 1996.

90. Bacman S, et al. Circulating antibodies against neurotransmitter receptor activities in children with congenital heart block and their mothers. FASEB J 8 (14):1170–1176, 1994.

91. Mijares A, et al. From agonist to antagonist: Fab fragments of an agonist-like monoclonal anti-beta(2)-adrenoceptor antibody behave as antagonists. Mol Pharmacol 58 (2):373–379, 2000.

92. Quan CP, et al. High affinity serum-derived Fab fragments as another source of antibodies in the gut lumen of both neonates and adults. Scand J Immunol 44 (2):108–114, 1996.

93. Wedeking-Schohl H, Maisch B, Schonian UH. [Fetal arrhythmias—new immunologic studies and results]. Z Geburtshilfe Perinatol 197 (3):144–147, 1993.

94. Kleinman CS, Nehgme RA. Cardiac arrhythmias in the human fetus. Pediatr Cardiol 25 (3):234–251, 2004.

95. Moise KJ Jr. Management of rhesus alloimmunization in pregnancy. Obstet Gynecol 100 (3):600–611, 2002.

96. Lambin P, et al. IgG1 and IgG3 anti-D in maternal serum and on the RBCs of infants suffering from HDN: relationship with the severity of the disease. Transfusion 42 (12):1537–1546, 2002.

97. Fung Kee Fung K, et al. Prevention of Rh alloimmunization. J Obstet Gynaecol Can 25 (9):765–773, 2003.

98. Maayan-Metzger A, et al. Maternal anti-D prophylaxis during pregnancy does not cause neonatal haemolysis. Arch Dis Child Fetal Neonatal Ed 84 (1):F60–62, 2001.

99. Collinet P, et al. Successful treatment of extremely severe fetal anemia due to Kell alloimmunization. Obstet Gynecol 100 (5 Pt 2):1102–1105, 2002.

100. Denomme GA, et al. Maternal ABO-mismatched blood for intrauterine transfusion of severe hemolytic disease of the newborn due to anti-Rh17. Transfusion 44 (9):1357–1360, 2004.

101. Mundy CA. Intravenous immunoglobulin in the management of hemolytic disease of the newborn. Neonatal Netw 24 (6):17–24, 2005.

102. Miqdad AM, et al. Intravenous immunoglobulin G (IVIG) therapy for significant hyperbilirubinemia in ABO hemolytic disease of the newborn. J Matern Fetal Neonatal Med 16 (3):163–166, 2004.

103. Narang A, Jain N. Haemolytic disease of newborn. Indian J Pediatr 68 (2):167–172, 2001.

104. Sarici SU, et al. An early (sixth-hour) serum bilirubin measurement is useful in predicting the development of significant hyperbilirubinemia and severe ABO hemolytic disease in a selective high-risk population of newborns with ABO incompatibility. Pediatrics 109(4):e53.

105. Dinesh D. Review of positive direct antiglobulin tests found on cord blood sampling. J Paediatr Child Health 2005. 41 (9–10):504–507, 2002.

106. Dikshit SK, Gupta PK. Exchange transfusion in neonatal hyperbilirubinemia. Indian Pediatr 26 (11):1139–1145, 1989.

107. Amato M, et al. Effectiveness of single versus double volume exchange transfusion in newborn infants with AB0 hemolytic disease. Helv Paediatr Acta 43 (3):177–186, 1988.

108. Geifman-Holtzman O, et al. Female alloimmunization with antibodies known to cause hemolytic disease. Obstet Gynecol 89 (2):272–275, 1997.

109. Wenk RE, Goldstein P, Felix JK. Kell alloimmunization, hemolytic disease of the newborn, and perinatal management. Obstet Gynecol 66 (4):473–476, 1985.

110. Mochizuki K, et al. Hemolytic disease of the newborn due to anti-Di: a case study and review of the literature. Transfusion 46 (3):454–460, 2006.

111. Vaughan JI, et al. Inhibition of erythroid progenitor cells by anti-Kell antibodies in fetal alloimmune anemia. N Engl J Med 338 (12):798–803, 1998.

112. Grant SR, et al. The outcome of pregnancy in Kell alloimmunisation. Bjog 107 (4):481–485, 2000.

113. Dhodapkar KM, Blei F. Treatment of hemolytic disease of the newborn caused by anti-Kell antibody with recombinant erythropoietin. J Pediatr Hematol Oncol 23 (1):69–70, 2001.

114. Uhrynowska M, Maslanka K, Zupanska B. Neonatal thrombocytopenia: incidence, serological and clinical observations. Am J Perinatol 14 (7):415–418, 1997.

115. Kaplan C, et al. Fetal and neonatal alloimmune thrombocytopenia: current trends in diagnosis and therapy. Transfus Med 2 (4):265–271, 1992.

116. Manno CS. Management of bleeding disorders in children. Hematology (Am Soc Hematol Educ Program), 2005:416–22.

117. Deaver JE, Leppert PC, Zaroulis CG. Neonatal alloimmune thrombocytopenic purpura. Am J Perinatol 3 (2):127–131, 1986.

118. Davoren A, et al. Neonatal neutropenia and bacterial sepsis associated with placental transfer of maternal neutrophil-specific autoantibodies. Transfusion 44 (7):1041–1046, 2004.

119. Maheshwari A, Christensen RD, Calhoun DA. Immune neutropenia in the neonate. Adv Pediatr 49:317–339, 2002.

120. Minchinton RM, McGrath KM. Alloimmune neonatal neutropenia–a neglected diagnosis? Med J Aust 147 (3):139–141, 1987.

121. Han TH, Chey MJ, Han KS. A case of neonatal alloimmune neutropenia associated with anti-human neutrophil antigen-1a (HNA-1a) antibody. J Korean Med Sci 21 (2):351–354, 2006.

122. Curtis BR, Reno C, Aster RH. Neonatal alloimmune neutropenia attributed to maternal immunoglobulin G antibodies against the neutrophil alloantigen HNA-1c (SH): a report of five cases. Transfusion 45 (8):1308–1313, 2005.

123. Hagimoto R, et al. A possible role for maternal HLA antibody in a case of alloimmune neonatal neutropenia. Transfusion 41 (5):615–620, 2001.

124. Tomicic M, et al. Severe neonatal neutropenia due to anti-human leucocyte antigen B49 alloimmunization only: a case report. Transfus Med 13 (4):233–237, 2003.

125. Kameoka J, et al. Autoimmune neutropenia in pregnant women causing neonatal neutropenia. Br J Haematol 114 (1):198–200, 2001.

126. Lee LA. Neonatal lupus: clinical features and management. Paediatr Drugs 6 (2):71–78, 2004.

127. Kanagasegar S, et al. Neonatal lupus manifests as isolated neutropenia and mildly abnormal liver functions. J Rheumatol 29 (1):187–191, 2002.

128. Fung YL, et al. Managing passively acquired autoimmune neonatal neutropenia: a case study. Transfus Med 15 (2):151–155, 2005.

129. Bastian JF, et al. Maternal isoimmunisation resulting in combined immunodeficiency and fatal graft-versus-host disease in an infant. Lancet 1 (8392):1435–1437, 1984.

130. Fu J, et al. Risk factors of primary thyroid dysfunction in early infants born to mothers with autoimmune thyroid disease. Acta Paediatr 94 (8):1043–1048, 2005.

131. Dussault JH, Fisher DA. Thyroid function in mothers of hypothyroid newborns. Obstet Gynecol 93 (1):15–20, 1999.

132. Lazarus JH. Thyroid disease in pregnancy and childhood. Minerva Endocrinol 30 (2):71–87, 2005.

133. Svensson J, et al. Thyroid autoantibodies in cord blood sera from children and adolescents with autoimmune thyroiditis. Thyroid 16 (1):79–83, 2006.

134. Pop VJ, et al. Maternal thyroid peroxidase antibodies during pregnancy: a marker of impaired child development? J Clin Endocrinol Metab 80 (12):3561–3566, 1995.

135. Biro E, et al. Association of systemic and thyroid autoimmune diseases. Clin Rheumatol 25 (2):240–245, 2006.

136. McDonagh JE, Isenberg DA. Development of additional autoimmune diseases in a population of patients with systemic lupus erythematosus. Ann Rheum Dis 59 (3):230–232, 2000.

137. Ruggeri RM, et al. Thyroid hormone autoantibodies in primary Sjogren syndrome and rheumatoid arthritis are more prevalent than in autoimmune thyroid disease, becoming progressively more frequent in these diseases. J Endocrinol Invest 25 (5):447–454, 2002.

138. Spence D, et al. Increased risk of complete congenital heart block in infants born to women with hypothyroidism and anti-Ro and/or anti-La antibodies. J Rheumatol 33 (1):167–170, 2006.

139. Alexander EK, et al. Timing and magnitude of increases in levothyroxine requirements during pregnancy in women with hypothyroidism. N Engl J Med 351 (3):241–249, 2004.

140. Polak M. Hyperthyroidism in early infancy: pathogenesis, clinical features and diagnosis with a focus on neonatal hyperthyroidism. Thyroid 8 (12):1171–1177, 1998.

141. Zimmerman D. Fetal and neonatal hyperthyroidism. Thyroid 9 (7):727–733, 1999.

142. Kung AW, Lau KS, Kohn LD. Epitope mapping of TSH receptor-blocking antibodies in Graves' disease that appear during pregnancy. J Clin Endocrinol Metab 86 (8):3647–3653, 2001.

143. Luton D, et al. Management of Graves' disease during pregnancy: the key role of fetal thyroid gland monitoring. J Clin Endocrinol Metab 90 (11):6093–6098, 2005.

144. Nachum Z, et al. Graves' disease in pregnancy: prospective evaluation of a selective invasive treatment protocol. Am J Obstet Gynecol 189 (1):159–165, 2003.

145. Kamishlian A, et al. Different outcomes of neonatal thyroid function after Graves' disease in pregnancy: patient reports and literature review. J Pediatr Endocrinol Metab 18 (12):1357–1363, 2005.

146. Chertow BS, et al. The effects of human insulin on antibody formation in pregnant diabetics and their newborns. Obstet Gynecol 72 (5):724–728, 1988.

147. Naserke HE, Bonifacio E, Ziegler AG. Immunoglobulin G insulin autoantibodies in BABYDIAB offspring appear postnatally: sensitive early detection using a protein A/G-based radiobinding assay. J Clin Endocrinol Metab 84 (4):1239–1243, 1999.

148. Di Mario U, et al. Insulin-anti-insulin complexes in diabetic women and their neonates. Diabetologia 27 (Suppl):83–86, 1984.

149. Dotta F, et al. Humoral and cellular immune abnormalities in neonates of diabetic mothers: any pathological role? Exp Clin Endocrinol 89 (3):333–339, 1987.

150. Poletaev AB, et al. Possible mechanisms of diabetic fetopathy. Hum Antibodies 9 (4):189–197, 2000.

151. Koczwara K, Ziegler AG, Bonifacio E. Maternal immunity to insulin does not affect diabetes risk in progeny of non obese diabetic mice. Clin Exp Immunol 136 (1):56–59, 2004.

152. Greeley SA, et al. Elimination of maternally transmitted autoantibodies prevents diabetes in non-obese diabetic mice. Nat Med 8 (4):399–402, 2002.

153. Melanitou E, et al. Early and quantal (by litter) expression of insulin autoantibodies in the nonobese diabetic mice predict early diabetes onset. J Immunol 173 (11):6603–6610, 2004.

154. Naserke HE, Bonifacio E, Ziegler AG. Prevalence, characteristics and diabetes risk associated with transient maternally acquired islet antibodies and persistent islet antibodies in offspring of parents with type 1 diabetes. J Clin Endocrinol Metab 86 (10):4826–4833, 2001.

155. Ludvigsson J, Wahlberg J. Diabetes-related autoantibodies in cord blood from children of healthy mothers have disappeared by the time the child is one year old. Ann N Y Acad Sci 958:289–292, 2002.

156. Hamalainen AM, et al. Disease-associated autoantibodies during pregnancy and at birth in families affected by type 1 diabetes. Clin Exp Immunol 126 (2):230–235, 2001.

157. Lindsay RS, et al. Type 1 diabetes-related antibodies in the fetal circulation: prevalence and influence on cord insulin and birth weight in offspring of mothers with type 1 diabetes. J Clin Endocrinol Metab 89 (7):3436–3439, 2004.

158. Weiss PA, et al. Anti-insulin antibodies and birth weight in pregnancies complicated by diabetes. Early Hum Dev 53 (2):145–154, 1998.

159. Gamlen TR, et al. Immunological studies in the neonate of a mother with Addison's disease and diabetes mellitus. Clin Exp Immunol 28 (1):192–195, 1977.

160. Betterle C, et al. Assessment of adrenocortical function and autoantibodies in a baby born to a mother with autoimmune polyglandular syndrome Type 2. J Endocrinol Invest 27 (7):618–621, 2004.

161. Eymard B, et al. Anti-acetylcholine receptor antibodies in neonatal myasthenia gravis: heterogeneity and pathogenic significance. J Autoimmun 4 (2):185–195, 1991.

162. Lefvert AK, et al. Determination of acetylcholine receptor antibody in myasthenia gravis: clinical usefulness and pathogenetic implications. J Neurol Neurosurg Psychiatry 41 (5): 394–403, 1978.

163. Sisman J, Ceri A, Nafday SM. Seronegative neonatal myasthenia gravis in one of the twins. Indian Pediatr 41 (9):938–940, 2004.

164. Podciechowski L, et al. Pregnancy complicated by Myasthenia gravis – twelve years experience. Neuro Endocrinol Lett 26 (5):603–608, 2005.

165. Lefvert AK, Osterman PO. Newborn infants to myasthenic mothers: a clinical study and an investigation of acetylcholine receptor antibodies in 17 children. Neurology 33 (2):133–138, 1983.

166. Cantagrel S, et al. Akinesia, arthrogryposis, craniosynostosis: a presentation of neonatal myasthenia with fetal onset. Am J Perinatol 19 (6):297–301, 2002.

167. Riemersma S, et al. Association of arthrogryposis multiplex congenita with maternal antibodies inhibiting fetal acetylcholine receptor function. J Clin Invest 98 (10):2358–2363, 1996.

168. Hesselmans LF, et al. Development of innervation of skeletal muscle fibers in man: relation to acetylcholine receptors. Anat Rec 236 (3):553–562, 1993.

169. Gardnerova M, et al. The fetal/adult acetylcholine receptor antibody ratio in mothers with myasthenia gravis as a marker for transfer of the disease to the newborn. Neurology 48 (1):50–54, 1997.

170. Eymard B, et al. Assay of anti-acetylcholine receptor antibodies in myasthenic syndromes of newborn infants. Presse Med 15 (22):1019–1022, 1986.

171. Rieder AA, Conley SF, Rowe L. Pediatric myasthenia gravis and velopharyngeal incompetence. Int J Pediatr Otorhinolaryngol 68 (6):747–752, 2004.

172. Barnes PR, et al. Recurrent congenital arthrogryposis leading to a diagnosis of myasthenia gravis in an initially asymptomatic mother. Neuromuscul Disord 5 (1):59–65, 1995.

173. Ferrero S, et al. Myasthenia gravis: management issues during pregnancy. Eur J Obstet Gynecol Reprod Biol 121 (2):129–138, 2005.

174. Verspyck E, et al. Myasthenia gravis with polyhydramnios in the fetus of an asymptomatic mother. Prenat Diagn 13 (6):539–542, 1993.

175. Donat JF, Donat JR, Lennon VA. Exchange transfusion in neonatal myasthenia gravis. Neurology 31 (7):911–912, 1981.

176. Tagher RJ, Baumann R, Desai N. Failure of intravenously administered immunoglobulin in the treatment of neonatal myasthenia gravis. J Pediatr 134 (2):233–235, 1999.

177. Hamrock DJ. Adverse events associated with intravenous immunoglobulin therapy. Int Immunopharmacol 6 (4):535–542, 2006.

178. Siegel J. Safety considerations in IGIV utilization. Int Immunopharmacol 6 (4):523–527, 2006.

179. Schmidt-Ott R, et al. Improved serological diagnosis stresses the major role of campylobacter jejuni in triggering Guillain-Barre syndrome. Clin Vaccine Immunol 13 (7):779–783, 2006.

180. Caporale CM, et al. Susceptibility to Guillain-Barre syndrome is associated to polymorphisms of CD1 genes. J Neuroimmunol 2006.

181. Jackson AH, Baquis GD, Shah BL. Congenital Guillain-Barre syndrome. J Child Neurol 11 (5):407–410, 1996.

182. Bamford NS, et al. Congenital Guillain-Barre syndrome associated with maternal inflammatory bowel disease is responsive to intravenous immunoglobulin. Eur J Paediatr Neurol 6 (2):115–119, 2002.

183. Buchwald B, et al. Neonatal Guillain-Barre syndrome: blocking antibodies transmitted from mother to child. Neurology 53 (6):1246–1253, 1999.

184. Attarian S, et al. Neonatal lower motor neuron syndrome associated with maternal neuropathy with anti-GM1 IgG. Neurology 63 (2):379–381, 2004.

185. Bansal PJ, Tobin MC. Neonatal microscopic polyangiitis secondary to transfer of maternal myeloperoxidase-antineutrophil cytoplasmic antibody resulting in neonatal pulmonary hemorrhage and renal involvement. Ann Allergy Asthma Immunol 93 (4):398–401, 2004.

186. Lee BH, et al. Adverse neonatal outcomes associated with antenatal dexamethasone versus antenatal betamethasone. Pediatrics 117 (5):1503–1510, 2006.

187. Finer NN, et al. Prospective evaluation of postnatal steroid administration: a 1-year experience from the California Perinatal Quality Care Collaborative. Pediatrics 117 (3):704–713, 2006.

188. Mildenhall LF, et al. Exposure to repeat doses of antenatal glucocorticoids is associated with altered cardiovascular status after birth. Arch Dis Child Fetal Neonatal Ed 91 (1):F56–60, 2006.

189. Bakker JM, et al. Neonatal dexamethasone treatment increases susceptibility to experimental autoimmune disease in adult rats. J Immunol 165 (10):5932–5937, 2000.

190. Dolfin T, et al. Acute renal failure in a neonate caused by the transplacental transfer of a nephrotoxic paraprotein: successful resolution by exchange transfusion. Am J Kidney Dis 34 (6):1129–1131, 1999.

191. Laugel V, et al. Neonatal management of symptomatic transplacental cryoglobulinaemia. Acta Paediatr 93 (4):556–558, 2004.

192. Tissot JD, et al. Monoclonal gammopathy in a 30 weeks old premature infant. Appl Theor Electrophor 3 (2):67–68, 1992.

193. Rosenblatt DS, Cooper BA. Inherited disorders of vitamin B12 metabolism. Blood Rev 1 (3):177–182, 1987.

194. Rothenberg SP, et al. Autoantibodies against folate receptors in women with a pregnancy complicated by a neural-tube defect. N Engl J Med 350 (2):134–142, 2004.

195. Whittingham S, Mackay IR. Autoimmune gastritis: historical antecedents, outstanding discoveries, and unresolved problems. Int Rev Immunol 24 (1–2):1–29, 2005.

196. Bar-Shany S, Herbert V. Transplacentally acquired antibody to intrinsic factor with vitamin B12 deficiency. Blood 30 (6):777–784, 1967.

197. Kondo H, Imamura T. Pernicious anemia (PA) subsequent to insulin-dependent diabetes mellitus and idiopathic thrombocytopenic purpura, and effects of oral cobalamin on PA. Am J Hematol 62 (1):61–62, 1999.

198. Perros P, et al. Prevalence of pernicious anaemia in patients with Type 1 diabetes mellitus and autoimmune thyroid disease. Diabet Med 17 (10):749–751, 2000.

199. Durand JM, et al. Systemic lupus erythematosus associated with pernicious anemia. Clin Exp Rheumatol 12 (2):233, 1994.

200. Hertl M, Veldman C. Pemphigus–paradigm of autoantibody-mediated autoimmunity. Skin Pharmacol Appl Skin Physiol 14 (6):408–418, 2001.

201. Mahoney MG, et al. Delineation of diversified desmoglein distribution in stratified squamous epithelia: implications in diseases. Exp Dermatol 15 (2):101–109, 2006.

202. Wu H, et al. Protection against pemphigus foliaceus by desmoglein 3 in neonates. N Engl J Med 343 (1):31–35, 2000.

203. Parlowsky T, et al. Neonatal pemphigus vulgaris: IgG4 autoantibodies to desmoglein 3 induce skin blisters in newborns. J Am Acad Dermatol 48 (4):623–625, 2003.

204. Campo-Voegeli A, et al. Neonatal pemphigus vulgaris with extensive mucocutaneous lesions from a mother with oral pemphigus vulgaris. Br J Dermatol 147 (4):801–805, 2002.

205. Fenniche S, et al. Neonatal pemphigus vulgaris in an infant born to a mother with pemphigus vulgaris in remission. Pediatr Dermatol 23 (2):124–127, 2006.

206. Diaz LA, et al. Anti-desmoglein-1 antibodies in onchocerciasis, leishmaniasis and Chagas disease suggest a possible etiological link to Fogo selvagem. J Invest Dermatol 123 (6):1045–1051, 2004.

207. Nagasaka T, et al. Defining the pathogenic involvement of desmoglein 4 in pemphigus and staphylococcal scalded skin syndrome. J Clin Invest 114 (10):1484–1492, 2004.

208. Chiossi MP, Costa RS, Roselino AM. Dermal dendritic cell number correlates with serum autoantibody titers in Brazilian pemphigus foliaceus patients. Braz J Med Biol Res 37 (3):337–341, 2004.

209. Shieh S, et al. Pemphigus, pregnancy, and plasmapheresis. Cutis 73 (5):327–329, 2004.

210. Fainaru O, et al. Pemphigus vulgaris in pregnancy: a case report and review of literature. Hum Reprod 15 (5):1195–1197, 2000.

211. Nguyen VT, et al. Pemphigus vulgaris acantholysis ameliorated by cholinergic agonists. Arch Dermatol 140 (3):327–334, 2004.

212. Ortiz-Urda S, et al. The plant lectin wheat germ agglutinin inhibits the binding of pemphigus foliaceus autoantibodies to desmoglein 1 in a majority of patients and prevents pathomechanisms of pemphigus foliaceus in vitro and in vivo. J Immunol 171 (11):6244–6250, 2003.

213. Burch JM, et al. Autoantibodies in mothers of children with neonatal liver disease. J Pediatr Gastroenterol Nutr 37 (3):262–267, 2003.

214. Whitington PF, Kelly S, Ekong UD. Neonatal hemochromatosis: fetal liver disease leading to liver failure in the fetus and newborn. Pediatr Transplant 9 (5):640–645, 2005.

215. Kelly AL, et al. Classification and genetic features of neonatal haemochromatosis: a study of 27 affected pedigrees and molecular analysis of genes implicated in iron metabolism. J Med Genet 38 (9):599–610, 2001.

216. Ekong UD, Kelly S, Whitington PF. Disparate clinical presentation of neonatal hemochromatosis in twins. Pediatrics 116 (6):e880–e884, 2005.

217. Whitington PF, Malladi P. Neonatal hemochromatosis: is it an alloimmune disease? J Pediatr Gastroenterol Nutr 40 (5):544–549, 2005.

218. Whitington PF, Hibbard JU. High-dose immunoglobulin during pregnancy for recurrent neonatal haemochromatosis. Lancet 364 (9446):1690–1698, 2004.

219. Pall H, Jonas MM. Pediatric hepatobiliary disease. Curr Opin Gastroenterol 21 (3):344–347, 2005.

220. Flynn DM, et al. Progress in treatment and outcome for children with neonatal haemochromatosis. Arch Dis Child Fetal Neonatal Ed 88 (2):F124–127, 2003.

221. Gleicher N. Autoantibodies and pregnancy loss. Lancet 343 (8900):747–748, 1994.

222. Wallukat G, et al. Agonistic autoantibodies directed against the angiotensin II AT1 receptor in patients with preeclampsia. Can J Physiol Pharmacol 81 (2):79–83, 2003.

223. Xia Y, et al. Maternal autoantibodies from preeclamptic patients activate angiotensin receptors on human trophoblast cells. J Soc Gynecol Investig 10 (2):82–93, 2003.

224. Bobst SM, et al. Maternal autoantibodies from preeclamptic patients activate angiotensin receptors on human mesangial cells and induce interleukin-6 and plasminogen activator inhibitor-1 secretion. Am J Hypertens 18 (3):330–336, 2005.

225. Dechend R, et al. Agonistic autoantibodies to the AT1 receptor in a transgenic rat model of preeclampsia. Hypertension 45 (4):742–746, 2005.

226. Dragun D, et al. Angiotensin II type 1-receptor activating antibodies in renal-allograft rejection. N Engl J Med 352 (6):558–569, 2005.

227. Kutteh WH, Rote NS, Silver R. Antiphospholipid antibodies and reproduction: the antiphospholipid antibody syndrome. Am J Reprod Immunol 41 (2):133–152, 1999.

228. Nishiguchi T, Kobayashi T. Antiphospholipid syndrome: characteristics and obstetrical management. Curr Drug Targets 6 (5):593–605, 2005.

229. Wu S, Stephenson MD. Obstetrical antiphospholipid syndrome. Semin Reprod Med 24 (1):40–53, 2006.

230. Zurgil N, et al. Detection of anti-phospholipid and anti-DNA antibodies and their idiotypes in newborns of mothers with anti-phospholipid syndrome and SLE. Lupus 2 (4):233–237, 1993.

231. el-Roeiy A, et al. A common anti-DNA idiotype and other autoantibodies in sera of offspring of mothers with systemic lupus erythematosus. Clin Exp Immunol 68 (3):528–534, 1987.

232. Silver RK, et al. Fetal stroke associated with elevated maternal anticardiolipin antibodies. Obstet Gynecol 80 (3 Pt 2):497–499, 1992.

233. Pierangeli SS, et al. Requirement of activation of complement C3 and C5 for antiphospholipid antibody-mediated thrombophilia. Arthritis Rheum 52 (7):2120–2124, 2005.

234. Girardi G, Redecha P, Salmon JE. Heparin prevents antiphospholipid antibody-induced fetal loss by inhibiting complement activation. Nat Med 10 (11):1222–1226, 2004.

235. Inagaki J, et al. Pregnancy loss and endometriosis: pathogenic role of anti-laminin-1 autoantibodies. Ann N Y Acad Sci 1051:174–184, 2005.

236. Klaffky EJ, Gonzales IM, Sutherland AE. Trophoblast cells exhibit differential responses to laminin isoforms. Dev Biol 292 (2):277–289, 2006.

237. Matalon ST, et al. Immunization of naive mice with mouse laminin-1 affected pregnancy outcome in a mouse model. Am J Reprod Immunol 50 (2):159–165, 2003.

238. Inagaki J, et al. IgG anti-laminin-1 autoantibody and recurrent miscarriages. Am J Reprod Immunol 45 (4):232–238, 2001.

239. Ludvigsson JF, Falth-Magnusson K, Ludvigsson J. Tissue transglutaminase auto-antibodies in cord blood from children to become celiacs. Scand J Gastroenterol 36 (12):1279–1283, 2001.

240. Eliakim R, Sherer DM. Celiac disease: fertility and pregnancy. Gynecol Obstet Invest 51 (1):3–7, 2001.

241. Hager H, et al. Developmental regulation of tissue transglutaminase during human placentation and expression in neoplastic trophoblast. J Pathol 181 (1):106–110, 1997.

242. Robinson NJ, et al. Tissue transglutaminase expression and activity in placenta. Placenta 27 (2–3):148–157, 2006.

243. Hoff JM, Daltveit AK, Gilhus NE. Myasthenia gravis: consequences for pregnancy, delivery, and the newborn. Neurology 61 (10):1362–1366, 2003.

244. Hoff JM, Daltveit AK, Gilhus NE. Asymptomatic myasthenia gravis influences pregnancy and birth. Eur J Neurol 11 (8):559–562, 2004.

245. Ghafoor F, et al. Role of thyroid peroxidase antibodies in the outcome of pregnancy. J Coll Physicians Surg Pak 16 (7):468–471, 2006.

246. Mecacci F, et al. Thyroid autoimmunity and its association with non-organ-specific antibodies and subclinical alterations of thyroid function in women with a history of pregnancy loss or pre-eclampsia. J Reprod Immunol 46 (1):39–50, 2000.

247. Peleg D, et al. The relationship between maternal serum thyroid-stimulating immunoglobulin and fetal and neonatal thyrotoxicosis. Obstet Gynecol 99 (6):1040–1043, 2002.

248. Viskari H, et al. Relationship between the incidence of type 1 diabetes and maternal enterovirus antibodies: time trends and geographical variation. Diabetologia 48 (7):1280–1287, 2005.

249. Sadeharju K, et al. Enterovirus infections as a risk factor for type I diabetes: virus analyses in a dietary intervention trial. Clin Exp Immunol 132 (2):271–277, 2003.

250. Harkonen T, et al. Enterovirus infection may induce humoral immune response reacting with islet cell autoantigens in humans. J Med Virol 69 (3):426–440, 2003.

251. Green I, Inkelas M, Allen LB. Hodgkin's disease: a maternal-to-fetal lymphocyte chimaera? The Lancet, 1960:30–32.

252. Desai RG, Creger WP. Maternofetal passage of leukocytes and platelets in man. Blood 21:665–673, 1963.

253. Lo ES, et al. Transfer of nucleated maternal cells into fetal circulation during the second trimester of pregnancy. Br J Haematol 100 (3):605–606, 1998.

254. Piotrowski P, Croy BA. Maternal cells are widely distributed in murine fetuses in utero. Biol Reprod 54 (5):1103–1110, 1996.

255. Berry SM, et al. Association of maternal histocompatibility at class II HLA loci with maternal microchimerism in the fetus. Pediatr Res 56 (1):73–78, 2004.

256. Lambert NC, et al. Quantification of maternal microchimerism by HLA-specific real-time polymerase chain reaction: studies of healthy women and women with scleroderma. Arthritis Rheum 50 (3):906–914, 2004.

257. Zarou DM, Lichtman HC, Hellman LM. The transmission of chromium-51 tagged maternal erythrocytes from mother to fetus. Am J Obstet Gynecol 88:565–571, 1964.

258. Petit T, et al. A highly sensitive polymerase chain reaction method reveals the ubiquitous presence of maternal cells in human umbilical cord blood. Exp Hematol 23 (14):1601–1605, 1995.

259. Socie G, et al. Search for maternal cells in human umbilical cord blood by polymerase chain reaction amplification of two minisatellite sequences. Blood 83 (2):340–344, 1994.

260. Lo YM, et al. Two-way cell traffic between mother and fetus: biologic and clinical implications. Blood 88 (11):4390–4395, 1996.

261. Lo YM. Fetal DNA in maternal plasma. Ann N Y Acad Sci 906:141–147, 2000.

262. Loubière LS, et al. Maternal microchimerism in healthy adults in lymphocytes, monocyte/macrophages, and NK cells. Lab Invest 86:1185–1192, 2006.

263. Reed AM, et al. Does HLA-dependent chimerism underlie the pathogenesis of juvenile dermatomyositis? J Immunol 172 (8):5041–5046, 2004.

264. Artlett CM, et al. Chimeric cells of maternal origin in juvenile idiopathic inflammatory myopathies. Childhood Myositis Heterogeneity Collaborative Group. Lancet 356 (9248):2155–2156, 2000.

265. Keller MA, et al. Transfer of tuberculin immunity from mother to infant. Pediatr Res 22 (3):277–281, 1987.

266. Osada S, et al. A case of infantile acute monocytic leukemia caused by vertical transmission of the mother's leukemic cells. Cancer 65 (5):1146–1149, 1990.

267. Catlin EA, et al. Transplacental transmission of natural-killer-cell lymphoma. N Engl J Med 341 (2):85–91, 1999.

268. Tolar J, Coad JE, Neglia JP. Transplacental transfer of small-cell carcinoma of the lung. N Engl J Med 346 (19):1501–1502, 2002.

269. Alexander A, et al. Metastatic melanoma in pregnancy: risk of transplacental metastases in the infant. J Clin Oncol 21 (11):2179–2186, 2003.

270. Stevens AM, et al. Differentiated Maternal and Fetal Cells in Tissues from Patients with and without Autoimmune Disease. Arthritis Rheum 48:S511, 2003.

271. Khosrotehrani K, et al. Presence of chimeric maternally derived keratinocytes in cutaneous inflammatory diseases of children: the example of pityriasis lichenoides. J Invest Dermatol 126 (2):345–348, 2006.

272. Sugimoto H, et al. Bone-marrow-derived stem cells repair basement membrane collagen defects and reverse genetic kidney disease. Proc Natl Acad Sci USA 103 (19):7321–7326, 2006.

273. Holzgreve W, et al. Disturbed feto-maternal cell traffic in preeclampsia. Obstet Gynecol 91 (5 Pt 1):669–672, 1998.

274. Smid M, et al. Quantitative analysis of fetal DNA in maternal plasma in pathological conditions associated with placental abnormalities. Ann NY Acad Sci 945:132–137, 2001.

275. Zhong XY, et al. Elevation of both maternal and fetal extracellular circulating deoxyribonucleic acid concentrations in the plasma of pregnant women with preeclampsia. Am J Obstet Gynecol 184 (3):414–419, 2001.

276. Bianchi DW, et al. Significant fetal-maternal hemorrhage after termination of pregnancy: implications for development of fetal cell microchimerism. Am J Obstet Gynecol 184 (4):703–706, 2001.

277. Lo YM, et al. Increased fetal DNA concentrations in the plasma of pregnant women carrying fetuses with trisomy 21. Clin Chem 45 (10):1747–1751, 1999.

278. Kaplan J, Land S. Influence of maternal-fetal histocompatibility and MHC zygosity on maternal microchimerism. J Immunol 174 (11):7123–7128, 2005.

279. Lambert NC, et al. Cutting edge: persistent fetal microchimerism in T lymphocytes is associated with HLA-DQA1*0501: implications in autoimmunity. J Immunol 164 (11):5545–5548, 2000.

280. Stevens AM, et al. Maternal microchimerism in the human thymus. Arthritis Rheum 44 (9):S340, 2001.

281. Marrack P, Kappler J. Control of T cell viability. Annu Rev Immunol 22:765–787, 2004.

282. van Dijk BA, Boomsma DI, de Man AJ. Blood group chimerism in human multiple births is not rare. Am J Med Genet 61 (3):264–268, 1996.

283. Kuhl-Burmeister R, et al. Equal distribution of congenital blood cell chimerism in dizygotic triplets after in-vitro fertilization. Hum Reprod 15 (5):1200–1204, 2000.

284. Hall JG. Twinning. Lancet 362 (9385):735–743, 2003.

285. Stevens AM, et al. Maternal and sibling microchimerism in twins and triplets discordant for neonatal lupus syndrome-congenital heart block. Rheumatology (Oxford) 44 (2):187–191, 2005.

286. Sudik R, et al. Chimerism in a fertile woman with 46,XY karyotype and female phenotype. Hum Reprod 16 (1):56–58, 2001.

287. Bianchi DW, et al. Male fetal progenitor cells persist in maternal blood for as long as 27 years postpartum. Proc Natl Acad Sci USA 93 (2):705–708, 1996.

288. Lambert NC, et al. Male microchimerism in women with systemic sclerosis and healthy women who have never given birth to a son. Ann Rheum Dis 64 (6):845–848, 2005.

289. Yan Z, et al. Male microchimerism in women without sons: quantitative assessment and correlation with pregnancy history. Am J Med 118 (8):899–906, 2005.

290. Guettier C, et al. Male cell microchimerism in normal and diseased female livers from fetal life to adulthood. Hepatology 42 (1):35–43, 2005.

291. Carrier E, et al. Induction of tolerance in nondefective mice after in utero transplantation of major histocompatibility complex-mismatched fetal hematopoietic stem cells. Blood 86 (12):4681–4690, 1995.

292. Hayward A, et al. Microchimerism and tolerance following intrauterine transplantation and transfusion for alpha-thalassemia-1. Fetal Diagn Ther 13 (1):8–14, 1998.

293. Peranteau WH, et al. High-level allogeneic chimerism achieved by prenatal tolerance induction and postnatal nonmyeloablative bone marrow transplantation. Blood 100 (6):2225–2234, 2002.

294. Vietor HE, et al. Survival of donor cells 25 years after intrauterine transfusion. Blood 95 (8):2709–2714, 2000.

295. Kim HB, etal. In utero bone marrow transplantation induces donor-specific tolerance by a combination of clonal deletion and clonal anergy. J Pediatr Surg 34(5):726-9; discussion 729-30, 1999.

296. Carrier E, et al. Microchimerism does not induce tolerance after in utero transplantation and may lead to the development of alloreactivity. J Lab Clin Med 136 (3):224–235d, 2000.

297. van der Veen FM, Rolink AG, Gleichmann E. Autoimmune disease strongly resembling systemic lupus erythematosus (SLE) in F1 mice undergoing graft-versus-host reaction (GVHR). Adv Exp Med Biol 149:669–677, 1982.

298. Parkman R, et al. Graft-versus-host disease after intrauterine and exchange transfusions for hemolytic disease of the newborn. N Engl J Med 290 (7):359–363, 1974.

299. Donahue J, et al. Microchimerism does not induce tolerance and sustains immunity after in utero transplantation. Transplantation 71 (3):359–368, 2001.

300. Moustafa ME, et al. Chimerism and tolerance post-in utero transplantation with embryonic stem cells. Transplantation 78 (9):1274–1282, 2004.

301. Andrassy J, et al. Tolerance to noninherited maternal MHC antigens in mice. J Immunol 171 (10):5554–5561, 2003.

302. Molitor ML, et al. HLA class I noninherited maternal antigens in cord blood and breast milk. Hum Immunol 65 (3):231–239, 2004.

303. Davis MK. Breastfeeding and chronic disease in childhood and adolescence. Pediatr Clin North Am 48 (1):125–141, ix, 2001.

304. Bertotto A, et al. Lymphocytes bearing the T cell receptor gamma delta in human breast milk. Arch Dis Child 65 (11):1274–1275, 1990.

305. Bertotto A, et al. Human breast milk T lymphocytes display the phenotype and functional characteristics of memory T cells. Eur J Immunol 20 (8):1877–1880, 1990.

306. Wirt DP, et al. Activated and memory T lymphocytes in human milk. Cytometry 13 (3):282–290, 1992.

307. Goldman AS. The immune system of human milk: antimicrobial, antiinflammatory and immunomodulating properties. Pediatr Infect Dis J 12 (8):664–671, 1993.

308. Losonsky GA, Ogra PL. Maternal-neonatal interactions and human breast milk. Prog Clin Biol Res 70:171–182, 1981.

309. Shimamura M, Huang YY, Goji H. Antibody production in early life supported by maternal lymphocyte factors. Biochim Biophys Acta 1637 (1):55–58, 2003.

310. Vernochet C, et al. Affinity-dependent alterations of mouse B cell development by noninherited maternal antigen. Biol Reprod 72 (2):460–469, 2005.

311. Reber AJ, Hippen AR, Hurley DJ. Effects of the ingestion of whole colostrum or cell-free colostrum on the capacity of leukocytes in newborn calves to stimulate or respond in one-way mixed leukocyte cultures. Am J Vet Res 66 (11):1854–1860, 2005.

312. Reber AJ, et al. Colostrum induced phenotypic and trafficking changes in maternal mononuclear cells in a peripheral blood leukocyte model for study of leukocyte transfer to the neonatal calf. Vet Immunol Immunopathol 109 (1–2):139–150, 2006.

313. Tuboly S, Bernath S. Intestinal absorption of colostral lymphoid cells in newborn animals. Adv Exp Med Biol 503:107–114, 2002.

314. Pollack MS, et al. Identification by HLA typing of intrauterine-derived maternal T cells in four patients with severe combined immunodeficiency. N Engl J Med 307 (11):662–666, 1982.

315. Pollack MS, et al. DR-positive maternal engrafted T cells in a severe combined immunodeficiency patient without graft-versus-host disease. Transplantation 30 (5):331–334, 1980.

316. Thompson LF, R.D. O'Connor RD, Bastian JF. Phenotype and function of engrafted maternal T cells in patients with severe combined immunodeficiency. J Immunol 133 (5):2513–2517, 1984.

317. Knobloch C, Goldmann SF, Friedrich W. Limited T cell receptor diversity of transplacentally acquired maternal T cells in severe combined immunodeficiency. J Immunol 146 (12):4157–4164, 1991.

318. Muller SM, et al. Transplacentally acquired maternal T lymphocytes in severe combined immunodeficiency: a study of 121 patients. Blood 98 (6):1847–1851, 2001.

319. Wahn V, et al. Expansion of a maternally derived monoclonal T cell population with CD3+/CD8+/ T cell receptor-gamma/delta+ phenotype in a child with severe combined immunodeficiency. J Immunol 147 (9):2934–2941, 1991.

320. Zhou M, Mellor AL. Expanded cohorts of maternal CD8+ T-cells specific for paternal MHC class I accumulate during pregnancy. J Reprod Immunol 40 (1):47–62, 1998.

321. Lambert N, Erickson T. Fetal and maternal microchimerism are simultaneously present in multiple organs in systemic sclerosis: a quantitative study. Arthritis Rheum 46 (9S), 2003.

322. Morse JH, et al. Isolated pulmonary hypertension in the grandchild of a kindred with scleroderma (systemic sclerosis): "neonatal scleroderma"? J Rheumatol 16 (12):1536–1541, 1989.

323. Barba A, et al. Morphoea in a newborn boy. Br J Dermatol 140 (2):365–366, 1999.

324. Ohtaki N, et al. Concurrent multiple morphea and neonatal lupus erythematosus in an infant boy born to a mother with SLE. Br J Dermatol 115 (1):85–90, 1986.

325. Sato S, Ishida W, Takehara K. A case of juvenile systemic sclerosis with disease onset at six months old. Clin Rheumatol 22 (2):162–163, 2003.

326. Brucato A, et al. Pregnancy outcome in 100 women with autoimmune diseases and anti-Ro/SSA antibodies: a prospective controlled study. Lupus 11 (11):716–721, 2002.

327. Reed A, et al. Chimerism in children with juvenile dermatomyositis. Lancet 356:2156–2157, 2000.

328. Harney S, et al. Non-inherited maternal HLA alleles are associated with rheumatoid arthritis. Rheumatology (Oxford) 42 (1):171–174, 2003.

329. Kowalzick L, et al. Chronic graft-versus-host-disease-like dermopathy in a child with CD4+ cell microchimerism. Dermatology 210 (1):68–71, 2005.

330. Vajsar J, Jay V, Babyn P. Infantile myositis presenting in the neonatal period. Brain Dev 18 (5):415–419, 1996.

331. McNeil SM, et al. Congenital inflammatory myopathy: a demonstrative case and proposed diagnostic classification. Muscle Nerve 25 (2):259–264, 2002.

332. Morrow J, et al. In: Morrow J, ed. Autoimmune rheumatic disease. New York: Oxford University Press; 1999.

333. Stevens AM, et al. Maternal HLA class II compatibility in men with systemic lupus erythematosus. Arthritis Rheum 52 (9):2768–2773, 2005.

334. Barrera P, et al. Noninherited maternal antigens do not increase the susceptibility for familial rheumatoid arthritis. European Consortium on Rheumatoid Arthritis Families (ECRAF). J Rheumatol 28 (5):968–974, 2001.

335. van Rood JJ, Claas F. Noninherited maternal HLA antigens: a proposal to elucidate their role in the immune response. Hum Immunol 61 (12):1390–1394, 2000.

336. Barrera P, et al. Noninherited maternal antigens do not play a role in rheumatoid arthritis susceptibility in Europe. European Consortium on Rheumatoid Arthritis Families. Arthritis Rheum 43 (4):758–764, 2000.

337. van der Horst-Bruinsma IE, et al. Influence of non-inherited maternal HLA-DR antigens on susceptibility to rheumatoid arthritis. Ann Rheum Dis 57 (11):672–675, 1998.

338. Lee LA, et al. Immunogenetics of the neonatal lupus syndrome. Ann Intern Med 99 (5):592–596, 1983.

339. Watson RM, et al. Neonatal lupus erythematosus. A clinical, serological and immunogenetic study with review of the literature. Medicine (Baltimore) 63 (6):362–378, 1984.

340. Brucato A, et al. Isolated congenital complete heart block: longterm outcome of mothers, maternal antibody specificity and immunogenetic background. J Rheumatol 22 (3):533–540, 1995.

341. Siren MK, et al. Role of HLA in congenital heart block: susceptibility alleles in mothers. Lupus 8 (1):52–59, 1999.

342. Colombo G, et al. DNA typing of maternal HLA in congenital complete heart block: comparison with systemic lupus erythematosus and primary Sjogren's syndrome. Arthritis Rheum 42 (8):1757–1764, 1999.

343. Matsuoka K, et al. Fetal tolerance to maternal antigens improves the outcome of allogeneic bone marrow transplantation by a CD4+ CD25+ T-cell-dependent mechanism. Blood 107 (1):404–409, 2006.

344. Owen RD, et al. Evidence for actively acquired tolerance to Rh antigens. Proc Natl Acad Sci USA 40 (6):420–424, 1954.

345. Claas FH, et al. Induction of B cell unresponsiveness to noninherited maternal HLA antigens during fetal life. Science 241 (4874):1815–1817, 1988.

346. van den Boogaardt DE, et al. The influence of inherited and noninherited parental antigens on outcome after transplantation. Transpl Int 19 (5):360–371, 2006.

347. Opelz G. Analysis of the "NIMA effect" in renal transplantation. Collaborative Transplant Study. Clin Transpl:63–67, 1990.

348. Sakaguchi S. Naturally arising Foxp3-expressing CD25+CD4+ regulatory T cells in immunological tolerance to self and non-self. Nat Immunol 6 (4):345–352, 2005.

349. Maggi E, et al. Thymic regulatory T cells. Autoimmun Rev 4 (8):579–586, 2005.

350. Chatila TA. Role of regulatory T cells in human diseases. J Allergy Clin Immunol 116(5):949-59; quiz 960, 2005.

351. Cupedo T, et al. Development and activation of regulatory T cells in the human fetus. Eur J Immunol 35 (2):383–390, 2005.

352. Thornton CA, et al. Functional maturation of CD4+CD25+CTLA4+CD45RA+ T regulatory cells in human neonatal T cell responses to environmental antigens/allergens. J Immunol 173 (5):3084–3092, 2004.

353. Piccirillo CA, et al. CD4(+)CD25(+) regulatory T cells can mediate suppressor function in the absence of transforming growth factor beta1 production and responsiveness. J Exp Med 196 (2):237–246, 2002.

354. Schaub B, et al. Neonatal immune responses to TLR2 stimulation: influence of maternal atopy on Foxp3 and IL-10 expression. Respir Res 7:40, 2006.

355. Somerset DA, et al. Normal human pregnancy is associated with an elevation in the immune suppressive CD25+ CD4+ regulatory T-cell subset. Immunology 112 (1):38–43, 2004.

356. Godfrey WR, et al. Cord blood CD4(+)CD25(+)-derived T regulatory cell lines express FoxP3 protein and manifest potent suppressor function. Blood 105 (2):750–758, 2005.

357. Wing K, et al. CD4+ CD25+ FOXP3+ regulatory T cells from human thymus and cord blood suppress antigen-specific T cell responses. Immunology 115 (4):516–525, 2005.

Chapter 10

What Insights Into Human Cord Blood Lymphocyte Function Can Be Gleaned From Studying Newborn Mice?

Cheri D. Landers, MD • Subbarao Bondada, PhD

Human Newborn Susceptibility to Infection

Human Newborn Immune Response

Murine Newborn Immune Response

Correlates in the Human Neonate

Human and Mouse Differences

Clinical Implications and Future Investigation Needs

Animal models for human conditions allow in vitro and in vivo research with more control over variables than enrolling human subjects. By minimizing genetic variation between animals and creating transgenic or knockout animals using targeted mutations and specific breeding along with strict control of environmental and research conditions, complex systems and diseases can be studied one component at a time down to the molecular level. Animal models also allow studying potentially toxic interventions and therapies prior to trials in the human population. The disadvantages of using animal models to study the pathophysiology and treatment of human disease processes include physiologic variation between animal and human species and the genetic variability between humans that is not present in most research animal species. This means that extrapolation of data from animal models to the human is not always possible but it does allow a reasonable starting point for investigation in humans. The mouse is a common mammal used for human physiology and disease modeling. Mice reproduce reliably, require little space for housing and have established genetic characteristics. Murine models for human disease are currently being used to study a variety of processes, including immune regulation (1), neurologic development and disease (2–5), vascular diseases (6), drug therapy (7, 8), pulmonary disease mechanisms (9, 10), congenital diseases and malformations (2, 11), cancer physiology, etiology and treatment (7, 12–14), and therapies for infectious diseases (15, 16).

Knowledge of the human immune system has grown immensely due to the utilization of animal models. The complex human immune system consists of primary and secondary lymphoid organs, with bone marrow as a source of immune cells and the secondary lymphoid organs such as the spleen and other lymphoid organs being the sites of the immune response. Lymphoid organ architecture, cytokines and chemokines play a critical role in the nature of the immune response. The normal human immune system response changes with age, maturing from neonate to adult and then declining again as humans get older. Similar changes occur throughout the life span of the mouse. In addition, the newborn mouse has one of the most immature mammalian immune systems at birth and mice require about 1/15th of their life span to reach full immune competence (17). Therefore, murine models for the normal human neonatal immune response are of assistance in increasing our knowledge of the developing human system. Specifically, the immune response of newborn mouse lymphocytes can be used as a model for the human neonatal immune response and allows more focused research when moving onto studies involving human neonates and cord blood (18–21). This chapter will briefly review the human neonate's susceptibility to infection, describe the deficiencies in the immune system of the human neonate and then focus on the neonate's insufficient B cell immunoglobulin response to specific antigens, compare this to what is seen in the newborn mouse and describe studies in the newborn mouse that have led to progress in improving the response of neonatal lymphocytes to antigen.

HUMAN NEWBORN SUSCEPTIBILITY TO INFECTION

Neonates are more susceptible than adults to a multitude of infections. This susceptibility is due to an immature acute inflammatory response, poor T and B cell cooperation and immunologic memory capability, lower mucosal antibody production and decreased reticuloendothelial clearance, leading to increased susceptibility to *Escherichia coli*, *Staphylococcus aureus*, *Streptococcus pneumoniae*, *Haemophilus influenza* type b, *Neisseria meningitidis*, viruses, and Candidal infections in the first 6 months of life (22). In particular, infants and young children are susceptible to infection from polysaccharide-encapsulated bacteria due to the infant's lack of antibody response to the polysaccharide antigen. This includes infections from the bacteria *H. influenza*, *S. pneumoniae* and *N. meningitidis* (23, 24). These organisms can cause very severe, invasive disease such as pneumonia, sepsis and meningitis that carries a significant risk of death in young children. Antibody to the capsular polysaccharides of these organisms is critical for elimination of these extracellular bacteria. Once antibody attaches to its target antigen, the antigen–antibody complex decreases the infectivity of the bacteria and initiates one of several responses that lead to release of inflammatory mediators, complement activation, opsonization and phagocytosis (25).

Until approximately 4–6 months of age, infant immunity benefits from immunoglobulin received from maternal placental transmission of IgG. After placentally derived maternal antibodies are depleted, children from age 6 months to 2 years are susceptible to serious infection caused by encapsulated bacteria (22, 26–28). Later in childhood (at age 2–5 years), children begin to respond immunologically to polysaccharide antigens. To achieve immunity to serious diseases between 6 months and 5 years of age, vaccines are administered to infants during the first 6 months of life for polioviruses, *Corynebacterium diphtheriae*, *Clostridium tetani*, *Haemophilus influenza* type b, hepatitis B virus, *Bordetella pertussis*, and *Streptococcus pneumoniae*, thereby protecting the child from polio, diphtheria, tetanus, hepatitis, whooping cough and some causes of severe pneumonia, sepsis and meningitis.

Prior to the introduction of the *H. influenza* (Hib) protein conjugate vaccination, Hib was the most common bacterial infection in young children of industrialized nations (29). It caused diseases that ranged from relatively mild (otitis media) to very severe (sepsis and meningitis). Neonates less than 6 months of age were rarely affected, due to transmission of maternal antibody across the placenta, with peak infection rates between 6 and 12 months occurring after placental antibodies disappeared and prior to the infant's ability to produce its own immunoglobulin (29). Natural immunity to Hib occurs from nasopharyngeal colonization or infection but neither natural nor pure polysaccharide vaccine-acquired immunity can develop until after 24 months of age. In addition, there is no memory or booster response following natural or pure polysaccharide vaccine-initiated polysaccharide antibody response. Hence, the protein conjugate vaccine was developed.

Following the success of the Hib protein conjugate vaccine, S. pneumoniae emerged as a prominent infectious organism in the infant and child. The highest rate of invasive pneumococcal disease occurs in the child under 2 years of age, then declines into adolescence, following which the rate gradually increases in older adults (30). Recently a conjugate vaccine for S. pneumoniae has been developed and is being administered to infants.

The current vaccines for H. influenza type b and heptavalent S. pneumoniae vaccine Prevnar® from Wyeth pharmaceuticals are effective because the bacteria-specific capsular polysaccharide is conjugated to a protein such as tetanus toxoid or mutant diphtheria toxin, among others. Conjugated vaccines lead to immunologic memory and booster responses and have caused a dramatic decrease in serious Hib infection and an up to 75% decrease in invasive cases of pneumococcal infection caused by the seven serotypes included in the vaccine (31) (Table 10-1). There are, however, 90 total individual S. pneumoniae serotypes. Because of this, the development of a comprehensive conjugate vaccine has been challenging and the current vaccine only contains seven of the most common and invasive serotypes. The remaining 83 serotypes not included in the conjugate pneumococcal vaccine can still cause disease and there are data that the incidence of pneumococcal disease due to non-vaccine serotypes 15 and 33 is increasing (31). Conjugate vaccines are an excellent example of studies from murine model systems leading to an effective vaccines in the human neonate (32–37).

The peak incidence of the third polysaccharide-encapsulated bacteria, N. meningitidis, occurs between 6 and 15 months of age, the presentation of which can be as benign as asymptomatic nasopharyngeal carriage to fulminant shock leading to death within hours (38). There is currently no vaccine for N. meningitidis that is approved for children less than 2 years of age. The existing N. meningitidis vaccines used to immunize adolescents and adults are composed of the Neisserial capsular polysaccharide alone (39).

Table 10-1 Polysaccharide Encapsulated Bacteria and Available Vaccines

Bacteria	Vaccines	Comments
Haemophilus influenza	Protein conjugate	Administered starting at 2 months of age; multiple available licensed vaccines with various protein conjugates; serious infection almost eliminated
Streptococcus pneumoniae	Polysaccharide (23 valent)	Not effective in infants
	Protein conjugate (7 valent)	Effective in infants; administered starting at 2 months of age; infection due to non-vaccine serotypes are emerging
Neisseria meningitidis	Polysaccharide	Not effective in infants; covers Types A, C Y and W-135 (not Type B)

HUMAN NEWBORN IMMUNE RESPONSE

The human newborn and young child are more susceptible to infection than the adult due to multiple factors. Both innate and adaptive immunity are immature or poorly responsive to invasion by virus, bacteria or fungi. Neutrophils, macrophages, dendritic cells, $\gamma\delta$ T cells and B-1 cells are major mediators of innate immunity, while T cells, B cells, dendritic cells and macrophages are required for adaptive immune responses (40).

Neutrophil Function

Neutrophils are one component of innate immunity characterized by rapid response to invasion with no modification upon repeated exposure to the same microbe. Neutrophils and mononuclear phagocytes are the first line of defense against bacteria, fungi and protozoa. These cells have surface receptors for antibodies and complement, which leads to recognition of the pathogen-bound antibody and/or complement to enhance phagocytosis of the microorganism (40). Compared with adults, infants have a deficient bone marrow storage pool of neutrophils to be mobilized during infection even though their circulating neutrophil numbers are actually somewhat higher than adult (41). There is also a decreased ability of neonatal neutrophils to adhere and migrate across endothelium under both normal and stimulated conditions (42–45), decreased complement receptor cell content and surface expression (46–48), poor bactericidal activity when stressed by infection (49), poor opsonin activity, and reduced oxidative metabolism, chemotaxis (directed cell movement) (50), chemokinesis (random cell movement), and intracellular killing by neutrophils (51–55). This leaves the newborn susceptible to neutropenia after circulating neutrophils are depleted, decreased microbial isolation and killing by neutrophils when the body is invaded by microorganisms (Table 10-2).

Adaptive Immunity

The body's first exposure to a pathogen generates an adaptive immune response, also called a primary immune response, which requires participation of several immune cells such as T cells, B cells, dendritic cells and macrophages. The adaptive immune response can be further subdivided into cell-mediated immunity and the humoral immune response. An important hallmark of the adaptive immune response is memory, which helps the host to respond faster and in a more specific manner to a second exposure to the same pathogen encountered in the primary response.

T Lymphocyte Immunity

One component of adaptive immunity is cell-mediated and occurs via T lymphocytes. Cell-mediated immunity is designed to battle intracellular microbes (56). T-cell-mediated immunity can be via T helper lymphocytes (CD4$^+$) or cytotoxic T lymphocytes (CD8$^+$, cytotoxic lymphocytes [CTL]). Naïve T helper cells are stimulated by antigens to differentiate into two subsets characterized by the cytokines produced by each subset. T_H1 cells secrete IFN-γ and IL-12, for example, and T_H2 cells secrete IL-4 and IL-5 (40). T_H1 cells are critical for cell-mediated immunity, which is required for control of intracellular bacteria such as Mycobacteria species or parasites such as Leishmania. T_H2 cells promote humoral immune responses which are better suited to control infections with extracellular bacteria and helminths. To both atopic and non-atopic antigens, human neonates produce

Table 10-2   Characteristics of Adult and Neonatal Immunity

Immune cell	Adult characteristics	Neonate
Neutrophil	Rapid response	Rapid response
	No memory	No memory
	Bone marrow pool	Decreased reserves in bone marrow
	Cell surface complement and antibody receptors	Decreased
	Migrate to site of infection	Decreased adherence and migration
	Phagocytosis and intracellular killing	Decreased
T cell	Memory	Memory
	T_H1 and T_H2 cells	T_H2 response more than T_H1
	Cytotoxic lymphocytes	CTL achieves adult response only under certain conditions
B cells/Ig	Memory	Shorter duration of memory
	Antibody secretion against:	
	TD antigens	Delayed, with lower peaks and affinity
	TI antigens	Deficient
	IgM, IgG1 and IgG2 and IgA secretion	IgM, IgG1, little IgA
	Adult amounts of IgG	Maternal IgG degrades over time, IgG nadir at 3–4 months of age
Accessory cells	Cytokine secretion	Anti-inflammatory/pro-inflammatory balance
	Intracellular killing	Decreased
	Antigen presentation	Decreased number of cells

T_H, T helper cells; CTL, cytotoxic lymphocytes; TD, thymus-dependent; TI, thymus-independent; Ig, immunoglobulin.

less T_H1 response and a more profound T_H2 response (57, 58). However, adult-level T_H1 cell responses can be achieved in the neonate under certain specific conditions such as immunization with the *Mycobacterium bovis* bacillus Calmette-Guerin (BCG) vaccine (59–61). The T_H2 type response is predominant when the fetus is exposed in utero to environmental antigens (59, 62, 63). Similarly, CTL activity can reach adult levels only under specific conditions such as congenital infection with cytomegalovirus or *Trypanosoma cruzi* (64, 65) (Table 10-2).

B Lymphocyte Immunity

The other component of adaptive immunity is humoral immunity mediated by B cells that secrete specific antibodies to an antigen/microbe. Like cell-mediated immunity, active humoral immunity requires exposure to the microbe but, in the case of humoral immunity, the microbe must be extracellular. Antibodies specifically recognize microbial antigens, decreasing their infectivity and initiating removal of the pathogen from the body (25). Humoral immunity can be passive or active. Passive immunity is obtained from maternal antibody (class IgG but not IgM) that crosses the placenta via a transport mechanism. These placental antibodies degrade over time and, because the infant is unable to make adult amounts of IgG, infant IgG levels reach a nadir at 3–4 months (66, 67).

The active humoral immune response develops gradually over the first years of life. Neonatal antigen-specific antibody production is impaired against certain types of antigens (polysaccharides and lipopolysaccharides among others) and the neonatal IgG response is restricted to certain subclasses. The polysaccharide antigen antibody response in humans of all ages is IgG, IgA and IgM but infants produce primarily IgG_1 while adults produce both IgG_1 and IgG_2 (68, 69). A major reason for the defective polysaccharide response in the neonate is B cell immaturity. As the phenotype and location of B cell subpopulations change with age, the child becomes able to produce antibody to polysaccharide antigen like the adult (22). Each immunoglobulin subclass reaches adult levels at different ages up until age 12 years, when all finally reach adult levels (70) (Table 10-2).

In addition to a poor response to natural infection, neonates and young children respond differently than adults to vaccination. Neonates are often unable to mount an effective immune response to immunizations with pure polysaccharides that are effective in young adults (24). Polysaccharide antigens alone stimulate a thymus-independent (TI) response since these polysaccharides are poorly processed or not at all by antigen-presenting cells, resulting in their inability to generate polysaccharide-specific T helper cells. TI antigens were first defined as those that could produce an immune response in athymic nude mice (71). However, TI antigens are more complicated to define as it was discovered that athymic nude mice actually have a small number of $CD4^+$ and $CD8^+$ T cells (72). The protein conjugate vaccines (e.g., polysaccharide from *H. influenza* and *S. pneumoniae* coupled to proteins such as tetanus and diphtheria toxins) stimulate thymus-dependent (TD) responses and produce better immunity in the neonate than the pure polysaccharide. TD responses require major histocompatibility complex (MHC) class II-restricted presentation of the processed antigen to T cells. Types of TD antigens include proteins, viruses, nucleic acids and red blood cells. Unlike TI antigens, TD antigens elicit some response in the neonate. However, TD responses in neonates are delayed, reach lower peaks, are of shorter duration, have lower affinity and reduced heterogeneity than adults and differ in the type of IgG subclass, with human neonates showing lower IgG2 (73) (Table 10-2). These poor responses are at least partly due to incomplete development of lymphoid tissue until the age of 4 months (74).

TI antibody responses do not require MHC class II-restricted presentation to T cells. The thymus-independent response requires participation by B cells and macrophages. Macrophages provide a source of cytokines that promote B cell maturation and differentiation. In the neonate, this thymus-independent response is poor; TI antigens are more slowly degraded than TD antigens, have poor or no induction of immunologic memory and an antibody response that does not occur until later in life. TI antibody responses are further broken down into TI-1 and TI-2 classification. Examples of TI-1 antigens are lipopolysaccharides (LPS), *Brucella abortus*, *Nocardia* extract, *N. meningitidis* heat-killed bacteria and outer membrane protein. TI-2 antigens include TNP-Ficoll and bacterial polysaccharides from *H. influenza*, *S. pneumoniae* and *N. meningitidis* (75) (Table 10-3). TI-2 antigens can cross-link B cell receptors, which can lead to B cell activation. Although TI-2 antigen responses are not dependent on MHC class II-restricted presentation, they are dependent on antigen non-specific T cells and/or cytokines produced by T cells and accessory cells (76, 77).

Possible etiologies for the human neonate's inability to respond to TI-2 antigens such as the polysaccharides include an immature B cell population (78), deficiency of B cell subsets involved in TI-2 responses (75), increased susceptibility of neonatal B cells to tolerance induction (79), improper balance of suppressor and amplifier T cells (80) and accessory cell defects, including inadequate production of stimulatory cytokines and an excess production of inhibitory cytokines (81).

At the same time that the young child becomes able to respond to polysaccharide antigens, there is a change in the phenotype and location of B cell subpopulations. Neonatal B cells express both IgM and IgD as well as either IgG or IgA,

Table 10-3   Thymus-Independent Immune Response Characteristics

	TI		TD
	TI-1	TI-2	
MHC class II presentation required	No	No	Yes
Requires B cells and macrophages	Yes	Yes	No
Neonate	Poor response	Poor response	Adequate response
Antigen degradation	Slower	Slower	Faster
Memory	Poor or none	Poor or none	Yes
Antigen examples	LPS	TNP-Ficoll	Proteins
	Brucella abortus	Bacterial polysaccharides	Viruses
	Nocardia extract		Lipoproteins
	N. meningitidis heat-killed bacteria and outer membrane protein		Red blood cells

suggesting incomplete heavy-chain isotype class switching at that age (78). In addition, neonatal B cells are predominantly $CD5^+$ (a marker for a B lymphocyte subpopulation that develops early in ontogeny) and change to predominantly CD5- with age (40, 82–85). Neonatal B cells also have fewer cytokine receptors for IL-2 (with IL-4 stimulates proliferation of activated B cells), IL-4, IL-6 (stimulates B cells to mature into plasma cells and produce antibodies) and IL-7 (stimulates proliferation of immature B cells) and a decreased ability to up-regulate the IL-2 receptor with stimulation (86–88).

The spleen plays an important role in B cell immunity; as evidenced by patients who have either functional or surgical splenectomies and become susceptible to infection from polysaccharide-encapsulated bacteria (89). The receptor for complement component C3 (CD21) is a marker of mature B cells; the B cells that reside in splenic marginal zone express high levels of CD21. CD21 is the complement receptor for breakdown products of C3b and is complexed with two other receptors (90). Co-ligation of B cell receptor and CD21 enhances B cell responses and reduces the threshold of antigen level required for B cell stimulation by several orders of magnitude. Binding of B cell receptors to microbes on which complement component C3b is deposited enhances their response (91). Neonatal spleens lack the $CD21^+$ marginal zone B cells. In addition, the spleen is the source for IgM memory B cells, which appear to be the B cell population responsible for antibody response to polysaccharide antigens. In children up to age 2 years, there is a lack of IgM memory B cells. At the time this population appears in circulating blood, the child also becomes able to respond to polysaccharide antigen (92).

Accessory Cell Function (macrophages/monocytes and dendritic cells)

Some monocyte/macrophage functions are also incomplete in the infant. Infant macrophages respond less to serum chemotactic factors, are unable to function efficiently due to reduced opsonic activity, and are more susceptible to metabolic stress due to reduced pyruvate kinase activity and ATP content (93, 94). They produce less G-CSF, contributing to neutropenia under stress conditions, less IL-6 and decreased activation upon exposure to interferon-γ (95–98).

Dendritic cells are antigen-presenting cells that prime naïve T cells to initiate an immune response or to develop tolerance to self-antigens. They are derived from the monocytic lineage in the presence of GM-CSF and/or IL-4 and are sentinel cells located in areas of likely microbial invasion to pick up antigen and present it to naïve T helper cells (99). Stimulated dendritic cells or mononuclear cells from cord blood produce reduced levels of IL-12p70 and IL-12p35 (subunits of the stimulatory cytokine IL-12) compared to adults (100–105). Monocyte-derived macrophages and plasmacytoid dendritic cells from the neonate show reduced activation and cytokine production capabilities when stimulated with IFN-γ or CpG DNA (CpG DNA discussed in detail later) (106, 107) (Table 10-2).

Cytokine Production

Cytokines are soluble mediators produced mainly by immune cells but also by non-immune cells. They have profound effects on the functions of T cells, B cells, dendritic cells, and macrophages as well as some non-immune cells. Conflicting data exist in humans regarding the relative amounts of cytokine production by neonatal immune cells. The majority of studies show that cord blood monocytes produce less TNF-α than adult monocytes (108–112). For IL-1, a single study found that human neonatal monocytes produce less IL-1 than adult monocytes after LPS stimulation (110). Other studies have found no difference in IL-1 production after LPS or IFN-γ stimulation of monocytes (108, 109, 111, 113). There is also conflicting evidence with regard to IL-6 production by human neonatal monocytes. Some authors have found a deficit compared to adult monocytes (96, 98, 108), others have found no difference (109, 114, 115), whereas others have demonstrated an increased production of IL-6 from cord mononuclear cells at baseline (116) and in response to stimulus (116–118). Cord and neonatal peripheral blood mononuclear cells (PBMCs) produce less IFN-γ than adult PBMCs after stimulation (119, 120). One study evaluated IL-8 production in cord/neonatal blood versus adult. With LPS stimulation IL-8 production was higher in cord blood than adult; baseline levels of IL-8 were also higher in the cord after incubation without stimulus (118). One study showed that mRNA and intracytoplasmic production of the anti-inflammatory cytokine IL-10 was less in LPS-stimulated cord blood than adult (121), while another showed similar production across age groups when cells were incubated with Gram-positive and -negative bacteria (117). Possible reasons for conflicting results in these human studies are the different cell populations studied (peripheral whole blood vs. mononuclear cells vs. monocytes/macrophages), the stimulus used (LPS vs. phytohemagglutinin vs. bacteria, etc.), method of measurement (mRNA vs. intracellular vs. supernatant) and limited numbers of donors studied.

MURINE NEWBORN IMMUNE RESPONSE

Like humans, the newborn mouse has a diminished immune capacity that improves by the time the mouse reaches adulthood. Murine models have, therefore, been used to gather knowledge from neonatal mice that could illuminate reasons and possible interventions for the human neonatal immune response. Populations of immune cells to study in mice are usually obtained from the spleen, lymph node, thymus, lung or peritoneum rather than peripheral blood, which, as described later, may contribute to some of the differences seen when the murine model is applied to the human system.

T Lymphocyte Immunity

The number of T cells is reduced in neonatal mice by 1–2 log fold compared to adults, perhaps contributing to the limited protective response that develops after exposure to antigen, yet a subset of neonatal T cells are able to proliferate (122). In neonatal mice, CD4$^+$ cells originate from both fetal and adult hematopoietic precursors. After immunization, the fetal-derived T cells produce a primarily T_H2 cell response upon re-exposure to the immunized antigen (123). Fetal origin T cells are present in the human as well and in utero exposure to environment antigens leads to a T_H2 skewed response (57, 59, 62, 63). Early studies found that neonatal T cells are especially prone to tolerance when examined in transplant models. Recent studies have shown this to be due to an imbalance in the ratio of T cells to dendritic cells (124) and also may be due to a lack of regulatory CD4 and CD8 T cells (59). Neonatal mice can be induced to mount adult-level T cell responses under the right circumstances if provided with adequate numbers of dendritic cells (59, 124). Neonatal T cell responses are biased toward the T_H2 cell lineage but can be converted to T helper (T_H1) cell responses when antigen exposure is coordinated with agents that promote T_H1 cell response such as DNA vaccines or oligonucleotides containing CpG motifs. This T_H2 bias in newborn mice is not quite as noticeable in human neonates and both T_H1 and T_H2 responses are reduced in some human neonatal situations such as malaria infection (125). The origin or location of the neonatal T cells may contribute to the response elicited to infection. For example, neonatal murine lymph node cells remain deficient in their T_H1 response when transplanted into adult mice, whereas neonatal splenic cells were able to develop mature T_H1 functions that could resolve *Pneumocystis carnii* infection when transferred to an adult murine environment (126, 127). Neonatal cytotoxic T lymphocytes have strong primary and/or memory functions when exposed to strong T_H1 promoting agents such as those noted above (59). Recent studies found that CD8$^+$ cytotoxic T cell function in the neonates is comparable to that in the adult in both mice and humans, especially when examined soon after immunization (59).

B Lymphocyte Immunity

Like human neonates, TD and TI responses are less in neonatal mice than adult mice. Phenotypic differences have been demonstrated in the neonatal mouse with immature IgM$^+$/IgD$^{low/-}$ B cells predominating the murine spleen B cell population. Immature B cells are negatively signaled when the B cell receptor is ligated; they do not up-regulate co-stimulatory molecules or MHC class II molecules that allow interaction with T cells for the TD response (128–130). The concept of TI responses came from extensive studies in murine model systems such as nude mice that are congenitally athymic. Subsequently modern cell-separation techniques have established that highly purified B cells from the adult but not neonate can respond to TI antigens in the complete absence of T cells. However, accessory cells or cytokines derived from T cells or accessory cells are essential for B cells to respond to TI antigens. In vivo studies using B cell receptor transgenic mice have shown that the TI response is primarily elicited from marginal zone B cells found in the spleen, with participation from blood dendritic cells and peritoneal B-1 cells (131, 132). Mouse data suggest that development of B-1a B cells that have a role in antibody responses to polysaccharides requires the presence of the spleen (133). As in humans, in mice also there are low numbers of marginal-zone B cells at birth and the appearance of these B cells later in life corresponds to the ability to respond to TI antigens (134).

Recent studies have shown that bacterial deoxyribonucleic acid (DNA), once thought to be immunologically inert, can produce a stimulatory immune response (135, 136). Bacterial DNA differs from mammalian DNA by its increased frequency of CpG dinucleotide sequences and by a lower number of these dinucleotides being methylated in bacteria (137). These differences may form a means by which mammalian organisms recognize foreign DNA and are thereby able to respond immunologically. In neonatal mice, stimulation with CpG ODN but not B cell receptor cross-linking alone can induce proliferation of B cells. Furthermore, CpG ODN stimulation can overcome the unresponsiveness of neonatal murine B cells to signals provided by the B cell receptor (BCR), as low concentrations of CpG and anti-IgM can induce a robust B cell proliferation response. Normally neonatal B cells undergo apoptosis in response to BCR ligation; the apoptosis is overcome by the CpG ODN. In addition, CpG ODNs stimulate neonatal murine B cells to produce polyclonal IgM in an amount comparable to adult murine B cells (81, 138).

Cytokines Needed for Neonatal Mouse Response

When neonatal B cell responses were studied using TNP-Ficoll or TNP-LPS as model TI antigens, it was found that highly purified neonatal B cells responded well to these stimuli only when supplemented with the cytokines IL-1 and IL-6 (139). In this system the neonatal responses were comparable to those in the adult. Both cytokines were required for optimal responses. The avidity of the response induced by TNP-Ficoll in the presence of cytokines was similar in the neonate and the adult (139). Cytokines IL-4 and IL-5 were effective when the TI stimulus was dextran-coupled-antibody to the BCR (140). In this later system neonatal B cell responses required stimulation via CD40L also. In either system neonatal B cells alone failed to respond to the TI antigen. In vivo studies demonstrated that the cytokine IL-12 can also augment polysaccharide responses in the murine neonate (141).

These studies demonstrate that intrinsic defects in neonatal B cells in their response to polysaccharide antigens can be overcome with a proper combination of signals from cytokines and CD40. Kinetic studies demonstrated that cytokines had to be added during the early phase of B cell activation. They were able to overcome the defect in BCR-induced proliferation of neonatal B cells as well as antigen-induced differentiation (139).

In mouse, the neonatal B cells are predominantly transitional-type in nature, which are the B cells that have recently emigrated from the bone marrow. Transitional-type B cells are defined by high levels of IgM, low levels of IgD and CD23 and by expression of the marker AA4.1 (142, 143). Such transitional B cells have also been identified recently in adult humans and cord blood; although such cells are present in the adult mouse also but in a very small number compared to the neonate. It is the presence of these transitional B cells that accounts for increased susceptibility of the neonate to B cell tolerance and decreased responses to the polysaccharide antigens. Interestingly, the transitional phenotype is not altered by the cytokines IL-1 and IL-6 that induce polysaccharide-specific responses from neonatal B cells. BAFF (also know as BLyS), a cytokine belonging to the TNF family, has been shown to be required for maturation of the transitional B cells into follicular B cells. In transgenic models that over-express BAFF, there was an increase of both marginal-zone B cells and B-1 cells (two subsets involved in polysaccharide responses) and such mice develop autoantibodies (144). In adults, BAFF supplementation has enhanced antibody responses to pneumococcal polysaccharides. Currently there are no studies that have examined the effect of BAFF on neonatal B cell responses.

CpG-Assisted Mouse Response

Oligonucleotides that contain CpG motifs have been shown to be powerful stimulants of immune response due to their action on B cells, dendritic cells and macrophages. We tested whether CpG stimulation can overcome neonatal B cell unresponsiveness to BCR cross-linking or to polysaccharide antigens. Indeed, supplementation with CpG enabled neonatal murine B cells to proliferate in response to anti-IgM antibodies. Moreover, CpG stimulation enabled neonatal B cells to produce antibodies in response to TNP-Ficoll, a TI-2 polysaccharide antigen. The effect of CpG appeared to be on B cell survival as shown by apoptosis assays and by measuring survival proteins such as Bcl-X$_L$ (138). In these experiments, highly purified neonatal B cells were utilized, suggesting that CpG ODNs were acting directly on B cells via the TLR9 receptor. Kovarik et al. tested in vivo immunization with CpG ODN with only marginal effects on polysaccharide responses (145). This could be related to the in vivo half-life of CpG.

Macrophage Cytokine Secretion

As noted above, TI responses require participation from both macrophages and B cells. The role of macrophages was investigated in a cell-mixing experiment wherein adult B cells were cultured with purified macrophages from neonatal or adult mice in the presence of TI stimuli (TNP-LPS). In this system, neonatal macrophages were unable to help adult B cells generate a TI antigen response whereas the adult macrophages induced the B cells to make excellent antibody responses. The inability of neonatal macrophages to induce neonatal B cells to respond to TI stimuli is due to a reduction in secretion of two cytokines, IL-1 and IL-6, which are important for B cell activation. The neonatal macrophages appear to have a global defect in the production of pro-inflammatory cytokines as they also make less TNF-α and IL-12 than adult macrophages when stimulated with TNP-LPS. Interestingly, the neonatal murine macrophages do not exhibit a similar defect in production of the anti-inflammatory cytokine IL-10, but make more of it than their adult counterparts. This increased IL-10 production by neonatal macrophages has a causal role in the reduced production of pro-inflammatory cytokines, since the production of IL-1, IL-6 and TNF-α was restored when anti-IL-10 was added to the culture or when neonatal macrophages were obtained from IL-10 gene knockout mice. Not only did anti-IL-10 restore production of IL-6 by the neonatal macrophages, but it also enabled neonatal spleen cells to make anti-TNP-LPS antibodies in culture (146, 147).

Mitogenic stimuli such as bacterial-derived LPS have recently been shown to be recognized by the family of Toll-like receptors (TLR), in particular TLR-4. Many of the TLR ligands are derived from bacteria; for example, TLR-2 is stimulated by peptidoglycan, TLR-5 by bacterial flagellin and TLR-9 by bacterial DNA that contains CpG motifs. Neonatal macrophages exhibit a similar cytokine dysregulation phenotype whether stimulated with the TLR-2 ligand, peptidoglycan or the TLR-9 ligand, CpG ODN, suggesting that they may have a global defect in the TLR signaling pathway leading to down-regulation of pro-inflammatory cytokines and up-regulation of anti-inflammatory cytokines such as IL-10. Expression of TLR receptors per se is not dramatically reduced in the neonatal macrophages although there are some quantitative differences between the two age groups. The molecular basis of the cytokine dysregulation phenotype of neonatal macrophages is not yet known. It is fascinating that macrophages from 2-year-old mice exhibit a similar cytokine dysregulation phenotype and are unable to support antibody responses to TNP-LPS like young adult B cells (147). Aged mice and humans are also hypo-responsive to pneumococcal polysaccharide antigens.

CORRELATES IN THE HUMAN NEONATE

Based on murine model data, interventions that modify the neonatal mouse's immune response have been evaluated in the human neonate (18, 20, 21, 100,

148–151). Most commonly, cord blood is the source of immune cells for research purposes in the neonate but, occasionally, peripheral blood is obtained from newborn infants. Immune cell populations are either studied within whole blood (19) or specific populations are separated from other cells by a variety of techniques such as density gradients (20, 21, 151), labeling cell surface markers with fluorescent antibody and separating by flow cytometry, labeling cell surface markers with magnetically tagged antibody and running the cells past a strong magnet (18, 20), or using the cells' own adhesive properties (151). Some of the most recent human discoveries with potential clinical relevance to newborns will be reviewed here.

Accessory Cells

Multiple studies have been done evaluating the effects of glucocorticoids on the murine immune response. Murine macrophage production and function are affected by steroids in a very complex manner depending on the timing of steroid exposure and the order in which antigens and the glucocorticoid are processed (152–159). Glucocorticoid administration post partum to maternal murine animals decreases the transmammary transfer of viral-specific IgG (160). Human neonatal macrophage function and surface marker expression were evaluated by Orlikowsky et al. in two studies. Cord blood macrophages were shown to express less of the macrophage activation markers CD80 and CD86 constitutively and increase these markers less than adults when stimulated with IFN-γ, cyclic adenosine monophosphate (cAMP), or CD40 ligand (binds to CD40 on B cells and promotes growth and maturation of B lymphocytes) (161, 162). The effect of dexamethasone on cord blood macrophages was evaluated to determine how treating premature labor in pregnant women with steroids might affect the premature infant's immune response (151). Cord blood macrophages were exposed to a stimulus (IFN-γ or cAMP) with and without the addition of dexamethasone. Cord blood macrophages again showed decreased baseline expression of CD80 and CD86; stimulation with IFN-γ increased CD80 and CD86 expression but less than on adult macrophages. The addition of dexamethasone inhibited the stimulus-mediated increase in both adults and cord blood macrophages but there was a greater degree of inhibition in the cord blood cells. cAMP stimulation results in similar effects, with the exception that CD80 was not increased but CD86 was (adult more than cord macrophages) and also was inhibited by dexamethasone treatment (more inhibition of cord cell response than adult) (151). These studies suggest that dexamethasone treatment of pregnant women in preterm labor may impair the newborn's ability to activate macrophages upon stimulation with inflammatory cytokines. Due to this, neonatal macrophages that are already in a relatively inactivated state will be less able to respond to infection by microbial phagocytosis and secrete cytokines necessary for cell-mediated and humoral immune responses.

Murine dendritic cell differentiation and function are also affected by steroid exposure (158, 159, 163, 164). In humans, Mainali et al. looked at the effect of dexamethasone on dendritic cell maturation in cord and adult blood (150). Dexamethasone was found to inhibit dendritic cell surface marker (CD1a) expression and increase the amount of macrophage marker (CD14) expression. This occurred to a much greater extent in the cord blood cells than in the adult. Dexamethasone altered the ratio of cytokine secretion by the dendritic/macrophage cells so that there was an increase in IL-10 (anti-inflammatory) over IL-12 (pro-inflammatory) secretion. The same cord cells that expressed the CD14 macrophage marker were also the ones that increased their endocytic ability with dexamethasone (150). Implications for the neonate either treated with steroids or born to a mother treated with steroids are fewer dendritic cells for antigen presentation to naïve T cells by maintaining the monocyte lineage rather than maturing into dendritic cells.

The dendritic cell phagocytizes apoptotic cells and necrotic cells, and the type of cell ingested leads to either an immune response (necrotic cells) or induction of tolerance (apoptotic cells). Tolerance is the condition of not responding to an antigen even though prior antigen exposure has occurred. Tolerance to self-antigens is important to prevent autoimmune diseases (40). Wong et al. evaluated whether neonatal dendritic cells responded differently to these two types of dying cells than adult dendritic cells (100). Both adult and cord dendritic cells were able to phago-cytose apoptotic and necrotic cells; however, adult dendritic cells phagocytosed a larger amount of each type of dying cell. Up-regulation of MHC-II, CD80, CD86 and CD83 surface markers was minimal in the cord dendritic cells, whereas it was significant for the adult cells that were exposed to the necrotic cells. Stimulated dendritic cells lead to naïve T-cell activation; however, cord blood dendritic cells exposed to necrotic cells or LPS were less able to stimulate T-cell proliferation than adults. LPS stimulation was able to increase the adult and cord dendritic cell expression of MHC-II, CD80, CD86, CD83 and CD40, but to a lesser degree in the cord.

The cytokines that dendritic cells produce upon stimulation (TNF-α, IL-10 and IL-12p70) are instrumental in modulating the type of T-cell response. Cord blood dendritic cells were able to increase TNF-α and IL-10 secretion but to a lesser degree than the adult. The adult significantly increased the amount of IL-12p70 secreted but the cord dendritic cells did not (100). IL-12 production is known to enhance T_H1 cell differentiation; whereas IL-10 can down-regulate T_H1 cell development. The T_H2 propensity of human neonates may be related to this dendritic cells phenotype. These studies are some of the first investigations into the role of the accessory cell in the human neonate.

B Lymphocytes

Synthetic CpG oligodeoxynucleotides (CpG ODNs) stimulate murine B-lymphocytes and dendritic cells to proliferate and produce cytokines and immu-noglobulins (136, 165–168). The stimulatory effect in mice is dependent on the presence of the CpG dinucleotide sequence as well as the surrounding nucleotides flanked by two 5' purines and 3' pyrimidines (CpG motif) (135, 169, 170). Human adult B cells are also stimulated by ODNs, but the CpG motif necessary for murine B cell activation is not mandatory (171).

CpG ODNs can be classified loosely by the types of cells they are able to stimulate. Some CpG ODNs induce highly purified human adult B cells to pro-liferate, produce IgM, IgG and IgA and increase cell surface expression of CD86 (a marker of B cell activation) and CD25 (the IL-2 receptor) (171). Maximal human B cell stimulation (cellular proliferation, CD80 and CD86 expression, immuno-globulin production and IL-6 secretion) is achieved with ODNs that possess a nuclease-resistant phosphorothioate-modified backbone with one or more CpG motifs and no polyG motif (172). The CpG ODNs that induce a Th-1 response and also stimulate B cells potently belong to the B class (also known as K type), while the A class (also known as D type) are potent in activating NK cells and human plasmacytoid dendritic cells to secrete interferon-α (173–175). A third class of CpG is known as the C class, which combines the properties of both A and B classes by being able to stimulate B cell and NK cell activation and IFN-α production (176, 177). The B-class CpG ODNs enhance the ability of den-dritic cells to produce IL-12 and help polarize T cell responses in the T_H1 direction. Several CpG ODNs are in clinical trials to enhance vaccine responses to infective agents and cancer cells (178–181).

As a natural offshoot of the murine neonate model, the role CpG ODNs could play in improving the human neonate's B cell response is beginning to be discovered. In one study, it was shown that cord blood B cells and dendritic cells in whole blood culture up-regulated CD40 in response to CpG stimulation but did so less effectively than adults (182). CpG ODNs can stimulate cord blood B cell proliferation and up-regulate expression of CD86 and HLA-DR, surface molecules important for T and B cell interaction. CpG ODN-induced cell surface marker up-regulation is similar in cord and adult B cells (18). Cord blood B cell proliferation is increased with CpG ODN stimulus but there are conflicting results as to whether cord cells proliferate to the same degree as adult B cells in response to CpG ODNs (18, 20). This proliferation effect was increased for both adult and cord B cells when anti-IgM was added to the CpG ODN-exposed cells (18). Cord blood polyclonal IgM production in response to CpG ODN stimulus was as robust as the adult; however, cord blood cells produced less IgG compared to adult cells and no IgA in response to CpG ODN stimulation (18, 20). CpG ODN can also induce chemokine secretion from cord and adult B cells (macrophage inflammatory protein [MIP]-1α and MIP-1β) which is further increased when anti-IgM is added (18). Importantly, the polyclonal B cell immunoglobulin response to CpG ODN contains antibodies specific for polysaccharide antigens (18, 20). Thus far it has not been demonstrated that CpG ODNs can amplify B cell antibody responses to polysaccharide antigens in a vaccine-like scenario rather than just a polyclonal response, perhaps due to an undetectable amount of polysaccharide-specific antibody or requirement for T cell or accessory cell cytokine. These studies support the possibility that the neonatal B cell can function like the adult but specific circumstances and conditions are important for maximal cord B cell response.

HUMAN AND MOUSE DIFFERENCES

Despite the murine neonatal spleen showing immature B cells compared to adult, studies in the human neonate typically involve peripheral blood, and the same deficits seen in the murine spleen are not seen in human peripheral blood lymphocytes (18). Indeed, murine lymph node B cells are more mature than splenic cells and splenectomy in mice does not influence IgG1 and IgG2a responses (59, 122). The polysaccharide antibody-antigen response in mice is predominantly IgM, whereas it is IgG, IgA and IgM in humans (183). TD responses in neonatal mice are low in IgG$_{2a}$, while human neonates are low in IgG$_2$ (73).

CLINICAL IMPLICATIONS AND FUTURE INVESTIGATION NEEDS

The identification of specific defects in the newborn's immune response can influence how physicians treat inflammatory processes and infections in the neonate. Already, CpG ODNs are being studied in adult mice as an adjuvant to polysaccharide vaccines to increase the antibody response to previously poor antigens (184). There is the potential that CpG ODNs could help the neonate's response to polysaccharide antigens, allowing the 23-valent pure polysaccharide S. pneumoniae vaccine now used in the elderly to also be effective in neonates. In addition, further data on CpG ODNs stimulatory capabilities in the neonate could aid in the development of an N. meningitidis vaccination program for infants. We speculate that CpG ODNs are likely to require a second stimulus to increase specific antigen responses as CpG ODNs alone were unable to stimulate increased amounts of polysaccharide antigen in cord blood in the laboratory setting.

Currently, once infection and the inflammatory cascade develop in the newborn infant, there is little therapy to counteract the effects other than antibiotics and supportive care. There have been many trials in adults evaluating the role of cytokine antagonists and other anti-inflammatory agents in treating septic shock (185–188). However, since the cytokine response in neonates is different from that in adults, different approaches to this type of therapy in the neonate may be needed. Since the newborn is relatively immune-suppressed and unable to respond to many infections with an adequate immune response, stimulatory cytokines might actually be of more benefit than the anti-inflammatory treatments evaluated in adults. Additionally, the preterm infant's immune system is different even from that of the term newborn (47, 95, 97, 108, 111, 118, 162, 189–194). For example, IL-8 baseline concentration is not dependent on gestational age but production by stimulated monocytes is lower in preterm cord blood than in term cord blood (97, 118). Further study is needed to delineate other immune response differences in the preterm infant.

REFERENCES

1. Pereira LE, Bostik P, Ansari AA, et al. The development of mouse APECED models provides new insight into the role of AIRE in immune regulation. Clin Dev Immunol 12:211–216, 2005.
2. Kamnasaran D. Agenesis of the corpus callosum: lessons from humans and mice. Clin Invest Med 28:267–282, 2005.
3. Meekins GD, Weiss MD. Electrodiagnostic studies in a murine model of demyelinating Charcot-Marie-Tooth disease. Phys Med Rehabil Clin N Am 16:967–979, ix, 2005.
4. Nico B, Roncali L, Mangieri D, Ribatti D. Blood-brain barrier alterations in MDX mouse, an animal model of the Duchenne muscular dystrophy. Curr Neurovasc Res 2:47–54, 2005.
5. Gibson KM, Jakobs C, Pearl PL, Snead OC. Murine succinate semialdehyde dehydrogenase (SSADH) deficiency, a heritable disorder of GABA metabolism with epileptic phenotype. IUBMB Life 57:639–644, 2005.
6. Ramirez F, Dietz HC. Therapy insight: aortic aneurysm and dissection in Marfan's syndrome. Nat Clin Pract Cardiovasc Med 1:31–36, 2004.
7. Kumar S, Anderson KC. Drug insight: thalidomide as a treatment for multiple myeloma. Nat Clin Pract Oncol 2:262–270, 2005.
8. Pomper MG, Lee JS. Small animal imaging in drug development. Curr Pharm Des 11:3247–3272, 2005.
9. Davies J, Turner M, Klein N. The role of the collectin system in pulmonary defence. Paediatr Respir Rev 2:70–75, 2001.
10. Doganci A, Sauer K, Karwot R, Finotto S. Pathological role of IL-6 in the experimental allergic bronchial asthma in mice. Clin Rev Allergy Immunol 28:257–270, 2005.
11. Chen J, Roop DR. Mouse models in preclinical studies for pachyonychia congenita. J Investig Dermatol Symp Proc 10:37–46, 2005.
12. Raja A, Engelhard HH. Animal models of leptomeningeal cancer. Cancer Treat Res 125:159–179, 2005.
13. Lallemand-Breitenbach V, Zhu J, Kogan S, et al. Opinion: how patients have benefited from mouse models of acute promyelocytic leukaemia. Nat Rev Cancer 5:821–827, 2005.
14. Keller C, Capecchi MR. New genetic tactics to model alveolar rhabdomyosarcoma in the mouse. Cancer Res 65:7530–7532, 2005.
15. Paul R, Koedel U, Pfister HW. Development of adjunctive therapies for bacterial meningitis and lessons from knockout mice. Neurocrit Care 2:313–324, 2005.
16. Hapfelmeier S, Hardt WD. A mouse model for S. typhimurium-induced enterocolitis. Trends Microbiol 13:497–503, 2005.
17. Solomon JB. Immunological milestones in the ontogeny of hamster, guinea pig, sheep, and man. Fed Proc 37:2028–2030, 1978.
18. Tasker L, Marshall-Clarke S. Functional responses of human neonatal B lymphocytes to antigen receptor cross-linking and CpG DNA. Clin Exp Immunol 134:409–419, 2003.
19. Halista SM, Johnson-Robbins LA, El-Mohandes AE, et al. Characterization of early activation events in cord blood B cells after stimulation with T cell-independent activators. Pediatr Res 43:496–503, 1998.
20. Landers CD, Bondada S. CpG oligodeoxynucleotides stimulate cord blood mononuclear cells to produce immunoglobulins. Clin Immunol 116:236–245, 2005.
21. Prescott SL, Irwin S, Taylor A, et al. Cytosine-phosphate-guanine motifs fail to promote T-helper type 1-polarized responses in human neonatal mononuclear cells. Clin Exp Allergy 35:358–366, 2005.
22. Pabst HF, Kreth HW. Ontogeny of the immune response as a basis of childhood disease. J Pediatr 97:519–534, 1980.

23. Douglas RM, Paton JC, Duncan SJ, Hansman DJ. Antibody response to pneumococcal vaccination in children younger than five years of age. J Infect Dis 148:131–137, 1983.

24. Broome CV, Breiman RF. Pneumococcal vaccine–past, present, and future. N Engl J Med 325:1506–1508, 1991.

25. Delves PJ, Roitt IM. The immune system. First of two parts. N Engl J Med 343:37–49, 2000.

26. Wald ER, Guerra N, Byers C. Upper respiratory tract infections in young children: duration of and frequency of complications. Pediatrics 87:129–133, 1991.

27. Gray BM, Dillon HC Jr. Clinical and epidemiologic studies of pneumococcal infection in children. Pediatr Infect Dis 5:201–207, 1986.

28. Klein JO. The epidemiology of pneumococcal disease in infants and children. Rev Infect Dis 3:246–253, 1981.

29. Cadoz M. Potential and limitations of polysaccharide vaccines in infancy. Vaccine 16:1391–1395, 1998.

30. Peter G, Klein JO. Streptococcus pneumoniae. In: Long SS, ed. Principles and practice of pediatric infectious diseases (2nd edn). New York: Churchill Livingstone; 2003:739–746.

31. Kaplan SL, Mason EO Jr, Wald ER, et al. Decrease of invasive pneumococcal infections in children among 8 children's hospitals in the United States after the introduction of the 7-valent pneumococcal conjugate vaccine. Pediatrics 113:443–449, 2004.

32. Dintzis RZ. Rational design of conjugate vaccines. Pediatr Res 32:376–385, 1992.

33. Seppala I, Makela O. Antigenicity of dextran-protein conjugates in mice. Effect of molecular weight of the carbohydrate and comparison of two modes of coupling. J Immunol 143:1259–1264, 1989.

34. Bixler GS Jr, Eby R, Dermody KM, et al. Synthetic peptide representing a T-cell epitope of CRM197 substitutes as carrier molecule in a Haemophilus influenzae type B (Hib) conjugate vaccine. Adv Exp Med Biol 251:175–180, 1989.

35. Tai JY, Vella PP, McLean AA, et al. Haemophilus influenzae type b polysaccharide-protein conjugate vaccine. Proc Soc Exp Biol Med 184:154–161, 1987.

36. Jennings HJ, Roy R, Gamian A. Induction of meningococcal group B polysaccharide-specific IgG antibodies in mice by using an N-propionylated B polysaccharide-tetanus toxoid conjugate vaccine. J Immunol 137:1708–1713, 1986.

37. Tsay GC, Collins MS. Preparation and characterization of a nontoxic polysaccharide-protein conjugate that induces active immunity and passively protective antibody against Pseudomonas aeruginosa immunotype 1 in mice. Infect Immun 45:217–221, 1984.

38. Gold R. Neisseria meningitidis. In: Long SS, ed. Principles and practice of pediatric infectious diseases (2nd edn). New York: Churchill Livingstone; 2003:748-756.

39. Pediatrics AA. Meningococcal Infections. In: Pickering LK, ed. Red Book: Report of the Committee on Infectious Diseases (26th edn). Elk Grove Village, IL: American Academy of Pediatrics; 2003:430–436.

40. Delves PJ, Roitt IM. The immune system. Second of two parts. N Engl J Med 343:108–117, 2000.

41. Engle WA, Schreiner RL, Baehner RL. Neonatal white blood cell disorders. Semin Perinatol 7:184–200, 1983.

42. Krause PJ, Maderazo EG, Scroggs M. Abnormalities of neutrophil adherence in newborns. Pediatrics 69:184–187, 1982.

43. Krause PJ, Malech HL, Kristie J, et al. Polymorphonuclear leukocyte heterogeneity in neonates and adults. Blood 68:200–204, 1986.

44. Anderson DC, Hughes BJ, Smith CW. Abnormal mobility of neonatal polymorphonuclear leukocytes. Relationship to impaired redistribution of surface adhesion sites by chemotactic factor or colchicine. J Clin Invest 68:863–874, 1981.

45. Anderson DC, Rothlein R, Marlin SD, et al. Impaired transendothelial migration by neonatal neutrophils: abnormalities of Mac-1 (CD11b/CD18)-dependent adherence reactions. Blood 76:2613–2621, 1990.

46. Abughali N, Berger M, Tosi MF. Deficient total cell content of CR3 (CD11b) in neonatal neutrophils. Blood 83:1086–1092, 1994.

47. McEvoy LT, Zakem-Cloud H, Tosi MF. Total cell content of CR3 (CD11b/CD18) and LFA-1 (CD11a/CD18) in neonatal neutrophils: relationship to gestational age. Blood 87:3929–3933, 1996.

48. Bruce MC, Baley JE, Medvik KA, Berger M. Impaired surface membrane expression of C3bi but not C3b receptors on neonatal neutrophils. Pediatr Res 21:306–311, 1987.

49. Quie PG, Mills EL. Bactericidal and metabolic function of polymorphonuclear leukocytes. Pediatrics 64:719–721, 1979.

50. Speer C, Johnston RBJ. Neutrophil function in newborn infants. In: Polin R, Fox W, eds. Fetal and neonatal physiology (2nd edn). Philadelphia: W.B. Saunders; 1997:1954–1960.

51. Davis CA, Vallota EH, Forristal J. Serum complement levels in infancy: age related changes. Pediatr Res 13:1043–1046, 1979.

52. Mills EL, Thompson T, Bjorksten B, et al. The chemiluminescence response and bactericidal activity of polymorphonuclear neutrophils from newborns and their mothers. Pediatrics 63:429–434, 1979.

53. Stoerner JW, Pickering LK, Adcock EW 3rd, Morriss FH Jr. Polymorphonuclear leukocyte function in newborn infants. J Pediatr 93:862–864, 1978.

54. Tono-Oka T, Nakayama M, Uehara H, Matsumoto S. Characteristics of impaired chemotactic function in cord blood leukocytes. Pediatr Res 13:148–151, 1979.

55. Miller MD. Natural defense mechanism: Development and characterization of innate immunity. In: Stiehm E, Fulginiti V, eds. Immunologic disorders of infants and children. Philadelphia: W.B. Saunders; 1973:127.

56. Abbas AK, Lichtman AH, Pober JS. B cell Activation and antibody production.In: Schmitt W, Hacker HN, Ehlers J, eds. Cellular and molecular immunology (4th edn). Philadelphia: W.B. Saunders; 2000:182-207.

57. Prescott SL, Macaubas C, Smallacombe T, et al. Development of allergen-specific T-cell memory in atopic and normal children. Lancet 353:196–200, 1999.

58. Prescott SL, Taylor A, King B, et al. Neonatal interleukin-12 capacity is associated with variations in allergen-specific immune responses in the neonatal and postnatal periods. Clin Exp Allergy 33:566–572, 2003.

59. Adkins B, Leclerc C, Marshall-Clarke S. Neonatal adaptive immunity comes of age. Nat Rev Immunol 4:553–564, 2004.

60. Hussey GD, Watkins ML, Goddard EA, et al. Neonatal mycobacterial specific cytotoxic T-lymphocyte and cytokine profiles in response to distinct BCG vaccination strategies. Immunology 105:314–324, 2002.

61. Vekemans J, Amedei A, Ota MO, et al. Neonatal bacillus Calmette-Guerin vaccination induces adult-like IFN-gamma production by CD4+ T lymphocytes. Eur J Immunol 31:1531–1535, 2001.

62. Prescott SL, Macaubes C, Yabuhara A, et al. Developing patterns of T cell memory to environmental allergens in the first two years of life. Int Arch Allergy Immunol 113:75–79, 1997.

63. Prescott SL, Macaubas C, Holt BJ, et al. Transplacental priming of the human immune system to environmental allergens: universal skewing of initial T cell responses toward the Th2 cytokine profile. J Immunol 160:4730–4737, 1998.

64. Marchant A, Appay V, Van Der Sande M, et al. Mature CD8(+) T lymphocyte response to viral infection during fetal life. J Clin Invest 111:1747–1755, 2003.

65. Hermann E, Truyens C, Alonso-Vega C, et al. Human fetuses are able to mount an adultlike CD8 T-cell response. Blood 100:2153–2158, 2002.

66. Morell A, Skvaril F, Hitzig WH, Barandun S. IgG subclasses: development of the serum concentrations in "normal" infants and children. J Pediatr 80:960–964, 1972.

67. Oxelius VA. IgG subclass levels in infancy and childhood. Acta Paediatr Scand 68:23–27, 1979.

68. Rijkers GT, Sanders EA, Breukels MA, Zegers BJ. Infant B cell responses to polysaccharide determinants. Vaccine 16:1396–1400, 1998.

69. Rijkers GT, Sanders LA, Zegers BJ. Anti-capsular polysaccharide antibody deficiency states. Immunodeficiency 5:1–21, 1993.

70. Schur PH, Rosen F, Norman ME. Immunoglobulin subclasses in normal children. Pediatr Res 13:181–183, 1979.

71. Andersson B, Blomgren H. Evidence for thymus-independent humoral antibody production in mice against polyvinylpyrrolidone and E. coli lipopolysaccharide. Cell Immunol 2:411–424, 1971.

72. Hale ML, Hanna EE, Hansen CT. Nude mice from homozygous nude parents show smaller PFC responses to sheep erythrocytes than nude mice from heterozygous mothers. Nature 260:44–45, 1976.

73. Siegrist CA. Neonatal and early life vaccinology. Vaccine 19:3331–3346, 2001.

74. Timens W, Rozeboom T, Poppema S. Fetal and neonatal development of human spleen: an immunohistological study. Immunology 60:603–609, 1987.

75. Bondada S, Garg M. Thymus-independent antigens. Handbook of B and T lymphocytes. Academic Press; 1994:343-370.

76. Bondada S, Wu H, Robertson DA, Chelvarajan RL. Accessory cell defect in unresponsiveness of neonates and aged to polysaccharide vaccines. Vaccine 19:557–565, 2000.

77. Mond JJ, Lees A, Snapper CM. T cell-independent antigens type 2. Annu Rev Immunol 13:655–692, 1995.

78. Gathings WE, Kubagawa H, Cooper MD. A distinctive pattern of B cell immaturity in perinatal humans. Immunol Rev 57:107–126, 1981.

79. Nossal GJ. Cellular mechanisms of immunologic tolerance. Annu Rev Immunol 1:33–62, 1983.

80. Baker PJ. T cell regulation of the antibody response to bacterial polysaccharide antigens: an examination of some general characteristics and their implications. J Infect Dis 165(Suppl 1):S44–S48, 1992.

81. Landers CD, Chelvarajan RL, Bondada S. The role of B cells and accessory cells in the neonatal response to TI-2 antigens. Immunol Res 31:25–36, 2005.

82. Abbas AK, Lichtman AH, Pober JS. Effector mechanisms of humoral immunity. In: Schmitt W, Hacker HN, Ehlers J, eds. Cellular and Molecular Immunology (4th edn). Philadelphia: W.B. Saunders; 2000:309-334.

83. Griffioen AW, Franklin SW, Zegers BJ, Rijkers GT. Expression and functional characteristics of the complement receptor type 2 on adult and neonatal B lymphocytes. Clin Immunol Immunopathol 69:1–8, 1993.

84. Barrett DJ, Sleasman JW, Schatz DA, Steinitz M. Human anti-pneumococcal polysaccharide antibodies are secreted by the CD5- B cell lineage. Cell Immunol 143:66–79, 1992.

85. Brooks DA, Beckman IG, Bradley J, et al. Human lymphocyte markers defined by antibodies derived from somatic cell hybrids. IV. A monoclonal antibody reacting specifically with a subpopulation of human B lymphocytes. J Immunol 126:1373–1377, 1981.

86. Ibelgaufts H (ed). COPE: Cytokines & cells online pathfinder encyclopaedia, vol 2005: Ibelgaufts H; 2006.

87. Saito S, Morii T, Umekage H, et al. Expression of the interleukin-2 receptor gamma chain on cord blood mononuclear cells. Blood 87:3344–3350, 1996.

88. Zola H, Fusco M, Macardle PJ, et al. Expression of cytokine receptors by human cord blood lymphocytes: comparison with adult blood lymphocytes. Pediatr Res 38:397–403, 1995.

89. Bohnsack JF, Brown EJ. The role of the spleen in resistance to infection. Annu Rev Med 37:49–59, 1986.

90. Timens W, Boes A, Rozeboom-Uiterwijk T, Poppema S. Immaturity of the human splenic marginal zone in infancy. Possible contribution to the deficient infant immune response. J Immunol 143:3200–3206, 1989.

91. Abbas AK, Lichtman AH, Pober JS. General properties of immune responses. In: Schmitt W, Hacker HN, Ehlers J, eds. Cellular and molecular immunology (4th edn). Philadelphia: W.B. Saunders; 2000:3–16.

92. Kruetzmann S, Rosado MM, Weber H, et al. Human immunoglobulin M memory B cells controlling Streptococcus pneumoniae infections are generated in the spleen. J Exp Med 197:939–945, 2003.

93. Graham CW, Saba TM, Lolekha S, Gotoff SP. Deficient serum opsonic activity for macrophage function in newborn infants. Proc Soc Exp Biol Med 143:991–994, 1973.

94. Das M, Henderson T, Feig SA. Neonatal mononuclear cell metabolism: further evidence for diminished monocyte function in the neonate. Pediatr Res 13:632–634, 1979.

95. Gessler P, Kirchmann N, Kientsch-Engel R, et al. Serum concentrations of granulocyte colony-stimulating factor in healthy term and preterm neonates and in those with various diseases including bacterial infections. Blood 82:3177–3182, 1993.

96. Schibler KR, Liechty KW, White WL, et al. Defective production of interleukin-6 by monocytes: a possible mechanism underlying several host defense deficiencies of neonates. Pediatr Res 31:18–21, 1992.

97. Schibler KR, Liechty KW, White WL, Christensen RD. Production of granulocyte colony-stimulating factor in vitro by monocytes from preterm and term neonates. Blood 82:2478–2484, 1993.

98. Pillay V, Savage N, Laburn H. Circulating cytokine concentrations and cytokine production by monocytes from newborn babies and adults. Pflugers Arch 428:197–201, 1994.

99. Kapenberg ML, Jansen MM. Antigen presentation and immunoregulation. In: Adkinson MF, Yunginger JW, Busse WW, et al., eds. Middleton's allergy: principles and practice (6th edn). Philidelphia: Mosby; 2003:178.

100. Wong OH, Huang FP, Chiang AK. Differential responses of cord and adult blood-derived dendritic cells to dying cells. Immunology 116:13–20, 2005.

101. Joyner JL, Augustine NH, Taylor KA, et al. Effects of group B streptococci on cord and adult mononuclear cell interleukin-12 and interferon-gamma mRNA accumulation and protein secretion. J Infect Dis 182:974–977, 2000.

102. Goriely S, Vincart B, Stordeur P, et al. Deficient IL-12(p35) gene expression by dendritic cells derived from neonatal monocytes. J Immunol 166:2141–2146, 2001.

103. Upham JW, Lee PT, Holt BJ, et al. Development of interleukin-12-producing capacity throughout childhood. Infect Immun 70:6583–6588, 2002.

104. Stefanovic V, Golubovic E, Vlahovic P, Mitic-Zlatkovic M. Age-related changes in IL-12 production by peripheral blood mononuclear cells (PBMC). J Intern Med 243:83–84, 1998.

105. Langrish CL, Buddle JC, Thrasher AJ, Goldblatt D. Neonatal dendritic cells are intrinsically biased against Th-1 immune responses. Clin Exp Immunol 128:118–123, 2002.

106. Marodi L, Goda K, Palicz A, Szabo G. Cytokine receptor signalling in neonatal macrophages: defective STAT-1 phosphorylation in response to stimulation with IFN-gamma. Clin Exp Immunol 126:456–460, 2001.

107. De Wit D, Olislagers V, Goriely S, et al. Blood plasmacytoid dendritic cell responses to CpG oligodeoxynucleotides are impaired in human newborns. Blood 103:1030–1032, 2004.

108. Bessler H, Komlos L, Punsky I, et al. CD14 receptor expression and lipopolysaccharide-induced cytokine production in preterm and term neonates. Biol Neonate 80:186–192, 2001.

109. Hebra A, Strange P, Egbert JM, et al. Intracellular cytokine production by fetal and adult monocytes. J Pediatr Surg 36:1321–1326, 2001.

110. Peters AM, Bertram P, Gahr M, Speer CP. Reduced secretion of interleukin-1 and tumor necrosis factor-alpha by neonatal monocytes. Biol Neonate 63:157–162, 1993.

111. Weatherstone KB, Rich EA. Tumor necrosis factor/cachectin and interleukin-1 secretion by cord blood monocytes from premature and term neonates. Pediatr Res 25:342–346, 1989.

112. Cohen L, Haziot A, Shen DR, et al. CD14-independent responses to LPS require a serum factor that is absent from neonates. J Immunol 155:5337–5342, 1995.

113. Glover DM, Brownstein D, Burchett S, et al. Expression of HLA class II antigens and secretion of interleukin-1 by monocytes and macrophages from adults and neonates. Immunology 61:195–201, 1987.

114. Muller K, Zak M, Nielsen S, et al. In vitro cytokine production and phenotype expression by blood mononuclear cells from umbilical cords, children and adults. Pediatr Allergy Immunol 7:117–124, 1996.

115. Berner R, Csorba J, Brandis M. Different cytokine expression in cord blood mononuclear cells after stimulation with neonatal sepsis or colonizing strains of Streptococcus agalactiae. Pediatr Res 49:691–697, 2001.

116. Schultz C, Rott C, Temming P, et al. Enhanced interleukin-6 and interleukin-8 synthesis in term and preterm infants. Pediatr Res 51:317–322, 2002.

117. Karlsson H, Hessle C, Rudin A. Innate immune responses of human neonatal cells to bacteria from the normal gastrointestinal flora. Infect Immun 70:6688–6696, 2002.

118. Dembinski J, Behrendt D, Heep A, et al. Cell-associated interleukin-8 in cord blood of term and preterm infants. Clin Diagn Lab Immunol 9:320–323, 2002.

119. Bryson YJ, Winter HS, Gard SE, et al. Deficiency of immune interferon production by leukocytes of normal newborns. Cell Immunol 55:191–200, 1980.

120. Hartel C, Adam N, Strunk T, et al. Cytokine responses correlate differentially with age in infancy and early childhood. Clin Exp Immunol 142:446–453, 2005.

121. Schultz C, Temming P, Bucsky P, et al. Immature anti-inflammatory response in neonates. Clin Exp Immunol 135:130–136, 2004.

122. Adkins B, Williamson T, Guevara P, Bu Y. Murine neonatal lymphocytes show rapid early cell cycle entry and cell division. J Immunol 170:4548–4556, 2003.

123. Adkins B, Bu Y, Vincek V, Guevara P. The primary responses of murine neonatal lymph node CD4+ cells are Th2-skewed and are sufficient for the development of Th2-biased memory. Clin Dev Immunol 10:43–51, 2003.

124. Ridge JP, Fuchs EJ, Matzinger P. Neonatal tolerance revisited: turning on newborn T cells with dendritic cells. Science 271:1723–1726, 1996.

125. Winkler S, Willheim M, Baier K, et al. Frequency of cytokine-producing T cells in patients of different age groups with Plasmodium falciparum malaria. J Infect Dis 179:209–216, 1999.

126. Adkins B, Bu Y, Guevara P. Murine neonatal CD4+ lymph node cells are highly deficient in the development of antigen-specific Th1 function in adoptive adult hosts. J Immunol 169:4998–5004, 2002.

127. Qureshi MH, Garvy BA. Neonatal T cells in an adult lung environment are competent to resolve Pneumocystis carinii pneumonia. J Immunol 166:5704–5711, 2001.

128. King LB, Norvell A, Monroe JG. Antigen receptor-induced signal transduction imbalances associated with the negative selection of immature B cells. J Immunol 162:2655–2662, 1999.

129. Marshall-Clarke S, Tasker L, Parkhouse RM. Immature B lymphocytes from adult bone marrow exhibit a selective defect in induced hyperexpression of major histocompatibility complex class II and fail to show B7.2 induction. Immunology 100:141–151, 2000.

130. Benschop RJ, Brandl E, Chan AC, Cambier JC. Unique signaling properties of B cell antigen receptor in mature and immature B cells: implications for tolerance and activation. J Immunol 167:4172–4179, 2001.

131. Balazs M, Martin F, Zhou T, Kearney J. Blood dendritic cells interact with splenic marginal zone B cells to initiate T-independent immune responses. Immunity 17:341–352, 2002.

132. Martin F, Kearney JF. Marginal-zone B cells. Nat Rev Immunol 2:323–335, 2002.

133. Wardemann H, Boehm T, Dear N, Carsetti R. B-1a B cells that link the innate and adaptive immune responses are lacking in the absence of the spleen. J Exp Med 195:771–780, 2002.

134. Mosier DE, Johnson BM. Ontogeny of mouse lymphocyte function. II. Development of the ability to produce antibody is modulated by T lymphocytes. J Exp Med 141:216–226, 1975.

135. Klinman DM, Yi AK, Beaucage SL, et al. CpG motifs present in bacteria DNA rapidly induce lymphocytes to secrete interleukin 6, interleukin 12, and interferon gamma. Proc Natl Acad Sci USA 93:2879–2883, 1996.

136. Krieg AM, Yi AK, Matson S, et al. CpG motifs in bacterial DNA trigger direct B-cell activation. Nature 374:546–549, 1995.

137. Bird AP. CpG-rich islands and the function of DNA methylation. Nature 321:209–213, 1986.

138. Chelvarajan RL, Raithatha R, Venkataraman C, et al. CpG oligodeoxynucleotides overcome the unresponsiveness of neonatal B cells to stimulation with the thymus-independent stimuli anti-IgM and TNP-Ficoll. Eur J Immunol 29:2808–2818, 1999.

139. Chelvarajan RL, Gilbert NL, Bondada S. Neonatal murine B lymphocytes respond to polysaccharide antigens in the presence of IL-1 and IL-6. J Immunol 161:3315–3324, 1998.

140. Snapper CM, Rosas FR, Moorman MA, Mond JJ. Restoration of T cell-independent type 2 induction of Ig secretion by neonatal B cells in vitro. J Immunol 158:2731–2735, 1997.

141. Buchanan RM, Arulanandam BP, Metzger DW. IL-12 enhances antibody responses to T-independent polysaccharide vaccines in the absence of T and NK cells. J Immunol 161:5525–5533, 1998.

142. Allman D, Lindsley RC, DeMuth W, et al. Resolution of three nonproliferative immature splenic B cell subsets reveals multiple selection points during peripheral B cell maturation. J Immunol 167:6834–6840, 2001.

143. Loder F, Mutschler B, Ray RJ, et al. B cell development in the spleen takes place in discrete steps and is determined by the quality of B cell receptor-derived signals. J Exp Med 190:75–89, 1999.

144. Gavin AL, Duong B, Skog P, et al. deltaBAFF, a splice isoform of BAFF, opposes full-length BAFF activity in vivo in transgenic mouse models. J Immunol 175:319–328, 2005.

145. Kovarik J, Bozzotti P, Tougne C, et al. Adjuvant effects of CpG oligodeoxynucleotides on responses against T-independent type 2 antigens. Immunology 102:67–76, 2001.

146. Chelvarajan L, Popa D, Liu Y, et al. Molecular mechanisms underlying anti-inflammatory phenotype of neonatal splenic macrophages. J Leukoc Biol 82:403–416; 2007.

147. Chelvarajan RL, Collins SM, Van Willigen JM, Bondada S. The unresponsiveness of aged mice to polysaccharide antigens is a result of a defect in macrophage function. J Leukoc Biol 77:503–512, 2005.

148. Li L, Godfrey WR, Porter SB, et al. CD4+CD25+ regulatory T-cell lines from human cord blood have functional and molecular properties of T-cell anergy. Blood 106:3068–3073, 2005.

149. Forster-Waldl E, Sadeghi K, Tamandl D, et al. Monocyte toll-like receptor 4 expression and LPS-induced cytokine production increase during gestational aging. Pediatr Res 58:121–124, 2005.

150. Mainali ES, Kikuchi T, Tew JG. Dexamethasone inhibits maturation and alters function of monocyte-derived dendritic cells from cord blood. Pediatr Res 58:125–131, 2005.

151. Orlikowsky TW, Dannecker GE, Spring B, et al. Effect of dexamethasone on B7 regulation and T cell activation in neonates and adults. Pediatr Res 57:656–661, 2005.

152. Szakacs J, Lazar G Jr, Lazar G, Husztik E. The effect of the glucocorticoid Oradexon on endotoxin-induced peritoneal cell response. Acta Physiol Hung 87:161–166, 2000.

153. Mlambo G, Sigola LB. Rifampicin and dexamethasone have similar effects on macrophage phagocytosis of zymosan, but differ in their effects on nitrite and TNF-alpha production. Int Immunopharmacol 3:513–522, 2003.

154. Willment JA, Lin HH, Reid DM, et al. Dectin-1 expression and function are enhanced on alternatively activated and GM-CSF-treated macrophages and are negatively regulated by IL-10, dexamethasone, and lipopolysaccharide. J Immunol 171:4569–4573, 2003.

155. Bradley LM, Mishell RI. Differential effects of glucocorticosteroids on the functions of helper and suppressor T lymphocytes. Proc Natl Acad Sci USA 78:3155–3159, 1981.

156. Evans GF, Zuckerman SH. Glucocorticoid-dependent and -independent mechanisms involved in lipopolysaccharide tolerance. Eur J Immunol 21:1973–1979, 1991.

157. Calandra T, Bernhagen J, Metz CN, et al. MIF as a glucocorticoid-induced modulator of cytokine production. Nature 377:68–71, 1995.

158. Kitajima T, Ariizumi K, Bergstresser PR, Takashima A. A novel mechanism of glucocorticoid-induced immune suppression: the inhibiton of T cell-mediated terminal maturation of a murine dendritic cell line. J Clin Invest 98:142–147, 1996.

159. Pan J, Ju D, Wang Q, et al. Dexamethasone inhibits the antigen presentation of dendritic cells in MHC class II pathway. Immunol Lett 76:153–161, 2001.

160. Yorty JL, Schultz SA, Bonneau RH. Postpartum maternal corticosterone decreases maternal and neonatal antibody levels and increases the susceptibility of newborn mice to herpes simplex virus-associated mortality. J Neuroimmunol 150:48–58, 2004.

161. Abbas AK, Lichtman AH, Pober JS. Lymphocyte maturation and expression of antigen receptor genes. In: Schmitt W, Hacker HN, Ehlers J, eds. Cellular and molecular immunology (4th edn). Philadelphia: W.B. Saunders; 2000:125–160.

162. Orlikowsky TW, Spring B, Dannecker GE, et al. Expression and regulation of B7 family molecules on macrophages (MPhi) in preterm and term neonatal cord blood and peripheral blood of adults. Cytometry B Clin Cytom 53:40–47, 2003.

163. Hoetzenecker W, Meingassner JG, Ecker R, et al. Corticosteroids but not pimecrolimus affect viability, maturation and immune function of murine epidermal Langerhans cells. J Invest Dermatol 122:673–684, 2004.

164. Aberer W, Stingl L, Pogantsch S, Stingl G. Effect of glucocorticosteroids on epidermal cell-induced immune responses. J Immunol 133:792–797, 1984.

165. Hartmann G, Krieg AM. CpG DNA and LPS induce distinct patterns of activation in human monocytes. Gene Ther 6:893–903, 1999.

166. Hartmann G, Weiner GJ, Krieg AM. CpG DNA: a potent signal for growth, activation, and maturation of human dendritic cells. Proc Natl Acad Sci USA 96:9305–9310, 1999.

167. Crabtree TD, Jin L, Raymond DP, et al. Preexposure of murine macrophages to CpG oligonucleotide results in a biphasic tumor necrosis factor alpha response to subsequent lipopolysaccharide challenge. Infect Immun 69:2123–2129, 2001.

168. Sweet MJ, Campbell CC, Sester DP, et al. Colony-stimulating factor-1 suppresses responses to CpG DNA and expression of toll-like receptor 9 but enhances responses to lipopolysaccharide in murine macrophages. J Immunol 168:392–399, 2002.

169. Krieg AM. An innate immune defense mechanism based on the recognition of CpG motifs in microbial DNA. J Lab Clin Med 128:128–133, 1996.

170. Krieg AM. Lymphocyte activation by CpG dinucleotide motifs in prokaryotic DNA. Trends Microbiol 4:73–76, 1996.

171. Liang H, Nishioka Y, Reich CF, et al. Activation of human B cells by phosphorothioate oligodeoxynucleotides. J Clin Invest 98:1119–1129, 1996.

172. Krieg AM. Now I know my CpGs. Trends Microbiol 9:249–252, 2001.

173. Krug A, Rothenfusser S, Hornung V, et al. Identification of CpG oligonucleotide sequences with high induction of IFN-alpha/beta in plasmacytoid dendritic cells. Eur J Immunol 31:2154–2163, 2001.

174. Ballas ZK, Rasmussen WL, Krieg AM. Induction of NK activity in murine and human cells by CpG motifs in oligodeoxynucleotides and bacterial DNA. J Immunol 157:1840–1845, 1996.

175. Verthelyi D, Ishii K, Gursel M, et al. Human peripheral blood cells differentially recognize and respond to two distinct CPG motifs. J Immunol 166:2372–2377, 2001.

176. Marshall JD, Fearon K, Abbate C, et al. Identification of a novel CpG DNA class and motif that optimally stimulate B cell and plasmacytoid dendritic cell functions. J Leukoc Biol 73:781–792, 2003.

177. Vollmer J, Weeratna R, Payette P, et al. Characterization of three CpG oligodeoxynucleotide classes with distinct immunostimulatory activities. Eur J Immunol 34:251–262, 2004.

178. Carpentier A, Laigle-Donadey F, Zohar S, et al. Phase 1 trial of a CpG oligodeoxynucleotide for patients with recurrent glioblastoma. Neuro-oncology 8:60–66, 2006.

179. Cooper CL, Davis HL, Angel JB, et al. CPG 7909 adjuvant improves hepatitis B virus vaccine seroprotection in antiretroviral-treated HIV-infected adults. Aids 19:1473–1479, 2005.

180. Broide DH. DNA vaccines: an evolving approach to the treatment of allergic disorders. Allergy Asthma Proc 26:195–198, 2005.

181. Friedberg JW, Kim H, McCauley M, et al. Combination immunotherapy with a CpG oligonucleotide (1018 ISS) and rituximab in patients with non-Hodgkin lymphoma: increased interferon-alpha/beta-inducible gene expression, without significant toxicity. Blood 105:489–495, 2005.

182. Pichyangkul S, Yongvanitchit K, Kum-arb U, et al. Whole blood cultures to assess the immunostimulatory activities of CpG oligodeoxynucleotides. J Immunol Methods 247:83–94, 2001.

183. Adderson EE. Antibody repertoires in infants and adults: effects of T-independent and T-dependent immunizations. Springer Semin Immunopathol 23:387–403, 2001.

184. Chu RS, McCool T, Greenspan NS, et al. CpG oligodeoxynucleotides act as adjuvants for pneumococcal polysaccharide-protein conjugate vaccines and enhance antipolysaccharide immunoglobulin G2a (IgG2a) and IgG3 antibodies. Infect Immun 68:1450–1456, 2000.

185. Bernard GR, Vincent JL, Laterre PF, et al. Efficacy and safety of recombinant human activated protein C for severe sepsis. N Engl J Med 344:699–709, 2001.

186. Das UN. Current advances in sepsis and septic shock with particular emphasis on the role of insulin. Med Sci Monit 9:RA181–RA192, 2003.

187. Freeman BD, Zehnbauer BA, Buchman TG. A meta-analysis of controlled trials of anticoagulant therapies in patients with sepsis. Shock 20:5–9, 2003.

188. Vincent JL, Abraham E, Annane D, et al. Reducing mortality in sepsis: new directions. Crit Care 6(Suppl 3):S1–S18, 2002.

189. Gengenbacher D, Salm H, Vogt A, Schneider H. Detection of cell surface determinants for anti-Leu M3 (CD14), MY9 (CD33) and MY4 (CD14) and phagocytic function of cord blood monocytes in the course of gestational age. Bone Marrow Transplant 22(Suppl 1):S48–S51, 1998.

190. Blahnik MJ, Ramanathan R, Riley CR, Minoo P. Lipopolysaccharide-induced tumor necrosis factor-alpha and IL-10 production by lung macrophages from preterm and term neonates. Pediatr Res 50:726–731, 2001.

191. Schibler KR, Trautman MS, Liechty KW, et al. Diminished transcription of interleukin-8 by monocytes from preterm neonates. J Leukoc Biol 53:399–403, 1993.

192. Dembinski J, Behrendt D, Martini R, et al. Modulation of pro- and anti-inflammatory cytokine production in very preterm infants. Cytokine 21:200–206, 2003.

193. Dembinski J, Behrendt D, Reinsberg J, Bartmann P. Endotoxin-stimulated production of IL-6 and IL-8 is increased in short-term cultures of whole blood from healthy term neonates. Cytokine 18:116-119, 2002.

194. Dembinski J, Martini R, Behrendt D, Bartmann P. Modification of cord blood IL-6 production with IgM enriched human immunoglobulin in term and preterm infants. Cytokine 26:25–29, 2004.

Chapter 11

Influence of Passive Antibodies on the Immune Response of Young Infants

W. Paul Glezen, MD

Measles and other Respiratory Viruses

Pertussis and Other Bacterial Vaccines

Summary

Examination of the effect of passively acquired antibody on active immunization of infants is important for multiple reasons, foremost being the consideration of boosting maternal antibodies for protection of neonates and young infants by delivering vaccine to pregnant women (1). The question is whether or not the enhanced maternal antibody levels will interfere with subsequent active immunization. This question will be addressed in this review along with some of the parameters of immune responsiveness that are related to this question.

First, it should be recognized that the pattern of transmission of naturally occurring passive immunity is changing. Extensive use of vaccines has altered the ecology of the diseases that the vaccines prevent. Examples of diseases with changing patterns of occurrence are measles and pertussis. For both diseases a major age shift in the incidence of serious disease to young infants has occurred that probably has resulted from a reduced endowment of maternal protection for the fetus. For pertussis and, perhaps, other diseases, boosting of maternal immunity is warranted both to increase protective antibody transmitted to the fetus and to reduce exposure of the infant by protecting the mother (and other household contacts) from infection with *Bordetella pertussis*. Other aspects of pertussis epidemiology will be discussed in the second section.

For many years it was assumed that the lower age limit for administration of measles vaccine was determined solely by the level of passively acquired maternal antibody. The changing ecology of measles has allowed dissection of the role of maternal antibody from immunologic immaturity of the infant as the determinants of the ability of the infant to respond to active immunization with a live virus vaccine. Examination of this relationship is relevant not only for measles virus but also for other paramyxoviruses, and orthomyxoviruses.

MEASLES AND OTHER RESPIRATORY VIRUSES

Measles

Measles vaccine was licensed in 1963 (2). The occurrence of natural measles infection declined as vaccine uptake increased. Originally, only a single dose of vaccine was recommended after the first year of life when maternal antibody had waned because it was recognized that even low levels of passively acquired antibody would interfere with infection with the attenuated measles virus and thereby limit the immune response. The early surge of vaccine uptake resulted in a significant reduction in exposure of the population to natural measles infection. As a consequence, starting in about 1985, infants born to women whose only exposure to measles infection was vaccination in early childhood had lower passively acquired antibody titers than were usually seen prior to the introduction of vaccine. For instance, Yeager et al. found a steady decline in measles antibody titers in cord blood specimens between 1969 and 1976, ranging from a geometric mean titer of 1:134 to 1:46, respectively (3). Infants immunized at 10 or 11 months of age were more likely to generate an immune response in 1976 compared to those born earlier. This resulted in earlier susceptibility of infants to natural infection and consideration of initiating active immunization at an earlier age. Lennon and Black estimated age of susceptibility of infants born to mothers in three birth cohorts, prior to 1957, 1958 through 1962 and >1963, by measuring maternal measles antibody titers (4). Projecting from the estimated half-life of passively acquired antibody, infants born to mothers born before 1958 were probably protected for an average of 11.5 months, while those whose mothers were born after 1962 were probably protected for only an average of 8.5 months.

As a consequence of these waning antibody levels and reduced exposure to natural infection, immunity of the population declined despite continued vaccination of children between 12 and 15 months of age (5). Despite an overall decline in reported measles, outbreaks continued to occur, culminating in a series of serious epidemics in 1987 and 1990. One feature of these outbreaks was the large proportion of cases in infants too young to receive vaccine. Hutchins et al. reported that 31% of those involved were <16 months of age (too young to receive vaccine by the existing recommendations) (6). Many of the children admitted to hospital with measles were <9 months of age, which was a rare finding before the introduction of vaccine.

Up to this time, the conventional wisdom was that maternal antibody was the limiting factor for successful immunization of infants. Therefore, the logical response to the occurrence of serious disease in infants <9 months of age was to administer the vaccine at an earlier age (7). Because of the variation in passive antibody levels, more potent vaccines were developed that would overcome low levels of maternal antibody present in some infants and the vaccines were delivered at <6 months of age. Follow-up of some of these infants detected increased mortality due to poorly defined causes by age 3 years and raised questions about the safety of high-dose vaccines administered at an early age (8). This experience led to re-examination of measles vaccine strategies.

Careful studies by Arvin and colleagues have helped to elucidate the immune responses of infants to measles vaccine (9–11). They compared antibody responses of infants at ages 6, 9 and 12 months with and without pre-existing measles antibody (9). At 6 months of age only 67% of antibody-negative infants had a 4-fold increase in neutralizing antibody titers and only 36% achieved "sero-protective" responses. Geometric mean titers of the 6-month-old infants were 27, compared to 578 and 972 for infants who were vaccinated at 9 and 12 months, respectively. The failure of the younger infants to respond to immunization in the absence of passively acquired antibody indicates a partial failure of maturation of the immune system. The limitation is partial because, in contrast to the neutralizing antibody responses, T-cell proliferation and cytokine responses to measles did not differ with age. These observations were extended by comparing the responses to mumps vaccine for the same age groups with essentially the same results (10, 11). Six-month-old infants had limited humoral responses to mumps virus vaccine, but the measures of cellular immunity were the same for all age groups. These infants – with and without pre-existing passive antibody – responded well to a second dose at 12 months of age. At that time all had protective titers (>120 mIU) to measles virus. This is evidence that immunologic priming occurred with the first dose of vaccine despite pre-existing passive antibody or immunologic immaturity (in the case of those 6 months of age at the time of the first vaccination).

Measles and mumps viruses belong to the *Paramyxoviridae* family. Mumps is closely related to the human parainfluenza viruses and less closely related to the pneumovirus (respiratory syncytial virus), orthomyxovirus (influenza viruses), and metapneumovirus (human metapneumovirus) (12). Longitudinal studies have shown that primary infections with most of these viruses will not generate a protective immune response in infants. This is true generally for both natural infection and infection with an attenuated vaccine virus. Protection is correlated with the level of neutralizing antibodies and has been demonstrated for passively acquired maternal antibody as well as antibody generated by natural infection. The evidence for these statements is summarized here.

Paramyxoviridae – Natural Infection

Longitudinal studies of infants followed from birth and correlation of maternal antibody levels to risk of infection have documented a negative correlation between severity of infection and pre-existing antibody against the common respiratory viruses – respiratory syncytial virus (RSV), parainfluenza virus type 3 and influenza A(H3N2) virus (13–15). Infections may occur in infants with relatively low levels of passively acquired neutralizing antibodies. When infection is documented by virus isolation or antigen detection, a neutralizing antibody response may not be measured. In some cases, maternal antibody may mask the response because the low titer will persist beyond the period when the passively acquired antibodies would normally persist. In other cases, a response is not evident for influenza and RSV. An unusual situation after parainfluenza type 3 infection in infants <6 months of age has been described. Kasel et al. found a gradual increase in neutralizing antibodies for several months after infection, documented by multiple cultures (16). Although it was not unusual to find repeated shedding up to 3 weeks after onset of illness, the increase in antibodies continued for months after consistently negative serial cultures. For infections with this group of viruses in young infants, it may be important to measure the antibody response for 6–8 weeks after infection because a significant rise may not be detectable by 3–4 weeks. At first, the pre-existing maternal antibody may mask the active antibody production or the immature immune mechanisms of the infant may require a longer time to mount a response.

Evidence for diminished protective immune response to infection in early infancy is the high frequency of re-infection during the first 2 years of life after primary infection occurs in early infancy (13–15). Infants who do not generate a neutralizing antibody response to the first infection have a very high risk of re-infection during the next season. This was especially true for RSV and parainfluenza type 3. For RSV, infants with neutralizing antibody titers <1:8 had re-infection rates of almost 83% in the second year compared to only 12% for those with titers of 1:128 or greater (14). For parainfluenza type 3, the rates were 88% and 40%, respectively (15). Both RSV and parainfluenza virus type 3 produce high infection rates and morbidity in young infants. Protection afforded by naturally acquired maternal antibodies against primary infection in the first months of life has been demonstrated for both of these viruses and influenza viruses (15, 17, 18). For the latter it has been shown that the age at the time of culture-positive influenza virus infection is inversely related to the level of neutralizing antibody present in cord sera at birth. In other words, the higher the titer at birth, the older the infant will be at the time of primary infection. This is important because younger infants are at greater risk for serious lower respiratory tract infections due to immunologic immaturity and small-caliber airways. In general, the longer that primary infection can be avoided, the better the outcome. Furthermore, it was demonstrated that infants with culture-positive infections had no detectable pre-existing antibody to the infecting virus strain at the time that they presented to the hospital (17).

Similar data are available for RSV infections in young infants (18, 19). Infants with culture-positive RSV infections during the first 8 weeks of life had significantly lower cord blood neutralizing titers than RSV-infected infants aged 9–18 weeks. It is important to note that the age of infants at the time of the largest proportion of hospital admissions for RSV disease is 4–8 weeks. Infants admitted to the hospital with neutralizing antibody titers of 1:16 or greater had significantly lower illness severity scores than those with titers <1:8. For parainfluenza type 3 virus, infants less than 5 months of age with cord blood titers <1:32 had infection rates of 33 per 100 compared to only 7 per 100 for infants with cord blood levels of 1:256 or higher (15). It is clear that maternal antibody will modify natural infection; therefore, it should be expected that it will affect the response to live, attenuated vaccine viruses.

Paramyxoviridae – Response to Vaccines

Influenza

Piedra et al. found that the response to inactivated influenza vaccine (two doses) was depressed by low levels of pre-existing antibodies – presumably of maternal origin – in young infants (20). This study also showed that antibody response may be delayed in young infants after administration of live attenuated vaccine; increased numbers of infants had significant increases in antibodies detected at 6–8 weeks after vaccination compared to 3–4 weeks. When two doses of live attenuated virus were given to young infants, only 20% of those vaccinated at 2 and 4 months of age achieved protective titers measure by hemagglutination inhibition, compared to 50% if the second dose was delayed until 6 months of age. Low levels of maternal antibody did not influence the results and the conclusion was that immaturity of the immune system was the main factor in determining the antibody response. Gruber et al. compared responses to bivalent A live attenuated vaccine in infants <6 and >6 months of age; 77% and 92% of seronegative infants >6 months of age seroconverted, while only 56% and 81% of those <6 months responded to a single-dose vaccine to influenza A(H1N1) and A(H3N2), respectively (21). The results for infants <6 months of age were similar for those with pre-existing (presumably maternal) antibody. Clements et al. were able to infect infants at 2 and 4 months of age with high-dose (10^7 $TCID_{50}$) monovalent influenza A(H1N1) attenuated vaccine; however, about 25% developed fever and 13% had cough as reactions to the vaccine, so that safety considerations were raised (22). Safety would be a greater concern for a trivalent preparation at this higher dose. In summary, for influenza vaccines maternal antibody may dampen the immune response to inactivated vaccines. The live attenuated vaccine does not appear to be affected by low levels of maternal antibody but the immune response is reduced by immunologic immaturity. High doses (10^7 tissue culture infective $dose_{50}$) of the attenuated virus vaccine may not be safe for infants <6 months of age.

The current approach to protection of infants <6 months of age is to vaccinate women who are pregnant during the influenza season (23, 24). Since the influenza vaccine formula is updated each year and is usually not available until early September, women can only receive the relevant vaccine after they are pregnant. Since women have increasing risk of complications of influenza as pregnancy progresses, the vaccine can serve a double purpose of protecting both the mother and her offspring.

RSV

The development of a vaccine for RSV has been more problematic than for influenza. Crowe has reviewed some of the difficulties in vaccine development that began with the experience of an alum-precipitated, formalin-inactivated preparation in the 1960s (25). This vaccine was given to infants 3–5 months of age and stimulated low levels of neutralizing antibodies. When these infants were challenged with natural infection they had a much higher hospitalization rate – near 50% – than did the controls. Two infants died of RSV disease at 14 and 16 months of age – an age when the consequences of infection are generally benign in otherwise healthy children. This experience had a chilling effect on the development of vaccine. In general, it has been decreed by the FDA that inactivated vaccines of any composition should not be used in infants before first natural priming with RSV infection. Limited studies of the purified F protein (PFP-2) RSV vaccine showed that even infants who have been born prematurely developed significant neutralizing antibody response to the PFP-2 vaccine after natural priming (26, 27). A whole series of live attenuated RSV vaccines have been studied. In general, the vaccines that are sufficiently attenuated to be given safely to young infants do not generate an immune response (28, 29). New recombinant strains are promising in that virus shedding at the time of re-challenge with the vaccine strain is limited in the first month after primary inoculation. However, antibody response is minimal and it is unlikely that this response would protect against wild RSV infection. In any event, multiple doses probably would be required to achieve any protection and this would be accomplished too late to protect the youngest infants, who are at greatest risk of serious disease. A better approach to protection of young infants may be to seek indirect protection by boosting the immunity of toddler-age children to reduce exposure of young infants (31). Immunization might be accomplished by either a potent subunit vaccine or a less attenuated live virus strain. Active immunization of young children >1 year of age could be combined with maternal immunization to boost the passive immunity of the infant, which should protect against lower respiratory disease in the first months of life (30, 32). Since immunologic immaturity limits an active immune response until after 6 months of age, maternal antibody will be degraded before active immunization is indicated. Therefore, enhanced maternal antibody present at birth would not interfere with active immunization after 6 months of age.

Studies in a primate model have yielded some intriguing results. Crowe et al. infected seronegative chimpanzees with a live attenuated RSV vaccine after pretreating half of the subjects with high-titered RSV immunoglobulin (33). The passive immunity blunted the antibody response after vaccination, but surprisingly, after challenge with a wild RSV strain, the protection was not different and the chimpanzees that were passively immunized prior to vaccination had enhanced neutralizing antibody responses that indicated priming with the vaccine under the cover of passive immunity. This study would certainly support the hypothesis that the principal limiting factor to immunization of young infants is not passively acquired antibody, but immunologic immaturity.

Parainfluenza Virus Type 3

Parainfluenza virus type 3 appears to be less sensitive to passively acquired maternal antibody than influenza virus or RSV (15). Infection rates in infants <5 months of age were inversely related to maternal antibody levels but the correlation was not as impressive; infection rates were 33.3%, 24.7% and 7.1% for infants with cord blood titers <1:32, 1:64–128, and >1:128, respectively. Overall the early infection rate was about half that seen for RSV and the frequency of lower respiratory tract illness was much less. Candidate vaccines have been developed by cold adaptation of human parainfluenza virus type 3 and by the Jennerian approach using bovine parainfluenza type 3 (12). Growth of the bovine strain is restricted in both non-human primates and in infants (34). The frequency of virus shedding was not related to preexisting antibodies. Studies in primates have shown that infection with the bovine virus protects against challenge with human parainfluenza type 3. Further studies are required to confirm the safety and efficacy of attenuated parainfluenza vaccines. The effect of maternal antibody appears to be minimal at this time.

Summary of Maternal Antibody and Infection with Paramyxoviridae

Measles virus is most sensitive to passively acquired antibody, and the other viruses in descending order are less sensitive: influenza, RSV and parainfluenza type 3. Although active antibody response to infection or vaccine may be dampened by maternal antibody, evidence of T cell priming is manifested by booster response to subsequent challenge. The main limiting factor to immunization in early infancy is immunologic immaturity and not maternal antibody. Passive immunity enhanced by boosting maternal antibody during pregnancy may provide the protection needed for the interval between birth and attainment of immunologic competency (1).

PERTUSSIS AND OTHER BACTERIAL VACCINES

Pertussis

Pertussis is a continuing public health problem despite the availability of effective vaccines that are safe and well-tolerated (35). Young infants less than 6 months of age develop life-threatening infections that require hospitalization and, often, intensive care. Between 1997 and 2000, over 7000 cases were reported in infants under 6 months of age and 63% were hospitalized (36). These infants comprised over 80% of those hospitalized, 90% of the deaths and over 50% of those with seizures or encephalopathy. At the same time the highest proportional increase in reported cases occurred among adolescents, 10–19 years of age; 30–40% of all cases were in this age group and about 2% were hospitalized. Adults constituted 20–30% of reported cases, of whom 3.5% were hospitalized and 2.6% had pneumonia. These distributions represent a shift in age to older adolescents and young adults, with most of the severe disease in infants too young to have developed immunity from active immunization.

Many of the adolescents and adults have cough illness that may not be recognized as pertussis (37). As a consequence, they may unknowingly expose young infants to infection. Many infants do not receive the primary series of acellular pertussis vaccine in a timely manner and are, therefore, vulnerable to infection. Even if they do receive vaccine at the recommended schedule of 2, 4 and 6 months, they may not have protection until after the third dose. Surveys have shown that women who are delivering babies currently have low levels of antibodies to pertussis antigens (38, 39). Although these antibodies are transmitted to their offspring, the levels are so low as to be undetectable by 2 months of age for almost all infants.

In order to reduce exposure of infants to pertussis, the Advisory Committee on Immunization Practices (ACIP) now recommends a routine pertussis vaccine booster at 10–11 years of age. The recommended vaccine is the combination of tetanus and diphtheria toxoids with acellular pertussis vaccine, Tdap. Any women presenting for prenatal care who have not had the recommended booster should receive Tdap (40). It is further recommended that all household contacts have Tdap boosters at the time of birth of the newborn.

In a large field trial comparing antibody responses to several acellular pertussis vaccines with a whole-cell vaccine in infants, residual maternal antibodies did not interfere with the responses to any of the components of the acellular preparations; however, maternal antibody did dampen the response to pertussis toxin in infants given the whole-cell pertussis vaccine (41). Since only potent acellular vaccines are currently used in practice, it is unlikely that maternal antibodies will interfere with active immunization of the infant; however, this question should be addressed by direct measurements of the antibody decay of maternally derived pertussis antibodies and the development of active responses to pertussis immunization in infants.

Bacterial Toxoids

Bacterial toxoids generally are very immunogenic. Both diphtheria and tetanus toxoids have been administered to pregnant women, resulting in high antibody titers. Bjorkholm et al. administered diphtheria toxoid to pregnant women during an outbreak; infants were actively immunized at 3 and 5 months of age (42). Infants with pre-existing titers of greater than 0.1 IU/ml had a lower response after the second dose but titers after the 12-month booster were indistinguishable from those of infants whose mothers had low titers. Infant response to active immunization with the tetanus toxoid conjugated to the capsular polysaccharide (PRP) of *Hemophilus influenzae* type b has been examined in infants whose mothers had received tetanus toxoid immunization during pregnancy (43). The antibody response to the PRP component was not affected by high maternal tetanus anti-toxin titers; however, the infant response to tetanus toxoid was dampened by high pre-existing anti-toxin levels. Despite this, all infants achieved protective levels of tetanus antitoxin – particularly after the booster dose of PRP-T.

Polysaccharide Vaccines

Meningococcal polysaccharide, pneumococcal polysaccharide and PRP (of *H. influenzae* type b) have been administered to pregnant women. During an epidemic in Brazil, several pregnant women received meningococcal polysaccharide vaccine (44). Responses of infants to active immunization at 6–8 months of age were the same for those whose mothers did or did not receive the vaccine during pregnancy for both serotypes A and C. No evidence of tolerance was found for infants exposed to maternal immunization with the meningococcal vaccine. A similar experience was reported for studies of PRP in pregnant women and subsequent active immunization of their infants. Amstey et al. found that infants of mothers who received PRP during pregnancy responded to active immunization at 18 months of age similarly to infants whose mothers were unvaccinated (45). Again no evidence of tolerance was found; this question had been raised by early studies of polysaccharide antigens in rodent models.

Conjugate Vaccines

Conjugate vaccines were developed because of the failure of infants to respond to the capsular polysaccharide antigens of important bacterial pathogens. Covalent binding of a polysaccharide to a carrier protein has been demonstrated to allow T cell-dependent processing of the polysaccharide antigen – even in young infants. Administration of conjugate vaccines to young infants potentially may be complicated by the presence of passive antibodies to either the carrier protein or to the capsular polysaccharide antigen of interest. Several vaccines against *Hemophilus influenzae* type b (Hib) have been developed by conjugation of the capsular polysaccharide, PRP, to a protein carrier. Most of these vaccines have employed protein carriers that are vaccine antigens or related to vaccine antigens. The most commonly used carrier proteins are tetanus toxoid, diphtheria toxoid or the mutant diphtheria toxin, CRM_{197}. PRP-T designates the Hib vaccine with PRP conjugated to tetanus toxoid. Neonatal immunization with PRP-T was found to be well-tolerated and infants who received the first dose in the newborn period followed by a booster at 4 months had higher doses after the 14-month booster than did infants who were vaccinated only at 4 months of age (46). Therefore, there was no evidence of tolerance to the antigen given in the newborn period. The initial response was dampened in infants with high passively acquired antibody titers but the 4-month dose elicited responses in all infants, indicating that priming occurred despite the high levels of pre-existing antibody. When the first dose of PRP-T was given at 1–2 months of age, maternal antibodies to tetanus toxoid did not interfere with the response to PRP (47). The authors concluded that infants with high levels of maternal anti-tetanus antibodies could be safely immunized with PRP-T. Furthermore, there was evidence that priming the infants with tetanus toxoid prior to the first dose of PRP-T enhanced the PRP antibody response (48).

Four different protein conjugates of PRP have been administered to women during pregnancy or to women of child-bearing age prior to conception (49). Compared to PRP alone, the conjugates give significantly higher titers and more IgG1 antibody that crosses the placenta more readily than IgG2 antibody. IgG2 antibody is usually preferentially produced in adults in response to polysaccharide antigens. Women in The Gambia received PRP-T or meningococcal polysaccharide vaccine during pregnancy (50). The infants were further subdivided to receive active immunization with either PRP-T or hepatitis B vaccines. All responded equally to active immunization and the infants whose mothers had received PRP-T were almost continuously protected against Hib during the first months of life before the active antibody response was evident after the second dose of PRP-T given at 3 months of age. Continuous protection may be important in developing countries where Hib infections are common in infants under 6 months of age.

Englund et al. showed that infants born with high titers of PRP antibody could respond to active immunization with a 10 µg dose of the HbOC vaccine consisting of PRP oligosaccharides conjugated to CRM_{197} (51). Infants immunized between 6 and 9 months of age had titers similar to those of infants whose mothers had not been vaccinated. The 10 µg dose of HbOC gave the highest titers in women of childbearing ag,e averaging 181 µg total PRP antibody (Farr assay) and 81 µg of IgG measured by ELISA. Subsequently a trial in pregnant women utilized a dose of only 2 µg of HbOC, one-fifth the infant dose, and generated an average level of 22.1 µg of total PRP antibody (49, 52). About one-half of this amount was transmitted to the infants, who responded well to active immunization with HbOC, allowing essentially continuous protective levels throughout infancy (Fig. 11-1 and Fig. 11-2). The infants received HbOC, 10 µg, at 2, 4, 6 and 15 months of age. Although their titers were lower than controls after the primary series, they all had

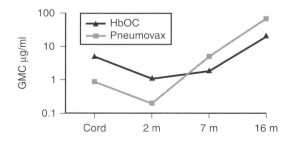

Figure 11-1 Total antibodies against the capsular polysaccharide (PRP) of *Hemophilus influenzae* type b (Hib) for infants after active immunization with the Hib conjugate vaccine, 10 µg, at 2, 4, 6 and 15 months of age are compared for those whose mothers had received the Hib conjugate vaccine, 2 µg, or pneumococcal polysaccharide vaccine during the third trimester of pregnancy.

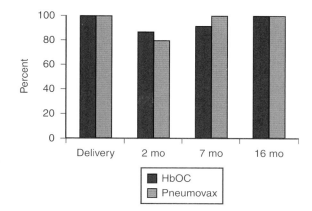

Figure 11-2 Proportion of infants with protective levels of anti-PRP antibodies at delivery, 2 months, 7 months and 16 months of age compared for those whose mothers had received HbOC vaccine or pneumococcal polysaccharide vaccine during the third trimester of pregnancy. All infants received HbOC vaccine at 2, 4, 6 and 15 months of age.

similar titers after the 15-month booster. It is evident that priming occurred even in the presence of high levels of passively acquired maternal antibody.

A pre-pregnancy trial in Native American women had similar results. In this trial, women of child-bearing age received either HbOC vaccine or the PRP-OMP vaccine 6–9 months prior to conception (53). (PRP-OMP utilizes the outer membrane protein of the group B meningococcus as the carrier protein.) Infants born to these women were actively immunized with PRP-OMP at 2, 4 and 12 months of age. Infants whose mothers received HbOC had higher anti-PRP titers before active immunization and their response to active immunization was suppressed after the primary series at 2 and 4 months of age; however, all responded equally to the booster at 12 months of age. This experience gives another example of strategies for maternal immunization that provide seamless protection for the mother and infant. The same pre-pregnancy schedule has been used for tetanus toxoid and has been effective for the prevention of both neonatal tetanus and puerperal tetanus.

SUMMARY

Passively acquired maternal antibody may dampen the antibody response to vaccines administered in the first months of life; however, studies indicate that helper T cell priming is usually present and brisk antibody responses will follow subsequent doses of vaccine. The main problem limiting early immunization is immaturity of the immune system. Strategies to provide protection of neonates and young infants include boosting of maternal antibody by vaccination either during pregnancy or prior to conception, indirect protection by immunizing older contacts of infants and passive immunization with antibody-rich preparations given monthly to high-risk infants. An example of the latter is the use of humanized monoclonal antibodies against RSV. For some vaccines, such as tetanus toxoid, immunization during pregnancy is necessary only if a woman presents for prenatal care without having had the recommended booster. For other vaccines, such as influenza vaccine, immunization can only occur during pregnancy because the vaccine is updated each year and the relevant vaccine is not available until after conception. These immunizations are effective and efficient because a single dose can protect two individuals at a vulnerable period of their lives.

REFERENCES

1. Glezen WP. Maternal vaccines. Primary Care: Clin Office Pract 28:791–806, 2001.
2. Atkinson WL, Markowitz LE. Measles and measles vaccine. Seminars Pediatr Infect Dis 2:100–107, 1991.

3. Yeager AS, Harvey B, Crosson FJ Jr, et al. Need for measles revaccination in adolescents: correlation with birth date prior to 1972. J Pediatr 102:191–195, 1983.

4. Lennon JL, Black FL. Maternally derived measles immunity in era of vaccine-protected mothers. J Pediatr 108:671–676, 1986.

5. Pabst HF, Sapdy DW, Marusyk RG, et al. Reduced measles immunity in infants in a well-vaccinated population. Pediatr Infect Dis J 11:525–529, 1992.

6. Hutchens S, Markowitz L, Atkinson W, et al. Measles outbreaks in the United States, 1987 through 1990. Pediatr Infect Dis J 15:31–38, 1996.

7. Markowitz LE, Sepulveda J, Diaz-Ortega JL, et al. Immunization of six-month-old infants with different doses of Edmonston-Zagreb and Schwarz measles vaccines. N Engl J Med 322:580–587, 1990.

8. Hussey GD, Goddard EA, Hughes J, et al. The effect of Edmonston-Zagreb and Schwarz measles vaccines on immune responses of infants. J Infect Dis 173:1320–1326, 1996.

9. Gans HA, Arvis AM, Galinus J, et al. Deficiency of the humoral immune response to measles vaccine in infants immunized at 6 months. JAMA 280:527–532, 1998.

10. Gans H, Yasulawa L, Rinki M, et al. Immune responses to measles and mumps vaccination of infants at 6, 9, and 12 months. J Infect Dis 184:817–826, 2001.

11. Gans H, DeHovitz R, Forghani B, et al. Measles and mumps vaccination as a model to investigate the developing immune system: passive and active immunity during the first year of life. Vaccine 21:3398–3405, 2003.

12. Piedra PA, Englund JA, Glezen WP. Respiratory syncytial virus and parainfluenza viruses. In: Richman DD, Whitley RJ, Hayden FG, eds. Clinical virology, 2nd edn. Washington DC: ASM Press; 2002:763–90.

13. Glezen WP, Taber LH, Frank AL, et al. Influenza virus infections in infants. Pediatr Infect Dis J 16:1065–1068, 1997.

14. Glezen WP, Taber LH, Frank AL, et al. Risk of primary infection and reinfection with respiratory syncytial virus. Am J Dis Child 140:543–546, 1986.

15. Glezen WP, Frank AL, Taber LH, et al. Parainfluenza virus type 3: seasonality and risk of infection and reinfection in young children. J Infect Dis 150:851–857, 1984.

16. Kasel JA, Frank AL, Keitel WA, et al. Acquisition of serum antibodies to specific viral glycoproteins of parainfluenza virus 3 in children. J Virol 52:828–832, 1984.

17. Puck JM, Glezen WP, Frank AL, et al. Protection of infants from infection with influenza A virus by transplacentally acquired antibody. J Infect Dis 142:844–849, 1980.

18. Glezen WP, Paredes A, Allison JE, et al. Risk of respiratory syncytial viurus infection for infants from low-income families in relationship to age, sex, ethnic group, and maternal antibody. J Pediatr 98:708–715, 1981.

19. Kasel JA, Walsh EE, Frank AL, et al. Relation of serum antibody to glycoproteins of respiratory syncytial virus with immunity to infection in children. Viral Immunol 1:199–205, 1987.

20. Piedra PA, Glezen WP, Mbawuike I, et al. Studies on reactogenicity and immunogenicity of attenuated bivalent cold recombinant influenza type A (CRA) and inactivated trivalent influenza (TI) vaccines in infants and young children. Vaccine 11:718–724, 1993.

21. Gruber WC, Darden PM, Lohr J, et al. Evaluation of bivalent live attenuated influenza A vaccines in children 2 months to 3 years of age: safety, immunogencity and dose-response. Vaccine 15:1379–1384, 1997.

22. Clements ML, Makhene MK, Karron RA, et al. Effective immunization with live attenuated influenza A virus can be achieved in early infancy. J Infect Dis 173:44–51, 1996.

23. Englund JA, Mbawuike IN, Hammill H, et al. Maternal immunization with influenza or tetanus toxoid vaccine for passive antibody protection in young infants. J Infect Dis 168:647–656, 1993.

24. Munoz FM, Greisinger AJ, Wehmanen OA, et al. Safety of influenza vaccination during pregnancy. Am J Obstet Gynecol 192:1098–1106, 2005.

25. Crowe JE Jr. Respiratory syncytial virus vaccine development. Vaccine 20:S32–S37, 2002.

26. Piedra PA, Glezen WP, Kasel JA, et al. Safety and immunogenicity of the PFP vaccine against respiratory syncytial virus (RSV): the Western blot assay aids in distinguishing immune responses of the PFP vaccine from RSV infection. Vaccine 13:1095–1101, 1995.

27. Groothuis JR, King SJ, Hogerman DA, et al. Safety and immunogenicity of a purified F protein respiratory syncytial virus (PFP-2) vaccine in seropositive children with bronchopulomonary dysplasia. J Infect Dis 177:467–469, 1998.

28. Karron RA, Wright PF, Belshe RB, et al. Identification of a recombinant live attenuated respiratory syncytial virus vaccine candidate that is highly attenuated in infants. J Infect Dis 191:1093–1104, 2005.

29. Kneyber MCJ, Kimpen JLL. Current concepts on active immunization against respiratory syncytial virus for infants and young children. Pediatr Infect Dis J 21:685–696, 2002.

30. Englund JA, Glezen WP, Piedra PA. Maternal immunization against viral disease. Vaccine 16:1456–1463, 1998.

31. Piedra AP, Jewell AM, Cron SG, et al. Correlates of immunity to respiratory syncytial virus (RSV) associated-hospitalization: establishment of minimal protective threshold levels of serum neutralizing antibodies. Vaccine 21:3479–3482, 2003.

32. Munoz FM, Piedra PA, Glezen WP. Safety and immunongenicity of respiratory syncytial virus purified fusion protein-2 vaccine in pregnant women. Vaccine 21:3465–3467, 2003.

33. Crowe JE Jr. Current approaches to the development of vaccines against disease caused by respiratory syncytial virus (RSV) and parainfluenza virus (PIV). Vaccine 13:415–421, 1995.

34. Karron RA, Makhene M, Gay K. Evaluation of a live attenuated bovine parainfluenza type 3 virus vaccine in two-to-six-month old infants. Pediatr Infect Dis J 15:650–654, 1996.

35. Rothstein E, Edwards K. Health burden of pertussis in infants and children. Pediatr Infect Dis J 24:S44–S47, 2005.

36. Centers for Disease control and Prevention. Pertussis: United States, 1997–2000. MMWR 51:73–76, 2002.

37. Bonhoeffer J, Bar G, Riffelmann M, et al. The role of *Bordetella* infections in patients with acute exacerbation of chronic bronchitis. Infection 33:13–17, 2005.

38. Healy CM, Munoz FM, Rench MA, et al. Prevalence of pertussis antibodies in maternal delivery, cord and infant serum. J Infect Dis 190:335–340, 2004.

39. Gonik B, Puder KS, Gonik N. Seroprevalence of *Bordetella pertussis* antibodies in mothers and their newborn infants. Infect Dis Obstet Gynecol 13:59–61, 2005.

40. Committee on Infectious Diseases. American Academy of Pediatrics. Pediatrics 117:965–977, 2006.

41. Englund JA, Anderson EL, Reed GF, et al. Effect of maternal antibody on the serologic response and incidence of adverse reactions after primary immunization with acellular and whole cell pertussis vaccines combined with diphtheria and tetanus toxoids. Pediatrics 96:580–584, 1995.

42. Bjorkholm B, Granstrom M, Taranger J, et al. Influence of high titers of maternal antibody on the serologic response of infants to diphtheria vaccination at 3, 5 and 12 months of age. Pediatr Infect Dis J 14:846–850, 1995.

43. Nohynek H, Gustafsson L, Capeding MRZ, et al. Effect of transplacentally acquired tetanus antibodies on the antibody responses to *Hemphilus influenzae* type b-tetanus toxoid conjugate and tetanus toxoid vaccines in Filipino infants. Pediatr Infect Dis J 18:25–30, 1999.

44. McCormick JB, Gusmao HH, Nakamura S, et al. Antibody response to sergroup A and C meningococcal polysaccharide vaccines in infants born to mothers vaccinated during pregnancy. J Clin Invest 65:1141–1145, 1980.

45. Amstey MS, Insel R, Munoz J, et al. Fetal-neonatal passive immunization against *Haemophilus influenzae* type b. Am J Obstet Gynecol 155:607–611, 1985.

46. Kurikka S, Kayhty H, Peltola H, et al. Neonatal immunization: response to *Haemophilus influenzae* type b-tetanus toxoid conjugate vaccine. Pediatrics 95:815–822, 1995.

47. Kurikka S, Olander R-M, Eskola J, et al. Passively acquired anti-tetanus and anti-*Haemophilus* antibodies and the response to *Haemophilus influenzae* type b-tetanus toxoid conjugate vaccine in infancy. Pediatr Infect Dis J 15:530–535, 1996.

48. Kurikka S. Priming with diphtheria-tetanus-pertussis vaccine enhances the response to the *Haemophilus influenzae* type b tetanus conjugate vaccine in infancy. Vaccine 14:1239–1242, 1996.

49. Englund JA, Glezen WP. Maternal immunization with *Haemophilus influenzae* type b vaccines in different populations. Vaccine 21:3455–3459, 2003.

50. Mulholland K, Suara RO, Siber G, et al. Maternal immunization with *Haemophilus influenzae* type b polysaccharide-tetanus protein conjugate vaccine in The Gambia. JAMA 275:1182–1188, 1996.

51. Englund JA, Glezen WP, Thompson C, et al. *Haemophilus influenzae* type b-specific antibody in infants after maternal immunization. Pediatr Infect Dis J 16:1122–1130, 1997.

52. Munoz FM, Englund JA, Cheesman CC, et al. Maternal immunization with pneumococcal polysaccharide vaccine in the third trimester of gestation. Vaccine 20:826–837, 2002.

53. Santosham M, Englund JA, McInnes P, et al. Safety and antibody persistence following *Haemophilus influenzae* type b conjugate or pneumococcal polysaccharide vaccines given before pregnancy in women of childbearing age and their infants. Pediatr Infect Dis J 20:931–940, 2001.

Chapter 12

Neonatal T-Cell Immunity and its Regulation by Innate Immunity and Dendritic Cells

David B. Lewis, MD

Thanks in large part to Rusian Medzhitov and Charlie Janeway Jr, who first identified Toll-like receptors (TLRs) in mammals (1), and to Ralph Steinman and his colleagues at the Rockefeller Institute, who were pioneers in studies of dendritic cells (DCs) (2), it is now abundantly clear that TLRs expressed by DCs are an important mechanism for the early detection of pathogen-derived molecules. This recognition in the context of other signals suggesting infection and tissue damage results in a DC maturation program that effectively presents antigen to and activates T cells in secondary lymphoid organs, such as draining lymph nodes and the spleen. Because there is substantial evidence that neonatal T-cell function, particularly that mediated by CD4 T cells, is reduced compared to that of the adult in response to infection (3), it is plausible that immaturity in DC function could be an important mechanism limiting such T-cell function in the neonate and fetus. This chapter will provide a brief overview of DCs, the role of TLRs in DC function and T-cell activation, summarize clinical and immunological studies indicating decreased T-cell immune function in the neonate, and discuss evidence that immaturity in TLR function by DCs may limit T-cell function in early post-natal life. Other recently identified non-TLR mechanisms for DC maturation and T-cell activation will also be mentioned, as these may be fruitful avenues for future investigation of neonatal immunity. This review will focus on immunity mediated by "conventional" CD4 and CD8 T cells expressing αβ-T-cell receptors, which account for >90% of T cells in peripheral lymphoid tissue. The developmental immunology of other human T-lineage cell populations, including gamma/delta T cells and NK T cells, has recently been reviewed elsewhere (3).

CONVENTIONAL (MYELOID) DENDRITIC CELLS

Conventional dendritic cells (cDCs), also referred to as myeloid or monocytoid DCs or DC1 cells, have been aptly considered the sentinels of the immune system because of their role in the early detection of infection (2) or danger (4) posed to extra-lymphoid tissues. They are bone marrow-derived cells that express the CD11c/CD18 β2 integrin protein and in their mature form display characteristic cytoplasmic protrusions or "dendrites". cDCs lack most or all cell surface molecules that characterize other bone-marrow derived cell lineages, a feature that is termed Lin⁻, including molecules that are typically expressed on T cells (e.g., CD3), monocytes or neutrophils (e.g., CD14), B cells (e.g., CD19 or CD20), natural killer (NK) cells (e.g., CD56). cDCs express MHC class II, which is involved in peptide antigen presentation to CD4 T cells, and, upon maturation, express greater amounts of MHC class II than any other cell type. cDCs also express relatively high levels of MHC class I, a virtually ubiquitous heterodimer protein that presents peptide antigen to CD8 T cells.

cDCs in the circulation and tissues are heterogeneous based on their surface phenotype and functional attributes. Interstitial cDCs are found in essentially all tissues and are highly effective in uptake of antigen in soluble or particulate form. cDCs in uninflamed tissues are immature in that they express only moderate levels of surface MHC class I and class II molecules. Immature cDCs are also found in the blood in relatively small numbers (0.2–0.4% of adult peripheral blood mononuclear cells (PBMCs) compared to monocytes (∼10% of PBMCs)) and are probably in transit to the uninflamed tissues from bone marrow sites of production. cDCs of the skin include Langerhans cells, which express CD1a and Birbeck granules but lack expression of the factor XIIIa coagulation factor, and interstitial cDCs of the dermis, which conversely lack Birbeck granules and are factor XIIIa-positive; both cell types express immunoglobulin-like transcript receptor-1 (ILT1) (5).

cDCs and mononuclear phagocytes (Mφ), which include circulating monocytes and tissue macrophages, appear to differentiate from a common bone marrow precursor cell termed the common Mφ and DC progenitor (MDP) (6). A more differentiated intrasplenic cDC precursor has also recently been identified in mice (7). Under certain conditions in vitro or in vivo, e.g., transendothelial differentiation, mature murine monocytes may give rise to cDCs, including Langerhans cells (8, 9). The extent to which this applies to humans in vivo remains unclear, but the

$CD16^+CD14^{mid}$ subset of human monocytes, which comprises about 20% of circulating monocytes in adults, more readily differentiates into cDCs in vitro than does the predominant $CD16^-CD14^{high}$ monocyte subset (10).

PLASMACYTOID DENDRITIC CELLS

Plasmacytoid dendritic cells (pDCs), also known as DC2 cells, and their immediate precursors constitute a cell lineage that appears to be distinct from cDCs, although the precursor product relationship between myeloid or lymphoid progenitor cells and pDCs remains controversial (11). Human pDC-lineage cells have a characteristic surface phenotype of high expression of the IL-3 receptor (CD123), low but detectable expression of CD4, low or absent CD11c, and a lack of ILT1 (12). Murine pDCs differ from human pDCs in that they express only low levels of CD123, have detectable expression of CD11, and, in contrast to cDCs, express B220 (an epitope of CD45 that predominates on murine B cells) and Ly6C, a protein that is recognized by a monoclonal antibody that cross-reacts with Ly6G of murine neutrophils (11). pDCs are found in the blood and secondary lymphoid organs, and the frequency of these cell in lymph nodes is markedly increased with inflammation (12). The difference in their pattern of localization from that of most immature cDCs is attributable to differences in the pattern of expression of adhesion molecules, such as L-selectin (CD62-L), which promotes entry into peripheral lymphoid tissue via high endothelial venules (11). In contrast to immature cDCs, immature pDCs have a limited capacity for antigen uptake and presentation but with maturation signals they acquire a substantial ability to present antigen and activate both CD4 and CD8 T cells (12). When appropriately stimulated, pDCs and their more mature derivatives also differ from cDCs in their markedly greater capacity to produce type I interferon (IFN). Type I IFN includes multiple types of IFN-α encoded by separate genes and a single IFN-β.

DENDRITIC CELLS MEDIATING NATURAL CYTOTOXICITY

A murine cell population with features of cDCs (CD11c expression and IL-12 production), pDCs (expression of B220 and type I IFN production) and NK cells (certain surface markers, natural cytotoxicity by a TRAIL-dependent mechanism against tumors, and IFN-γ production) have recently been described (13, 14). In contrast to NK cells, these IFN-producing killer dendritic cells (IKDCs) mature into DC-like cells that have increased expression of MHC class II and migrate to lymph nodes to present antigen to T cells (14). An analogous human cell population of IKDCs remains to be defined.

ACTIVATION OF DENDRITIC CELLS

cDC maturation and migration can be triggered by a variety of stimuli, including pathogen-derived products that are recognized through TLRs (discussed in detail in the next section), cytokines, such as interleukin (IL)-1, tumor necrosis factor (TNF)-α, and granulocyte macrophage-colony stimulating factor (GM-CSF), and by engagement of CD40 on the cDC surface by CD154 (CD40-ligand). Major sources of CD154 for this activation include activated CD4 T cells (15) and, at least in mice, by a subset of pDCs (ref. 16, and see below). Thus, the function and localization of cDCs can be rapidly modulated by direct recognition of microbes or their products, by cytokines produced by neighboring cDCs, pDCs (16), or other cells of the innate system (17), or by products of T cells to which they present antigens, e.g., CD154 (15). Exposure of immature cDCs to inflammatory stimuli prevents further antigen uptake and, instead, leads to the increased surface expression of MHC class II and class I molecules displaying antigenic peptides derived from previously internalized particles (18). Concurrently, cDC maturation results in their migration from non-lymphoid tissues to the T-cell dependent areas of secondary lymphoid organs, such as the lymph nodes and spleen. This migration is orchestrated, in part, by an increase in the cDC surface expression of the CCR7 chemokine receptor and decrease in expression of most other chemokine receptors. This favors migration of cDCs via lymphatics to T-cell rich areas of secondary lymphoid organs that express the CCR7 ligands, CCL19 (ELC) and CCL21 (SLC). Once cDCs home to these T-cell rich areas they can present foreign peptide/MHC complexes to antigenically naive T cells bearing cognate αβ-TCR for these peptides.

A recent study of herpes simplex virus (HSV) antigen presentation to CD8 T cells after skin infection suggests that cDCs that migrate to the lymph nodes may not directly present to T cells. Instead, these migratory DCs may rapidly transfer their antigen to cDCs that reside in the lymph nodes and that carry out such antigen presentation (19). The transfer of antigen from cDCs of the airways to cDCs resident in the mediastinal draining lymph nodes for CD8 T-cell antigen presentation also appears to occur following influenza A infection of the respiratory epithelium (20). Whether this sequential involvement of two cDC populations in antigen presentation to T cells applies to most antigens encountered for most infections remains to be determined. In cases of skin immunization of mice, both Langerhans cell and dermal cDCs are induced to migrate to draining lymph nodes. However, dermal DCs arrive in the lymph nodes first, at approximately 2 days post-immunization. In contrast, Langerhans cells, which probably must detach from adjacent keratinocytes, arrive in the lymph nodes at approximately 4 days post-immunization (21).

Like immature cDCs, activation of pDCs via TLR ligands, cytokines, or CD40-ligand results in their maturation, including acquisition of the cytoplasmic protrusions characteristic of immature or mature cDCs and an increased capacity to present antigen to naive T cells. A recent study suggests that human pDC after exposure to viruses or TLR ligands may also acquire cell-mediated cytotoxicity by TRAIL (22), a TNF-ligand family member expressed on the cytotoxic effector cell surface. The importance pDC-mediated cytotoxicity in vivo remains unknown.

TOLL-LIKE RECEPTORS AND DENDRITIC CELL ACTIVATION AND MATURATION

The TLR family of transmembrane proteins recognizes microbial structures, particularly those that are highly evolutionarily conserved and typically essential for the microbe's function. These microbial structures are relatively invariant and are not present in normal mammalian cells. For this reason, recognition of these "pathogen-associated molecular patterns" by TLRs provides infallible evidence for microbial invasion alerting the innate immune system to respond appropriately (1). Twelve different TLRs have been identified in humans, with distinct recognition specificities (23) and patterns of expression, and with both shared and unique downstream response pathways. For example, TLR-2 recognizes peptidoglycan, which is expressed at particularly high levels by Gram-positive bacteria; TLR-3 recognizes viral double-stranded RNA, a component of the life cycle of many viruses, and a synthetic mimic of double-stranded RNA, poly I:C; TLR-4 recognizes lipopolysaccharide (LPS) from Gram-negative bacteria and a protein encoded by respiratory syncytial virus (RSV); TLR-5 recognizes bacterial flagellin; human TLR-7 and TLR-8 can be activated by synthetic imidazoquinoline compounds with anti-viral activity (24), and TLR-8 can recognize single-stranded RNA (25), a characteristic of RNA viruses, such as influenza; TLR-9 recognizes DNA from bacteria, which contain unmethylated CpG dinucleotide residues (CpG DNA) and from DNA viruses, such as herpes simplex virus (HSV), in which these CpG residues are also unmethylated. Since TLR-9 does not recognize DNA containing methylated CpG residues, which predominate in human DNA, this receptor serves as a means to distinguish host from pathogen-related DNA. TLRs can also form heterodimers with distinct recognition properties, e.g., the TLR-1/TLR-2 and TLR-2/TLR-6 heterodimers recognize bacterial-derived triacyl and diacyl lipopeptides, respectively (26).

The efficient presentation by cDCs of peptide antigens to T cells requires that the foreign proteins that are internalized by cDCs be contained in phagosomes that also have TLR ligands (27). Signals from interaction of these TLR ligands with TLRs induce maturation and migration of DCs. Certain TLRs interact with their ligand on the cell surface, e.g., TLR-2 and TLR-4, while others, such as TLR-3, TLR-7, TLR-8, and TLR-9, interact with their ligands in endosomal compartments. The distribution of TLRs on cDCs and pDCs also differs markedly. Human cDCs express most TLRs that recognize bacterial, fungal and protozoan cell surface structures but do not express TLR-7, TLR-8, and TLR-9. Consequently, cDCs are not directly activated in response to either single-stranded RNA or unmethylated CpG DNA, but both are potent inducers of IFN-α production by pDCs, which express TLRs 7–9. However, cDCs express TLR-3 and therefore can produce type I IFN in response to dsRNA. They can also use RNA helicases for type I IFN induction, as discussed below. Most cytokine production by cDCs in response to TLR engagement requires the adaptor molecule MyD88 and the IRF-5 transcription factor (28). The production of type I IFN by pDCs by engagement of TLRs 7–9 is dependent on MyD88 and the IRF-7 transcription factor (29–31).

In mice, cDCs can upregulate their surface expression of MHC class II and T-cell co-stimulatory molecules, such as CD80 and CD86, by exposure to inflammatory mediators. However, these cDCs are not able to produce IL-12 and effectively drive naive CD4 T-cell differentiation towards Th1 cells unless they also receive a second signal by concurrent engagement of their TLRs (32). This "two-signal" requirement, which is reminiscent of T-cell activation needing both peptide/MHC and a separate co-stimulatory signal, may be important in preventing inappropriate T-cell activation by cDCs.

A recent study of murine infection with the Gram-positive intracellular bacterium *Listeria monocytogenes* suggests that the following sequence of interactions between pDCs and cDCs may be critical for protective immunity in response to unmethylated CpG DNA, a TLR-9 ligand: cDCs produce IL-15, which increases CD40 expression on cDCs; CD154 expressed by pDCs engages CD40 on cDCs, which markedly increases cDC IL-12 production (16). Whether this precise sequence of events also applies to viral infections that activate pDCs remains unclear. Recent studies of the murine HSV skin infection model have found that pDCs and cDCs both migrate to inflamed lymph nodes and are both required for the effective generation of HSV-specific CD8 T cells with cytotoxic activity (33). It will be of interest to determine whether pDC expression of CD154 and IL-15 produced by CD40 engagement of cDCs is also critical for viral antigen-specific CD8 T-cell immunity in this context.

TLRs expressed by T cells also play a role in the regulation of adaptive immunity. Human memory CD4 T cells express TLR-2 but not TLR-4 on the cell surface, and bacterial lipoprotein, a TLR-2 ligand, can directly enhance these cells' proliferation and production of T helper 1 (Th1) cytokines, e.g., IFN-γ (34). Memory CD4 T cells, particularly those that lack CCR7 and that are enriched in Th1 effector function, also can directly respond to ligands for TLR-2, TLR-5 (flagellin) and TLR-7/8 but not TLR-4 with increased proliferation and cytokine secretion (35, 36).

Naive CD4 T cells from cord blood lack surface expression of TLR-2 or TLR-4 but both receptors are expressed on the cell surface after activation by IFN-α and CD3 monoclonal antibody (34), which mimics engagement of the αβ-TCR/CD3 complex by peptide/MHC antigen. This activation stimulus allows cord blood naive CD4 T cells to become responsive to TLR-2 but not TLR-4 ligands as co-stimulators of increased T-cell proliferation and cytokine secretion (IFN-γ, IL-2, and TNF-α) (34). Thus, the TLR-2 pathway is functional in activated cord blood CD4 T cells, and it will be of interest to directly compare the function of this pathway in adult naive CD4 T cells.

TLR ligands also can influence the activity of a population of regulatory T cells (Tregs) that express high surface levels of CD25, a component of the high-affinity IL-2 receptor, and FoxP3, a transcription factor required for regulatory CD4 T-cell development and, possibly, regulatory function. Engagement of TLRs, such as TLR-5, enhances both FoxP3 expression and the ability of these cells to suppress the immune responses of effector T cells (36). Murine Tregs also express TLR-2 and in response to TLR-2 engagement proliferate and concurrently lose Treg activity in vitro and in vivo (37, 38). The loss of Treg activity is transient so that the expanded Treg population may then act to limit the effector T-cell response (37). Thus microbial-derived ligands may play a role in both the positive and negative regulation of adaptive immune responses.

TLR-INDEPENDENT INNATE IMMUNE MECHANISMS FOR DENDRITIC CELL ACTIVATION

Recently, several other families of receptors for microbial ligands have been identified, including the NOD (nucleotide-binding oligomerization domain) proteins, NALP (nacht domain-, leucine-rich repeat-, and pyrin domain-containing) proteins and two RNA helicases (39, 40). These receptors are cytoplasmic and, in contrast to TLRs, are not transmembrane proteins associated with lipid bilayers. With the exception of most NALPs, these cytoplasmic receptors contain CARD (N-terminal caspase recruitment domain) segments that activate the NF-κB pathway and NF-κB-dependent genes, such as those encoding pro-inflammatory cytokines (39).

NOD1 and NOD2 recognize γ-D-glutamyl-meso-diaminopimelic acid and muramyldipeptide (MDP), which are components of bacterial peptidoglycan (41, 42). NOD1 or NOD2 agonists strongly synergize with engagement of TLRs, such as TLR-4, in increasing the production of IL-12 by human MDDCs (43).

NALPS 1–3 are associated with other proteins making up an "inflammasome complex" that is involved in processing and activating precursor forms of IL-1β and IL-18 so that these are biologically active. These inflammasome complexes, particularly those containing NALP3, may be triggered not only by pathogen-derived products, such as bacterial RNA (44), but also by "danger" signals that are indicative of cell injury, such as uric acid crystals and low intracellular potassium concentrations that are triggered by extracellular ATP binding to purinergic receptors that mediate potassium efflux (39, 45).

The two RNA helicases, RIG-1 (retinoic acid-inducible gene-1) and MDA-5 (melanoma differentiation associated Gene 5), are able to trigger the production of type I IFN (40). RIG-1 appears to recognize nucleic acid from paramyxoviruses, influenza virus, and Japanese encephalitis virus, while MDA-5 detects RNA from picornaviruses (46). RIG-1 utilizes a downstream signaling adaptor molecule, variously called Cardif, MAVS, IPS-1, or VISA (39). RIG-1 and this downstream adaptor is important in inducing type I IFN production by cDCs and other cell types but not pDCs (47, 48). These RNA helicases are able to detect viral RNA found in the cytoplasm, while, in contrast, the recognition of viral nucleic acids by TLR-3, and TLRs 7–9 can only occur in the lumen of endosomes.

T-CELL ACTIVATION BY DENDRITIC CELLS

cDCs are poised to respond rapidly to microbial invasion by their secretion of cytokines and presentation of microbial antigens to T cells; this presentation leads to T-cell activation and functional differentiation. In steady-state conditions that prevail in uninfected individuals, cDCs play a central role in maintaining a state of tolerance to self antigens by presenting them to T cells in the absence of accessory signals required for T-cell activation. Upon maturation, mature cDCs express high levels of peptide-MHC complexes and molecules that act as co-stimulatory signals for T-cell activation, such as CD80 (B7–1) and CD86 (B7–2), and consequently are highly efficient for presenting antigen in a manner that effectively activates naive CD4 and CD8 T cells for clonal expansion. In the case of naive CD4 T-cell activation and differentiation into effector cells in vivo, TLR-induced cytokine production as well as TLR ligand maturation of cDCs is required. TLR signals act on cDCs to promote effector CD4 T-cell differentiation by enhancing effective antigen presentation and activation of naive CD4 but also by limiting the inhibitory effects of Tregs (49).

CD4 T cells recognize MHC class II-bound peptides, which are mainly derived from extracellular proteins or pathogens that have entered into intracellular lipid bilayer bound compartments in the APC, such as endosomes, by phagocytosis, pinocytosis, or internalization of the cell or nuclear membrane. cDCs also influence the quality of the T-cell response by producing cytokines that direct the differentiation of naive CD4 T cells into Th1 (capable of producing IFN-γ but not IL-4, IL-5, or IL-13), Th2 (capable of producing IL-4, IL-5, or IL-13 but not IFN-γ) and Th17 (capable of producing IL-17) (50, 51). The production by cDCs of IL-12p70, a heterodimeric cytokine consisting of a p35 and p40 chain, or of type I IFN by pDCs, skews differentiation towards the Th1 pathway, while the production of IL-23, which consists of a unique p19 chain and the IL-12 p40 chain, promotes Th17 differentiation, particularly when IFN-γ is absent (51).

Differential cytokine production by particular effector CD4 T cell populations is particularly important in orchestrating the overall immune response by providing stimulatory signals to other cells of the immune system. Th1 immunity is particularly important for the control of intracellular infections that occur in APCs, such as mononuclear phagocytes, including certain intracellular bacteria (e.g., *Mycobacteria*, *Salmonella*, *Listeria* (52), viruses (e.g., herpesviruses), fungi (e.g., *Candida*, *Pneumocystis*), and protozoa (e.g., *Toxoplasma*, *Plasmodium*). Th2 immunity is particularly important for promoting immune responses to pathogens such as extracellular pathogens that include antigen-specific IgE and cellular immunity by eosinophils, basophils, and mast cells. Th2 responses are also important in classic allergic disease. The role of Th17 responses in host defense largely remains to be defined, but appears to be important in controlling infection in which neutrophil activation is essential, such as infection with *Klebsiella* (53) and other bacteria that have an extracellular life style.

cDCs are also essential for activating CD8 T cells and have the unique ability among APCs to internally transfer proteins taken up from the external environment from an MHC class II antigen presentation pathway to the MHC class I pathway, a process called cross-presentation. How cross-presentation occurs in cDCs remains poorly understood, but recent genetic study indicates that a protein called UNC-93B, which is mainly found in the endoplasmic reticulum, is required for this process (54). Interestingly, UNC-93B is also required for intact signaling by TLRs 3, 7, and 9. A recent and unexpected finding is that cross-presentation may also be facilitated by the NADPH oxidase complex, which is critical for the oxidative mechanism killing of bacteria and fungi internalized intro neutrophils (55). Naive CD8 T cells that are effectively activated by cDCs expressing peptide/MHC class I complexes differentiate into effector cells expressing cytotoxins that are important for killing virally infected cells. CD8 T cells are also rich sources of cytokines, such as IFN-γ and TNF-α that have anti-viral activity and also may help overcome certain viral-mediated immunosubversive effects, such as the inhibition of antigen presentation.

The role of other innate immune receptors, such as the NOD, NALP, and RNA helicase families, in influencing the development of antigen-specific T-cell immunity remains unclear.

CLINICAL EVIDENCE FOR DEFICIENCIES OF T-CELL-MEDIATED IMMUNITY IN THE NEONATE AND YOUNG INFANT

Term newborns are highly vulnerable to severe infection with herpes simplex virus (HSV)-1 and -2, and neonatal infection frequently results in death or severe neurological damage, despite administration of high doses of anti-viral agents, such as acyclovir, to which HSV is susceptible (56, 57). Death from disseminated primary HSV infection is distinctly unusual after the neonatal period, except in cases of genetic T-cell immunodeficiency or in recipients of T-cell ablative chemotherapy or immunosuppression. Neonates with primary HSV infection have delayed and diminished appearance of HSV-specific Th1 responses, i.e., CD4 T-cell proliferation, secretion of IFN-γ and TNF-α, production of HSV-specific T-cell dependent antibody, compared to adults with primary infection (58, 59). These decreased responses ex vivo suggest that poor adaptive immune responses in vivo may allow HSV to disseminate and cause profound organ destruction for days to weeks after infection. Whether the post-infection appearance of HSV-specific CD8 T-cell immunity is also delayed in the neonate is unknown. It is also unclear by what age after birth the capacity to generate an HSV-specific CD4 T-cell immune response to primary infection becomes similar to that of adults.

The delayed Th1 immunity observed with neonatal HSV infection may also apply to other herpes viruses acquired during infancy. For example, we recently compared cytomegalovirus (CMV)-specific CD4 and CD8 T-cell immune responses in infants and young children versus adults following primary CMV infection, and found that infants and young children had persistently reduced Th1 immune responses (60). In contrast, CD8 T-cell responses were similar, including the expression of cytotoxin molecules (60, 61). Decreased CMV-specific CD4 T-cell responses were associated with persistent viral shedding in the urine (60), suggesting that CD4 T-cell immunity may be particularly important for the local control of viral replication in mucosae. It is likely that this selective decrease in CD4 T-cell immunity to CMV also applies to infection acquired perinatally and in the neonatal period, which is also characterized by persistent viral shedding. Interestingly, congenital CMV infection can result in a robust CMV-specific CD8 T-cell response in the fetus, suggesting that there may be major differences in the capacity for the generation of CD4 versus CD8 T-cell responses to CMV very early in ontogeny (62).

The otherwise healthy term newborn is also susceptible to severe infection from enteroviruses (63, 64), which have a relatively small RNA genome, indicating that limitations in anti-viral immunity are not unique to herpes viruses, which have a large DNA genome. The most severe form of infection, i.e., hepatic necrosis with disseminated intravascular coagulation and liver failure, is highly unusual outside the neonatal period except in cases of severe T-cell immunodeficiency, such as early after hematopoietic cell transplantation prior to T-cell reconstitution or in patients with severe combined immunodeficiency. This complication is particularly common in neonates with overt infection during the first week after birth (63), in contrast to HSV, which can present with severe disseminated infection up to several weeks of age (56, 57). It is not known whether the vulnerability of the neonate to severe enteroviral infection is paralleled by delayed or diminished T-cell responses compared to older children upon their first infection with this class of viruses.

The severity or persistence of non-viral infections for which T cells also play a critical role in control also suggests a general limitation in T-cell mediated immunity to pathogens in early human development. Examples include congenital infections, such as toxoplasmosis (65), which frequently disseminates to the retina, even when acquired during the last trimester of gestation. Mucocutaneous candidiasis, particularly thrush, is common during the first year of life (66). The high prevalence of thrush in early infancy may reflect, at least in part, decreased fungal-specific CD4 T-cell immunity, as thrush is also characteristic of adults with acquired defects in CD4 T-cell immunity, such as HIV-1 infection (67), as well as defects in innate immunity (68).

In the case of *M. tuberculosis* infection the tendency for the neonate and young infant to develop miliary disease and tuberculous meningitis is paralleled by decreased cell-mediated immunity compared to older children and young adults, as assessed by delayed-type sensitivity skin tests (69). The young infant is able to mount substantial levels of IFN-γ production by CD4 T cells following neonatal vaccination with bacillus Calmette-Guerin (BCG), a live attenuated strain of *Mycobacterium bovis* (70, 71). However, this does not rule out a reduced or delayed T-cell response to virulent *M. tuberculosis* or *bovis* in infants compared to adults.

MAJOR PHENOTYPES AND LEVELS OF CIRCULATING NEONATAL DENDRITIC CELLS

While most DCs are found in the tissues, small numbers, consisting of immature cDCs and pDCs and representing ~0.5% of circulating blood mononuclear cells, are found in the circulation. Several studies found that DCs with an immature pDC surface phenotype (Lin$^-$HLA-DR^{mid}CD11c$^-$CD33$^-$CD123^{hi}) predominated in cord blood and early infancy, constituting about 75% of the total Lin$^-$HLA-DR$^+$ DC (72) and ~0.75% of total blood mononuclear cells (73, 74). The remaining 25% of cells had a HLA-DR^{high}CD11c$^+$CD33$^+$CD123^{low} surface phenotype consistent with conventional cDCs found in adults, except that CD83 expression was absent (72).The "cocktail" of Lin (lineage) monoclonal antibodies (mAbs) used to enrich for DCs by negative selection included those for CD3 (T-cells), CD14 (monocytes), CD16 (NK cells), CD19 (B cells), CD34 (hematopoietic precursor cells), CD56 (NK cells), CD66b (granulocytes), and glycophorin A (erythroid cells).

More recent work has shown that circulating cDCs can be divided into four non-overlapping subsets that express either CD16, CD34, CD1c (BDCA-1), which is a non-classical antigen presentation molecule, or BDCA-3, a cDC marker with unknown function (75, 76). Moreover, a portion of the CD16 and CD1c cDC subsets may also express low levels of CD14 (76, 77). Thus, the inclusion of mAbs for CD16, CD34, and, perhaps, CD14, in lineage cocktails used for depletion will substantially reduce the final yield of cDCs. Another technical issue is that both cDCs and pDCs may also be lost by their forming complexes with T cells during the purification of mononuclear cells by density gradient centrifugation, e.g., with Ficoll-Hypaque (78).

More accurate determination of the circulating levels of DCs can be achieved by staining whole blood with mAbs, followed by red cell lysis, and flow cytometry. Using this whole blood approach and including CD16 as a marker for a subset of cDCs indicates that adult peripheral blood and cord blood have similar concentrations of Lin⁻CD11c⁺CD16⁻HLA-DR^{high} cDCs (~70–76 cells/μL) and Lin⁻CD11c⁺CD16⁺ DCs (~58–60 cells/μL). In contrast, the concentration of Lin⁻CD123^{high} pDCs in cord blood was significantly higher than in adult peripheral blood (~17.5 and 10.5 cells/μL, respectively)[78]. Other workers using the whole blood method and a Lin cocktail that removes both CD16⁺ and CD34⁺ cDCs have found that the levels of cord blood cDCs and pDCs are higher than those in adult peripheral blood [79]. After the neonatal period, the numbers of pDC lineage cells declines with increasing post-natal age, whereas the numbers of cDCs do not [80]. The biological significance of the predominance of pDCs in the neonatal circulation is uncertain but may reflect their relatively high rate of colonization of lymphoid tissue, which is undergoing rapid expansion at this age.

One study using the whole blood analytic technique found that cord blood may have an increased proportion of immature DCs with a distinct Lin⁻HLA-DR⁺CD11c⁻CD34⁻CD123^{mid} phenotype. These less differentiated (ld) DCs [81] may represent a precursor of more mature pDCs as they have been reported to stain with monoclonal antibody against BDCA-4, which is a marker of the pDC lineage [76]. In cord blood the concentration of ldDCs and CD123^{high} pDCs are similar. The concentration of ldDCs declines with age so that they are essentially absent by early adulthood. Confirmation of these results using additional markers that distinguish pDCs and cDCs and compares their function would be of interest.

CIRCULATING NEONATAL CONVENTIONAL DENDRITIC CELLS: TLR-DEPENDENT CHANGES IN SURFACE PHENOTYPE AND CYTOKINE PRODUCTION

Basal expression of MHC class II (HLA-DR) on cord blood and adult peripheral blood cDCs is similar (73, 82), although the level of the CD86 co-stimulatory molecule on both CD16- and CD16+ cDCs was lower in cord blood [83]. Stimulation with LPS (a TLR-4 ligand) and poly I:C (a TLR-3 ligand) increased the expression of HLA-DR and CD86 on cDCs to a similar extent by neonatal compared to adults cDCs. However, compared to adult peripheral blood cDCs, cDCs from cord blood had decreased upregulation of CD40 after incubation with ligands for TLR-2/6 (*Mycoplasma fermetans*), TLR-3 (poly I:C), TLR-4 (LPS), or TLR-7 (imiquimod) [82] and decreased upregulation of CD80 by TLR-3 and TLR-4 ligands (73, 82)

Neonatal blood cells produce less IFN-α than adult blood cells in response to poly I:C [82], and this most likely reflects decreased production by neonatal cDCs, which express TLR-3, rather than pDCs, which do not. The LPS-induced expression of TNF-α by cord blood cDCs was also reduced compared to adult cDCs both for the percentage of cells that expressed this cytokine as well as for the amount of cytokine produced among the cytokine-positive cells [84]; in contrast, the LPS-induced expression of IL-1α by cord blood and adult cDCs was similar. After stimulation with the combination of LPS and IFN-γ, cord blood CD16+ cDCs expressed less IL-1β and IL-6 compared to this cDC subset in adult peripheral blood [83]. TLR-4 surface expression was similar on cord blood and adult cDCs [84], consistent with the selective nature of diminished responses to LPS by cord blood DCs [84].

The production of bioactive IL-12p70 by cord blood mononuclear cells also appears to be reduced in response to LPS alone or in combination with IFN-γ or pertussis toxin, which also activates cDCs via TLR-4 [85], compared to older children or adults (86, 87). The cellular source of IL-12p70 in these in vitro cultures is probably cDC (86, 87). However, decreased IL-12 production by cord blood cDCs may not apply to all stimuli. For example, neonatal and adult blood mononuclear cells stimulated with *Staphylococcus aureus*, other Gram-positive and Gram-negative bacterial cells or meningococcal outer membrane proteins have been reported to produce equivalent amounts of IL-12 (88–91).

Interestingly, TLR-8 ligands, such as GU-rich single-stranded RNA, are particularly potent activators of both cord blood and adult cDCs, and these cell types also have similar levels of intracellular TLR-8 expression (92). This raises the possibility that TLR-8 ligands might be particularly effective at increasing cDC function in neonates compared to other TLR ligands, although it remains to be shown that TLR-8 engagement is also effective at inducing neonatal cDCs to produce pro-inflammatory cytokines and to allostimulate T cells for Th1 differentiation.

CIRCULATING NEONATAL PLASMACYTOID DENDRITIC CELLS: TLR-DEPENDENT CHANGES IN SURFACE PHENOTYPE AND CYTOKINE PRODUCTION

Like pDCs from the tonsils of older children (93, 94), cord blood pDCs are ineffective at uptake of either protein or peptide antigens (95). It is unclear whether maturation of pDCs in the neonate, e.g., by exposure to viruses, results in a similar increase in capacity for antigen presentation that is observed with adult pDCs. Stimulation with unmethylated CpG DNA (a TLR-9 ligand) increased the expression of HLA-DR on cord blood and adult pDCs to a similar extent (96), and, in combination with IL-3-containing medium, induced higher levels of CD80 and CD86 on cord blood pDCs than adult pDCs (97). The levels of CD80 and CD86 on cord blood pDCs after incubation with IL-3-containing medium alone for 20 h were also markedly lower than on adult pDCs (97), suggesting these differences are likely to apply to circulating pDCs in vivo.

Type I IFN production and the frequency of IFN-α-producing cells in response to HSV was diminished in cord blood mononuclear cells, particularly from prematurely born infants, compared to adult peripheral blood mononuclear cells (98). Similar results were obtained with whole blood preparations stimulated with unmethylated CpG DNA (73). It is likely that the decreased production of type I IFN by neonatal PBMCs or whole blood cells in response to viruses or unmethylated CpG DNA reflects decreased production by pDC lineage cells signaling through TLR-9 (73). Consistent with this idea, partially purified cord blood pDCs have been reported to have decreased production of IFN-α compared to adult pDCs after stimulation with unmethylated CpG DNA in IL-3-containing medium (97). However, this group did not confirm that these differences applied to the stimulation of whole blood preparations. This decreased production of IFN-α is not attributable to diminished TLR-9 expression by cord blood pDCs (97), suggesting that events downstream of engagement of intracellular TLR-9 may be involved. The extent to which the decreased cord blood pDC responses are due to the presence in cord blood of pDCs with CD123^{dim} staining (the ldDCs described above) (81) is unclear, but its is plausible that these phenotypically immature pDCs might also have reduced function compared to CD123^{high} pDCs.

ALLOSTIMULATION OF T CELLS BY CIRCULATING NEONATAL DENDRITIC CELLS

The first study to directly test the ability of cord blood DCs to activate T cells was done prior to the availability of markers that allow them to be isolated relatively rapidly and in high purity. In these studies cells cultured overnight in vitro were substantially less effective than adult cells in activating allogeneic T-cell proliferation (99, 100). This decreased activity was associated with reduced levels of expression of HLA-DR and the adhesion molecule ICAM-1 (99). In more recent studies cited above (73, 82), in which expression of HLA-DR was evaluated on uncultured DCs, HLA-DR expression on neonatal and adult cDCs and pDCs did not differ significantly. The lower level of HLA-DR expression by neonatal DC in the studies by Hunt and colleagues (99) probably reflects the overnight culture or the predominance of pDCs among DCs isolated from neonatal blood obtained using certain enrichment strategies. These pDCs express lower levels of HLA-DR than cDCs (72), and pDC lineage cells are highly prone to die during culture in vitro. Therefore, the use of an overnight protocol for cell isolation may adversely affect cord blood DCs, in which pDCs are predominant.

Several studies found that circulating DCs from cord blood can allogeneically stimulate cord blood T cells in vitro (72, 95, 101). However, their efficiency was not compared to adult DCs. Virtually all of the allostimulatory activity of partially purified cord blood DCs is mediated by the cDC subset rather than the pre-pDC subset (72). It should also be noted that activation of allogeneic T cells does not require uptake, processing and presentation of exogenous antigens, and, thus, is not as stringent a test of APC function as activation of foreign antigen-specific T cells.

As discussed above, DCs have a major influence on whether naive CD4 T cells differentiate into producers of Th1 cytokines, Th2 cytokines, or Th17 cytokines (i.e., IL-17) or into less committed cells that lack the capacity to produce any of these cytokines (51, 102). For example, antigen presentation by pDCs favors the differentiation of naive T cells into Th2 cells, unless these cells have been activated by viruses or unmethylated CpG DNA, which causes them to release IFN-α or IL-12 and, in turn, drive potent Th1 polarization (103). Thus, it is plausible that limitations in the production of IL-12 by neonatal cDCs and type I IFN by pDCs (via engagement of TLR-7 and TLR-9) and cDCs (via engagement of TLR-3) in the fetus and neonate may account for their tendency to have Th2 skewing of immune responses to environmental allergens, their limited responses to intracellular pathogens, the maintenance of fetal-maternal tolerance during pregnancy, and the lower risk of graft-versus-host disease following cord blood transplantation.

NEONATAL MONOCYTE-DERIVED DENDRITIC CELLS

Cells phenotypically similar to cDCs can be generated in vitro from a variety of precursor cell, including blood monocytes, immature pDCs, CD34$^+$ cells (104–106), and even granulocytes, depending on the cytokines and culture conditions employed. The generation of monocyte-derived dendritic cells (MDDCs) by culture of freshly isolated blood monocytes with GM-CSF and IL-4 has been a particularly useful experimental system for evaluating human DCs because a relatively large number of cells can be generated in vitro in a short period. These MDDCs have features of immature cDCs, and with further stimulation, e.g., incubation with LPS or TNF-α, acquire phenotypic and functional features characteristic of mature cDCs, e.g., increased expression of HLA-DR and co-stimulatory molecules. The expression of various DC markers, e.g., CD1a, as well as the functional capacity of MDDCs in vitro to produce cytokines, e.g., IL-12 p40, and to allostimulate T cells, is substantially influenced by the serum concentration of the growth media (107).

Both adult peripheral and cord blood MDDCs generated by GM-CSF and IL-4 incubation give rise to immature DCs similar to the cDC lineage. However, immature MDDCs from cord blood express less HLA-DR, co-stimulatory molecules (CD40 and CD80), and CD1a than do adult MDDCs (108, 109); the expression of CD11c, CD86, CCR5, and mannose receptor by cord blood MDDCs appears to be similar or only moderately lower than by adult MDDCs (108, 110). The internalization of FITC-dextran by cord blood MDDCs is substantially lower compared to adult peripheral blood MDDCs (109). LPS stimulation is also significantly less effective at increasing HLA-DR and CD86 expression by cord blood-derived MDDCs than those generated from adult peripheral blood (110).

Consistent with these reductions in HLA-DR and co-stimulatory molecules, MDDCs from cord blood matured by LPS stimulation have decreased allostimulatory activity for the production of IFN-γ by T cells compared to adult MDDCs (108, 110). The ability of neonatal MDDCs to allogeneically induce T-cell proliferation has been reported as reduced in one study (109) but not in two others (86, 108). The reduced IFN-γ production (110) during allostimulation of T cells is likely to be due to a markedly reduced capacity of immature neonatal MDDCs to produce IL-12p70. IL-12p70 production by isolated cord blood MDDCs was reduced compared to adult MDDCs after LPS stimulation (a TLR-4 ligand) in some studies (108, 110) but not all (86); the reasons for these discrepant results are not clear. Decreased IL-12p70 production by cord blood MDDCs was also observed after engagement of CD40 (which is the likely physiological stimulus for IL-12 production during allostimulation) or treatment with double-stranded RNA (poly (I:C)) (a TLR-3 ligand) (108, 110). The decreased IL-12 production by cord blood MDDCs is accounted for by a selective decrease in mRNA expression of the IL-12 (p35) chain component (108), a decrease that can be overcome by incubating these cells with the combination of LPS and IFN-γ. Decreased IL-12 p35 expression appears to be due to a chromatin configuration of the IL-12 p35 genetic locus in neonatal MDDCs that limits access to transcriptional activator proteins (111). In contrast to the results for IL-12p70, adult and cord blood MDDCs produce similar levels of TNF-α, IL-6, IL-8, and IL-10 after stimulation (108, 109, 112).

Cord blood MDDCs produce significantly higher levels of IL-23 than adult MDDCs after stimulation with either LPS or the TLR-8 ligand R-848 (resiquimod) (113). These two cell populations also produce similar amounts of IL-23 after incubation with PAM3CSK4 (S-[2,3-bis (palmitoyloxy)-(2-RS)-propyl]-N-palmitoyl-(R)-Cys-(S)-Ser-Lys4-OH trihydrochloride), a TLR-2 ligand, and poly (I:C) (113), indicating that signaling via TLR-2 and TLR-3 for IL-23 production is intact in cord blood MDDCs. Moreover, culture supernatants from LPS-stimulated cord blood or adult MDDCs are effective at inducing IL-17 production by neonatal T cells, especially those of the CD8 subset. This preferential induction of IL-17 by cord blood CD8 T cells rather than CD4 T cells is also observed after polyclonal activation and incubation with recombinant IL-23. These findings raise the possibility that the Th17 pathway of immunity might be intact in neonates. However, it should be pointed out that almost 1000-fold more IFN-γ is produced by polyclonally activated neonatal T cells treated with IL-12 compared to the production of IL-17 by these cells after treatment with IL-23 (114). Nevertheless, determining whether this IL-23/IL-17 pathway of T-cell differentiation is intact in vivo will be of interest, as Th17 immunity can compensate for limitations in Th1 immunity for certain pathogens (115).

These findings using MDDCs provide an explanation for limitations in Th1 immunity, such as delayed-type hypersensitivity skin reactions and antigen-specific CD4 T-cell IFN-γ production, which are discussed below. The relevance of these findings obtained with MDDCs is supported by observations in mice suggesting that myeloid DC can directly differentiate from monocytes when they undergo transendothelial trafficking (9). But it remains unclear whether the differentiation of monocytes into DCs using high doses of exogenous cytokines faithfully mimics DC differentiation from less mature precursors in vivo. A rigorous comparison of the gene and protein expression profiles and function of MDDCs with freshly isolated highly purified DC populations may help clarify this issue.

FETAL TISSUE DENDRITIC CELLS

Knowledge of tissue DCs in the human fetus and neonate is very limited. Immature cDC lineage cells have been identified in the interstitium of solid organs, including the kidney, heart, pancreas, and lung, but not the brain, by 12 weeks of gestation (116). The numbers of these cells in tissues other than the brain progressively increase by 21 weeks gestation. Epidermal Langerhans cells are found in the skin even earlier (7 weeks gestation) (117). In contrast to post-natal skin, these cells are uniformly CD1a$^-$ until 12–13 weeks of gestation (117), and CD1a$^+$ Langerhans cells do not predominate under about 27 weeks gestation (118). These findings indicate that colonization and differentiation of Langerhans cells in the fetal skin is developmentally regulated independently of exposure to inflammatory mediators.

Cells with the features of DCs, possibly of the pDC-lineage, are found in fetal lymph nodes between 19 and 21 weeks of gestation (93); they have an immature phenotype and are not recent emigrants from inflamed tissues. An early study found S100+ "T-zone histiocyte" cells, which had the histological appearance of pDCs, in the fetal liver between 2 and 3 months of gestation, a time when the liver is a major hematopoietic organ (119); this was followed by the appearance of these cells in the thymic medulla at 4 months and the spleen, lymph nodes, tonsils, and Peyer's patches by 4–5 months gestation. These findings need to be confirmed using better-characterized and more definitive histological markers.

POST-NATAL STUDIES OF TISSUE-ASSOCIATED DENDRITIC CELLS IN CHILDREN

A recent study of nasal wash samples obtained from children with acute viral respiratory infections demonstrated that both cDCs and pDCs can be identified as part of these secretions by multiparameter flow cytometry (120). Increased numbers of both DC populations were observed after acute infection with respiratory syncytial virus (RSV) or with other respiratory viral pathogens (parainfluenza and influenza). In the case of RSV infection, the number of these cells was correlated positively with the viral load, and persisted in the nasal mucosa for 2–8 weeks after acute infection. No CD83 expression by these DCs was detected, consistent with their being more tissue-associated DCs. Interestingly, infection with RSV but not parainfluenza/influenza resulted in decreased circulating levels of both cDCs and pDCs (120). It will be of interest to determine whether these DC populations accumulate to a similar degree in neonates and young infants, and the ability of these cells to function ex vivo.

POST-NATAL ONTOGENY OF MURINE DENDRITIC CELL FUNCTION

It is technically more difficult, particularly in humans, to assess the capabilities of dendritic cells that are resident in the peripheral tissues. To address this issue, we recently examined the impact of TLR-4 signaling on cDC in young mice (121). cDCs from the spleens of 6–12-week-old TLR-4-deficient (C3He/J) mice were similar to those of wild-type mice in the proportion of cells that were immature (MHC class II^{low}) compared to mature (MHC class II^{high}) (Fig. 12-1). However, mature splenic cDCs from TLR-4-deficient mice had reduced expression of B7 co-stimulatory proteins, e.g., CD86, in response to incubation with GM-CSF alone or together with CD40 engagement (Fig. 12-2). Moreover, myeloid cDCs from

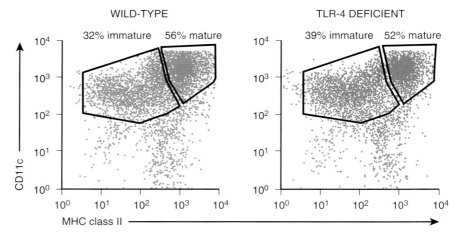

Figure 12-1 Wild-type and TLR-4-deficient mice have similar proportions of splenic conventional dendritic cells that are mature and immature as assessed by the level of MHC class II surface expression. CD11c and MHC class II surface expression was determined by flow cytometry, with the cell numbers shown expressed as the percent of total CD11c⁺ cells.

TLR-4-deficient mice also had significantly reduced capacity to produce IL-12 in response to CD40 engagement compared to those from wild-type mice (Fig. 12-3), a feature that would probably limit Th1 differentiation. It is interesting to speculate that cDCs from neonates, born from a sterile uterine environment, are functionally immature until they have had exposures to bacterial products in the extrauterine environment.

Consistent with this idea, the capacity of purified murine splenic cDCs, particularly those of the CD8-α-subset, to produce IL-12p70 increases between 1–2 weeks and 6 weeks of age in response to CpG (TLR-9 is expressed by cDCs in mice) and a combination of cytokines (122). Also supportive of this model, the expression of a number of surface markers on cDCs, e.g., CD8-α, CD11b, and F4/80, gradually increases after birth, achieving adult levels at approximately 4 weeks of age (123).

Interestingly, IFN-α production by purified murine splenic pDCs at 1–2 weeks of age was similar to or higher than these cells at 6 weeks of age (122), indicating that the developmental limitations in DC function may be limited to cDCs rather than pDCs. This is consistent with the robust induction of T-cell immunity in the neonatal mouse with the addition of unmethylated CpG DNA to protein vaccines (124). Moreover, in contrast to human neonatal cDCs, those of the neonatal mouse respond robustly to LPS, and are able to effectively activate naive T cells for differentiation into effector cells (125). Although it remains to be determined whether circulating cDCs in neonatal mice have reduced function compared to those in older mice, the available data in vivo strongly suggest that neonatal mice may not accurately model the apparent more prolonged and intrinsic limitations in cDC function in early post-natal life in humans. A recent murine neonatal study also suggests that the function of cDCs in vivo may be limited by a high level of production of IL-10 by the neonatal B1 B cell subset in response to TLR-9 engagement rather than an intrinsic limitation in cDC function (126). Whether a similar suppressive environment for cDC function is attributable to neonatal human B cells remains unclear.

A recent study by Kasper and co-workers in mice suggests that commensal bacterial-derived products, such as the bacterial polysaccharide of the anaerobic bacterium *Bacteroides fragilis*, can have a profound positive impact in early

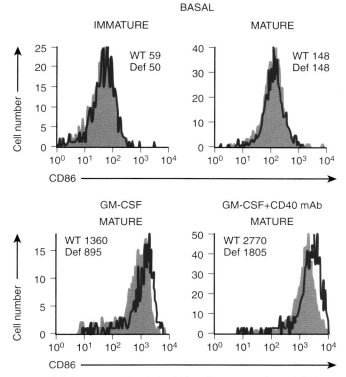

Figure 12-2 TLR-4-deficient conventional dendritic cells express substantially less surface CD86 (B72) co-stimulatory molecule after activation with GM-CSF either alone or in combination with CD40 engagement. CD86 expression was determined on immature (MHC class II^{low}) and mature (MHC class II^{high}) splenic dendritic cell populations immediately following purification (basal), and using gating, for the mature (MHC class II^{high}) cell population, 24 h after incubation with GM-CSF ± anti-CD40 mAb. The mean fluorescence index of positive cells is shown in the inserts for dendritic cells from wild-type (WT, clear histogram) and TLR-4-defective (Def, filled histogram) mice.

post-natal life in promoting lymphoid organogenesis, peripheral CD4 T-cell accumulation, and the capacity for CD4 T cells to produce Th1 cytokines. Moreover, this zwitterionic polysaccharide can be presented to T cells by cDCs in an MHC class II-restricted manner (127). Whether this impact of *Bacteroides fragilis* is dependent on TLRs or other innate immune mechanisms and whether the impact on CD4 T-cell expansion is truly polyclonal or limited to only a portion of CD4 T cells expressing a particular αβ-TCR repertoire remain to be determined.

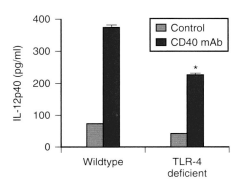

Figure 12-3 Splenic conventional dendritic cells from TLR-4-deficient mice produce less IL-12 compared to wild-type dendritic cells. The levels of IL-12p40 in supernatants of splenic conventional dendritic cells activated with anti-CD40 mAb for 48 h are shown. Data represent means ± SEM and are representative of three experiments. *$P < 0.05$ versus the wild-type CD40 mAb-treated group by the two-tailed unpaired Student's *t*-test.

It is also unclear whether this impact on CD4 T-lineage cells in vivo applies to humans, although *Bacteroides fragilis* is an abundant member of our gastrointestinal tracts.

NEONATAL CD4 T CELLS HAVE INTRINSIC LIMITATIONS IN Th1 DIFFERENTIATION

Numerous studies have demonstrated decreased Th1 function by human neonatal CD4 T cells (128–133). These findings can be accounted for by the increased numbers of differentiated memory T cells of the Th1 subset in adult blood compared to neonatal blood (131, 134, 135). Naive (CD45RA^{high}CD45R0^{low}) cells comprise approximately 60% of the CD4 T cells in most adults, but represent >90% of cells in infants (130). Thus any direct comparison of cord blood T cells to unfractionated adult cells compare a relatively pure population of naive cells to a mixed population containing both naive and memory cells. However, even when purified naive adult CD4$^+$ T cell are used for comparison, there appear to be major functional differences. For example, we recently investigated the capacity of neonatal T cells to mount Th1 responses (136). To avoid questions of inadequate antigen presentation by neonatal dendritic cells, a pool of allogeneic adult dendritic cells (MDDCs) were used as stimulators. Compared to purified adult naive CD4 T cells, neonatal naive CD4 T cells from cord blood secreted much less IL-2 and IFN-γ and expressed less CD154 on their cell surface (136). There was also a decrease in the IL-12p70 detected in the culture supernatants, indicating decreased induction of IL-12 secretion by dendritic cells by the neonatal CD4 T cells. This is probably due, in part, to decreased CD154/CD40 interactions. In addition, the neonatal CD4 T cells were impaired in their differentiation into Th1 cells because they expressed less STAT4 and had lower levels of STAT4 tyrosine phosphorylation, which is required for IL-12 signaling (136).

There was no evidence of increased skewing towards Th2 cells, based on the low level of IL-4 produced in both neonatal and adult CD4 T-cell cultures with the allogeneic dendritic cells. There was also no evidence of increased levels of immunosuppressive cytokines, such as IL-10, to account for reduced neonatal CD4 T-cell differentiation. We also found that the neonatal naive CD4 T cells in these experiments had a relatively reduced number of regulatory CD25^{high} CD4 T cells, based on their intracellular expression of the Foxp3 transcription factor (136). This strongly argues that the reduced ability of neonatal naive CD4 T cells to differentiate into Th1 cells in response to a potent allogeneic stimulus is not accounted for by an increased number of regulatory T cells, a cell population that is able to inhibit CD4 T-cell activation (137).

Epigenetic mechanisms may also regulate IFN-γ gene expression in neonatal T cells. Studies using methylation-sensitive restriction mapping demonstrated a hypermethylated CpG site in the IFN-γ promoter of neonatal and adult naive (CD45RA^{high}) CD4 T cells compared to memory/effector (CD45RO^{high}) CD4$^+$ T cells (138). This correlated with decreased IFN-γ expression in the cells with hypermethylation of the IFN-γ promoter. More recently, a more sensitive bisulfite sequencing technique was used by Holt and colleagues (139) to show that the IFN-γ promoter is hypermethylated at a number of sites in neonatal CD4 T cells compared to naive adult CD4 T cells. Interestingly, the IFN-γ promoter in neonatal CD8$^+$ T cells did not show the same degree of hypermethylation, and indeed, stimulated neonatal CD8 T cells were capable of making significant amounts of IFN-γ, albeit not as much as adult CD8 T cells. These differences in methylation of the IFN-γ gene in neonatal versus adult T cells are specific in that they are not associated with a general decrease in the overall level of methylation in T cells with aging (140).

REDUCED CD154 EXPRESSION

Interactions between CD154, which is expressed at high levels by activated CD4 T cells, and CD40, which is expressed by B cells, dendritic cells, and mononuclear phagocytes are critical for the induction of immunoglobulin class switching and memory formation by B cells, dendritic cell maturation and cytokine secretion, e.g., IL-12 secretion, and increased microbicidal activity by mononuclear phagocytes for pathogens, such as *Pneumocystis*. Patients with genetic deficiency of CD154 also lack vaccine-specific T cells that proliferate and produce IFN-γ, indicating the importance of the CD154/CD40 interaction in the accumulation of functional memory T cells, including those of the Th1 subset (141, 142). Part of the defect in Th1 differentiation probably lies in the inability of neonatal CD4 T cells to upregulate CD154, which in turn results in decreased IL-12 production from dendritic cells. We and others have shown that stimulated neonatal T cells fail to upregulate CD154 in spite of upregulation of other activation markers such as CD69 (143, 144). The decreased expression of CD154 was due to decreased transcription. This was linked to decreased calcium flux after TCR engagement, but even when the TCR was pharmacologically bypassed using ionomycin, transcription of CD154 remained low. As mentioned above, decreased CD154 expression was also observed when neonatal naive CD4$^+$ T cells were stimulated with fully mature allogeneic dendritic cells (136). This indicates that the defect in CD154 expression is intrinsic to the neonatal T cell and is likely to apply to activation in vivo that occurs in response to foreign antigens.

CONCLUSION

Immaturity of dendritic cells and the innate immune mechanisms that activate them, including Toll-like receptors and other innate immune receptor molecules, probably contributes to decreased T-cell immunity after birth. Although the circulating concentration of both conventional and plasmacytoid dendritic cells is similar in the neonate and the adult, some functions of both of these cell types may be selectively reduced in the neonate, including in response to certain Toll-like receptor ligands. The function of dendritic cells derived from neonatal monocytes in vitro is also reduced, particularly for the secretion of IL-12. However, it is unclear to what extent these in vitro decreases in dendritic cell function apply to cells found in the tissues where most dendritic cell interaction takes place with T cells. Studies of the phenotype and function of tissue-associated dendritic cells in the newborn has been limited for practical and ethical reasons, but in the future it should be possible to evaluate myeloid and plasmacytoid dendritic cells that are found in respiratory secretions during viral infections. Studies in mice also indicate that the exposure post-natally to commensal bacteria may play a role in conventional dendritic cell maturation, suggesting that early post-natal limitations in dendritic cells may be, in part, a normal physiologic consequence of a sterile intrauterine environment. In addition to potential limitations in dendritic cell function, intrinsic limitations in T-cell activation and Th1 differentiation, including in the production of CD40-ligand, the expression of the IFN-γ gene, and the cytokine-induced tyrosine phosphorylation of STAT4, may also contribute to an impaired ability of T cells in the neonate to respond to antigenic challenges. These limitations are likely to be important in explaining the increased vulnerability of the neonate to intracellular pathogens, the relatively low incidence of acute graft-versus-host disease when cord blood mononuclear cells are used for hematopoietic stem cell transplantation, and the inability of the neonate to reject allogeneic skin grafts.

REFERENCES

1. Medzhitov R, Janeway CA Jr. Decoding the patterns of self and nonself by the innate immune system. Science 296:298–300, 2002.
2. Steinman RM. Some interfaces of dendritic cell biology. Apmis 111:675–697, 2003.
3. Lewis DB, Wilson CB. Developmentalimmunology and role of host defenses in the fetal and neonatal susceptibility to infection. In: Remington JS, Klein JO, Wilson CB, Baker CJ, Infectious diseases of the fetus and newborn infant. Philadelphia: Elsevier; 2006: 87–210.
4. Gallucci S, Matzinger P. Danger signals: SOS to the immune system. Curr Opin Immunol 13:114–119, 2001.
5. Banchereau J, Briere F, Caux C, et al. Immunobiology of dendritic cells. Annu Rev Immunol 18:767–811, 2000.
6. Fogg DK, Sibon C, Miled C, et al. A clonogenic bone marrow progenitor specific for macrophages and dendritic cells. Science 311:83–87, 2006.
7. Naik SH, Metcalf D, A van Nieuwenhuijze, et al. Intrasplenic steady-state dendritic cell precursors that are distinct from monocytes. Nat Immunol 7:663–671, 2006.
8. Ginhoux F, Tacke F, Angeli V, et al. Langerhans cells arise from monocytes in vivo. Nat Immunol 7:265–273, 2006.
9. Randolph GJ, Inaba K, Robbiani DF, et al. Differentiation of phagocytic monocytes into lymph node dendritic cells in vivo. Immunity 11:753–761, 1999.
10. Randolph GJ, Sanchez-Schmitz G, Liebman RM, et al. The CD16(+) (FcgammaRIII(+)) subset of human monocytes preferentially becomes migratory dendritic cells in a model tissue setting. J Exp Med 196:517–527, 2002.
11. Colonna M, Trinchieri G, Liu YJ. Plasmacytoid dendritic cells in immunity. Nat Immunol 5:1219–1226, 2004.
12. Cella M, Jarrossay D, Facchetti F, et al. Plasmacytoid monocytes migrate to inflamed lymph nodes and produce large amounts of type I interferon. Nat Med 5:919–923, 1999.
13. Taieb J, Chaput N, Menard C, et al. A novel dendritic cell subset involved in tumor immunosurveillance. Nat Med 12:214–219, 2006.
14. Huang Y, Kucia M, Rezzoug F, et al. Flt3-ligand-mobilized peripheral blood, but not Flt3-ligand-expanded bone marrow, facilitating cells promote establishment of chimerism and tolerance. Stem Cells 24:936–948, 2006.
15. Quezada SA, Jarvinen LZ, Lind EF, et al. CD40/CD154 interactions at the interface of tolerance and immunity. Annu Rev Immunol 22:307–328, 2004.
16. Kuwajima S, Sato T, Ishida K, et al. Interleukin 15-dependent crosstalk between conventional and plasmacytoid dendritic cells is essential for CpG-induced immune activation. Nat Immunol 7:740–746, 2006.
17. Munz C, Steinman RM, Fujii S. Dendritic cell maturation by innate lymphocytes: coordinated stimulation of innate and adaptive immunity. J Exp Med 202:203–207, 2005.
18. Guermonprez P, Valladeau J, Zitvogel L, et al. Antigen presentation and T cell stimulation by dendritic cells. Annu Rev Immunol 20:621–667, 2002.
19. Allan RS, Waithman J, Bedoui S, et al. Migratory dendritic cells transfer antigen to a lymph node-resident dendritic cell population for efficient CTL priming. Immunity 25:153–162, 2006.
20. Belz GT, Smith CM, Kleinert L, et al. Distinct migrating and nonmigrating dendritic cell populations are involved in MHC class I-restricted antigen presentation after lung infection with virus. Proc Natl Acad Sci USA 101:8670–8675, 2004.
21. Kissenpfennig A, Henri S, Dubois B, et al. Dynamics and function of Langerhans cells in vivo: dermal dendritic cells colonize lymph node areas distinct from slower migrating Langerhans cells. Immunity 22:643–654, 2005.
22. Chaperot L, Blum A, Manches O, et al. Virus or TLR agonists induce TRAIL-mediated cytotoxic activity of plasmacytoid dendritic cells. J Immunol 176:248–255, 2006.
23. Ishii KJ, Coban C, Akira S. Manifold mechanisms of toll-like receptor-ligand recognition. J Clin Immunol 25:511–521, 2005.
24. Gorden KB, Gorski KS, Gibson SJ, et al. Synthetic TLR agonists reveal functional differences between human TLR7 and TLR8. J Immunol 174:1259–1268, 2005.
25. Heil F, Hemmi H, Hochrein H, et al. Species-specific recognition of single-stranded RNA via toll-like receptor 7 and 8. Science 303:1526–1529, 2004.
26. Kawai T, Akira S. Pathogenrecognition with Toll-like receptors. Curr Opin Immunol 17:338–344, 2005.
27. Blander JM, Medzhitov R. Toll-dependent selection of microbial antigens for presentation by dendritic cells. Nature 440:808–812, 2006.
28. Takaoka A, Yanai H, Kondo S, et al. Integral role of IRF-5 in the gene induction programme activated by Toll-like receptors. Nature 434:243–249, 2005.
29. Honda K, Yanai H, Mizutani T, et al. Role of a transductional-transcriptional processor complex involving MyD88 and IRF-7 in Toll-like receptor signaling. Proc Natl Acad Sci USA 101:15416–15421, 2004.
30. Tailor P, Tamura T, Ozato K. IRF family proteins and type I interferon induction in dendritic cells. Cell Res 16:134–140, 2006.
31. Akira S, Uematsu S, Takeuchi O. Pathogen recognition and innate immunity. Cell 124:783–801, 2006.
32. Sporri R, Reis e Sousa C. Inflammatory mediators are insufficient for full dendritic cell activation and promote expansion of CD4+ T cell populations lacking helper function. Nat Immunol 6:163–170, 2005.

33. Yoneyama H, Matsuno K, Toda E, et al. Plasmacytoid DCs help lymph node DCs to induce anti-HSV CTLs. J Exp Med 202:425–435, 2005.

34. Komai-Koma M, Jones L, Ogg GS, et al. TLR2 is expressed on activated T cells as a costimulatory receptor. Proc Natl Acad Sci USA 101:3029–3034, 2004.

35. Caron G, Duluc D, Fremaux I, et al. Direct stimulation of human T cells via TLR5 and TLR7/8: flagellin and R-848 up-regulate proliferation and IFN-gamma production by memory CD4+ T cells. J Immunol 175:1551–1557, 2005.

36. Crellin NK, Garcia RV, Hadisfar O, et al. Human CD4+ T cells express TLR5 and its ligand flagellin enhances the suppressive capacity and expression of FOXP3 in CD4+CD25+ T regulatory cells. J Immunol 175:8051–8059, 2005.

37. Liu H, Komai-Koma M, Xu D, et al. Toll-like receptor 2 signaling modulates the functions of CD4+ CD25+ regulatory T cells. Proc Natl Acad Sci USA 103:7048–7053, 2006.

38. Sutmuller RP, MH den Brok, Kramer M, et al. Toll-like receptor 2 controls expansion and function of regulatory T cells. J Clin Invest 116:485–494, 2006.

39. Meylan E, Tschopp J, Karin M. Intracellular pattern recognition receptors in the host response. Nature 442:39–44, 2006.

40. Kawai T, Akira S. Innate immune recognition of viral infection. Nat Immunol 7:131–137, 2006.

41. Chamaillard M, Hashimoto M, Horie Y, et al. An essential role for NOD1 in host recognition of bacterial peptidoglycan containing diaminopimelic acid. Nat Immunol 4:702–707, 2003.

42. Kobayashi KS, Chamaillard M, Ogura Y, et al. Nod2-dependent regulation of innate and adaptive immunity in the intestinal tract. Science 307:731–734, 2005.

43. Tada H, Aiba S, Shibata K, et al. Synergistic effect of Nod1 and Nod2 agonists with toll-like receptor agonists on human dendritic cells to generate interleukin-12 and T helper typ. 1 cells. Infect Immun 73:7967–7976, 2005.

44. Kanneganti TD, Ozoren N, Body-Malapel M, et al. Bacterial RNA and small antiviral compounds activate caspase-1 through cryopyrin/Nalp3. Nature 440:233–236, 2006.

45. Mariathasan S, Weiss DS, Newton K, et al. Cryopyrin activates the inflammasome in response to toxins and ATP Nature 440:228–232, 2006.

46. Kato H, Takeuchi O, Sato S, et al. Differential roles of MDA5 and RIG-I helicases in the recognition of RNA viruses. Nature 441:101–105, 2006.

47. Kato H, Sato S, Yoneyama M, et al. Cell type-specific involvement of RIG-I in antiviral response. Immunity 23:19–28, 2005.

48. Sun Q, Sun L, Liu HH, et al. The specific and essential role of MAVS in antiviral innate immune responses. Immunity 24:633–642, 2006.

49. Pasare C, Medzhitov R. Toll-dependent control mechanisms of CD4 T cell activation. Immunity 21:733–741, 2004.

50. Berenson LS, Ota N, Murphy KM. Issues in T-helper 1 development–resolved and unresolved. Immunol Rev 202:157–174, 2004.

51. Dong C. Diversification of T-helper-cell lineages: finding the family root of IL-17-producing cells. Nat Rev Immunol 6:329–333, 2006.

52. Picard C, Casanova JL. Inherited disorders of cytokines. Curr Opin Pediatr 16:648–658, 2004.

53. Happel KI, Zheng M, Young E, et al. Cutting edge: roles of Toll-like receptor 4 and IL-23 in IL-17 expression in response to Klebsiella pneumoniae infection. J Immunol 170:4432–4436, 2003.

54. Tabeta K, Hoebe K, Janssen EM, et al. The Unc93b1 mutation 3d disrupts exogenous antigen presentation and signaling via Toll-like receptors 3, 7 and 9. Nat Immunol 7:156–164, 2006.

55. Savina A, Jancic C, Hugues S, et al. NOX2 controls phagosomal pH to regulate antigen processing during crosspresentation by dendritic cells. Cell 126:205–218, 2006.

56. Whitley RJ. Herpes simplex virus infections of women and their offspring: implications for a developed society. Proc Natl Acad Sci USA 91:2441–2447, 1994.

57. Kimberlin DW. Neonatal herpes simplex infection. Clin Microbiol Rev 17:1–13, 2004.

58. Burchett SK, Weaver WM, Westall JA, et al. Regulation of tumor necrosis factor/cachectin and IL-1 secretion in human mononuclear phagocytes. J Immunol 140:3473–3481, 1988.

59. Sullender WM, Miller JL, Yasukawa LL, et al. Humoral and cell-mediated immunity in neonates with herpes simplex virus infection. J Infect Dis 155:28–37, 1987.

60. Tu W, Chen S, Sharp M, et al. Persistent and selective deficiency of CD4+ T cell immunity to cytomegalovirus in immunocompetent young children. J Immunol 172:3260–3267, 2004.

61. Chen SF, Tu WW, Sharp MA, et al. Antiviral CD8 T cells in the control of primary human cytomegalovirus infection in early childhood. J Infect Dis 189:1619–1627, 2004.

62. Marchant A, Appay V, Van Der Sande M, et al. Mature CD8(+) T lymphocyte response to viral infection during fetal life. J Clin Invest 111:1747–1755, 2003.

63. Lin TY, Kao HT, Hsieh SH, et al. Neonatal enterovirus infections: emphasis on risk factors of severe and fatal infections. Pediatr Infect Dis J 22:889–894, 2003.

64. Ventura KC, Hawkins H, Smith MB, et al. Fatal neonatal echovirus 6 infection: autopsy case report and review of the literature. Mod Pathol 14:85–90, 2001.

65. Rorman E, Zamir CS, Rilkis I, et al. Congenital toxoplasmosis–prenatal aspects of Toxoplasma gondii infection. Reprod Toxicol 21:458–472, 2006.

66. Marodi L. Neonatal innate immunity to infectious agents. Infect Immun 74:1999–2006, 2006.

67. de Repentigny L, Lewandowski D, Jolicoeur P. Immunopathogenesis of oropharyngeal candidiasis in human immunodeficiency virus infection. Clin Microbiol Rev 17:729–759, table of contents.

68. Marodi L. Innate cellular immune responses in newborns. Clin Immunol 118:137–144, 2006.

69. Smith S, Jacobs RF, Wilson CB. Immunobiology of childhood tuberculosis: a window on the on-togeny of cellular immunity. J Pediatr 131:16–26, 1997.

70. Marchant A, Goetghebuer T, Ota MO, et al. Newborns develop a Th1-type immune response to Mycobacterium bovis bacillus Calmette-Guerin vaccination. J Immunol 163:2249–2255, 1999.

71. Vekemans J, Amedei A, Ota MO, et al. Neonatal bacillus Calmette-Guerin vaccina-tion induces adult-like IFN-gamma production by CD4+ T lymphocytes. Eur J Immunol 31:1531–1535, 2001.

72. Borras FE, Matthews NC, Lowdell MW, et al. Identification of both myeloid CD11c+ and lymphoid CD11c- dendritic cell subsets in cord blood. Br J Haematol 113:925–931, 2001.

73. De Wit D, Olislagers V, Goriely S, et al. Blood plasmacytoid dendritic cell responses to CpG oligodeoxynucleotides are impaired in human newborns. Blood 103:1030–1032, 2004.

74. Teig N, Moses D, Gieseler S, et al. Age-related changes in human blood dendritic cell subpopula-tions. Scand J Immunol 55:453–457, 2002.

75. MacDonald KP, Munster DJ, Clark GJ, et al. Characterization of human blood dendritic cell subsets. Blood 100:4512–4520, 2002.

76. Dzionek A, Fuchs A, Schmidt P, et al. BDCA-2, BDCA-3, and BDCA-4: three markers for distinct subsets of dendritic cells in human peripheral blood. J Immunol 165:6037–6046, 2000.

77. Almeida J, Bueno C, Alguero MC, et al. Comparative analysis of the morphological, cytochemical, immunophenotypical, and functional characteristics of normal human peripheral blood lineage(-)/CD16(+)/HLA-DR(+)/CD14(-/lo) cells, CD14(+) monocytes, and CD16(-) dendritic cells. Clin Immunol 100:325–338, 2001.

78. Vuckovic S, Gardiner D, Field K, et al. Monitoring dendritic cells in clinical practice using a new whole blood single-platform TruCOUNT assay. J Immunol Methods 284:73–87, 2004.

79. Szabolcs P, Park KD, Reese M, et al. Absolute values of dendritic cell subsets in bone marrow, cord blood, and peripheral blood enumerated by a novel method. Stem Cells 21:296–303, 2003.

80. Vakkila J, Thomson AW, Vettenranta K, et al. Dendritic cell subsets in childhood and in children with cancer: relation to age and disease prognosis. Clin Exp Immunol 135:455–461, 2004.

81. Hagendorens MM, Ebo DG, Schuerwegh AJ, et al. Differences in circulating dendritic cell subtypes in cord blood and peripheral blood of healthy and allergic children. Clin Exp Allergy 33:633–639, 2003.

82. De Wit D, Tonon S, Olislagers V, et al. Impaired responses to toll-like receptor 4 and toll-like receptor 3 ligands in human cord blood. J Autoimmun 21:277–281, 2003.

83. Crespo I, Paiva A, Couceiro A, et al. Immunophenotypic and functional characterization of cord blood dendritic cells. Stem Cells Dev 13:63–70, 2004.

84. Drohan L, Harding JJ, Holm B, et al. Selective developmental defects of cord blood antigen-pre-senting cell subsets. Hum Immunol 65:1356–1369, 2004.

85. Kerfoot SM, Long EM, Hickey MJ, et al. TLR4 contributes to disease-inducing mechanisms result-ing in central nervous system autoimmune disease. J Immunol 173:7070–7077, 2004.

86. Upham JW, Lee PT, Holt BJ, et al. Development of interleukin-12-producing capacity throughout childhood. Infect Immun 70:6583–6588, 2002.

87. Tonon S, Goriely S, Aksoy E, et al. Bordetella pertussis toxin induces the release of inflammatory cytokines and dendritic cell activation in whole blood: impaired responses in human newborns. Eur J Immunol 32:3118–3125, 2002.

88. Lee SM, Suen Y, Chang L, et al. Decreased interleukin-12 (IL-12) from activated cord versus adult peripheral blood mononuclear cells and upregulation of interferon-gamma, natural killer, and lymphokine-activated killer activity by IL-12 in cord blood mononuclear cells. Blood 88:945–954, 1996.

89. Scott ME, Kubin M, Kohl S. Highlevel interleukin-12 production, but diminished interferon-gamma production, by cord blood mononuclear cells. Pediatr Res 41:547–553, 1997.

90. Perez-Melgosa M, Ochs HD, Linsley PS, et al. Carrier-mediated enhancement of cognate T cell help: the basis for enhanced immunogenicity of meningococcal outer membrane protein polysaccharide conjugate vaccine. Eur J Immunol 31:2373–2381, 2001.

91. Karlsson H, Hessle C, Rudin A. Innate immune responses of human neonatal cells to bacteria from the normal gastrointestinal flora. Infect Immun 70:6688–6696, 2002.

92. Levy O, Suter EE, Miller RL, et al. Unique efficacy of Toll-like receptor 8 agonists in activating human neonatal antigen-presenting cells. Blood 108:1284–1290, 2006.

93. Olweus J, BitMansour A, Warnke R, et al. Dendritic cell ontogeny: a human dendritic cell lineage of myeloid origin. Proc Natl Acad Sci USA 94:12551–12556, 1997.

94. Grouard G, Rissoan MC, Filgueira L, et al. The enigmatic plasmacytoid T cells develop into den-dritic cells with interleukin (IL)-3 and CD40-ligand. J Exp Med 185:1101–1111, 1997.

95. Sorg RV, Kogler G, Wernet P. Identification of cord blood dendritic cells as an immature CD11c-population. Blood 93:2302–2307, 1999.

96. Prescott SL, Irwin S, Taylor A, et al. Cytosine-phosphate-guanine motifs fail to promote T-helper typ. 1-polarized responses in human neonatal mononuclear cells. Clin Exp Allergy 35:358–366, 2005.

97. Gold MC, Donnelly E, Cook MS, et al. Purified neonatal plasmacytoid dendritic cells overcome intrinsic maturation defect with TLR agonist stimulation. Pediatr Res 60:34–37, 2006.

98. Cederblad B, Riesenfeld T, Alm GV. Deficien therpes simplex virus-induced interferon-alpha pro-duction by blood leukocytes of preterm and term newborn infants. Pediatr Res 27:7–10, 1990.

99. Hunt DW, Huppertz HI, Jiang HJ, et al. Studies of human cord blood dendritic cells: evidence for functional immaturity. Blood 84:4333–4343, 1994.

100. Petty RE, Hunt DW. Neonatal dendritic cells. Vaccine 16:1378–1382, 1998.
101. Sorg RV, Kogler G, Wernet P. Functional competence of dendritic cells in human umbilical cord blood. Bone Marrow Transplant 22(Supp. 1):S52–S54, 1998.
102. Kapsenberg ML. Dendritic-cell control of pathogen-driven T-cell polarization. Nat Rev Immunol 3:984–993, 2003.
103. Cella M, Facchetti F, Lanzavecchia A, et al. Plasmacytoid dendritic cells activated by influenza virus and CD40L drive a potent TH1 polarization. Nat Immunol 1:305–310, 2000.
104. Borras FE, Matthews NC, Patel R, et al. Dendritic cells can be successfully generated from CD34+ cord blood cells in the presence of autologous cord blood plasma. Bone Marrow Transplant 26:371–376, 2000.
105. Canque B, Camus S, Dalloul A, et al. Characterization of dendritic cell differentiation pathways from cord blood CD34(+)CD7(+)CD45RA(+) hematopoietic progenitor cells. Blood 96:3748–3756, 2000.
106. Dilioglou S, Cruse JM, Lewis RE. Function of CD80 and CD86 on monocyte- and stem cell-derived dendritic cells. Exp Mol Pathol 75:217–227, 2003.
107. Jakobsen MA, Moller BK, Lillevang ST. Serum concentration of the growth medium markedly affects monocyte-derived dendritic cells' phenotype, cytokine production profile and capacities to stimulate in MLR. Scand J Immunol 60:584–591, 2004.
108. Goriely S, Vincart B, Stordeur P, et al. Deficient IL-12(p35) gene expression by dendritic cells derived from neonatal monocytes. J Immunol 166:2141–2146, 2001.
109. Liu E, Tu W, Law HK, et al. Decreased yield, phenotypic expression and function of immature monocyte-derived dendritic cells in cord blood. Br J Haematol 113:240–246, 2001.
110. Langrish CL, Buddle JC, Thrasher AJ, et al. Neonatal dendritic cells are intrinsically biased against Th-1 immune responses. Clin Exp Immunol 128:118–123, 2002.
111. Goriely S, Van C Lint, Dadkhah R, et al. A defect in nucleosome remodeling prevents IL-12(p35) gene transcription in neonatal dendritic cells. J Exp Med 199:1011–1016, 2004.
112. Zheng Z, Takahashi M, Narita M, et al. Generation of dendritic cells from adherent cells of cord blood by culture with granulocyte-macrophage colony-stimulating factor, interleukin-4, and tumor necrosis factor-alpha. J Hematother Stem Cell Res 9:453–464, 2000.
113. Vanden Eijnden S, Goriely S, De Wit D, et al. Preferential production of the IL-12(p40)/IL-23(p19) heterodimer by dendritic cells from human newborns. Eur J Immunol 36:21–26, 2006.
114. Vanden Eijnden S, Goriely S, De Wit D, et al. IL-23 up-regulates IL-10 and induces IL-17 synthesis by polyclonally activated naive T cells in human. Eur J Immunol 35:469–475, 2005.
115. Cruz A, Khader SA, Torrado E, et al. Cutting edge: IFN-gamma regulates the induction and expansion of IL-17-producing CD4 T cells during mycobacterial infection. J Immunol 177:1416–1420, 2006.
116. Hofman FM, Danilovs JA, Taylor CR. HLA-DR (Ia)-positive dendritic-like cells in human fetal nonlymphoid tissues. Transplantation 37:590–594, 1984.
117. Foster CA, Holbrook KA. Ontogeny of Langerhans cells in human embryonic and fetal skin: cell densities and phenotypic expression relative to epidermal growth. Am J Anat 184:157–164, 1989.
118. Drijkoningen M, De Wolf-Peeters C, Van der Steen K, et al. Epidermal Langerhans' cells and dermal dendritic cells in human fetal and neonatal skin: an immunohistochemical study. Pediatr Dermatol 4:11–17, 1987.
119. Watanabe S, Nakajima T, Shimosato Y, et al. T-zone histiocytes with S100 protein. Development and distribution in human fetuses. Acta Pathol Jpn 33:15–22, 1983.
120. Gill MA, Palucka AK, Barton T, et al. Mobilization of plasmacytoid and myeloid dendritic cells to mucosal sites in children with respiratory syncytial virus and other viral respiratory infections. J Infect Dis 191:1105–1115, 2005.
121. Dabbagh K, Dahl ME, Stepick-Biek P, et al. Toll-like receptor 4 is required for optimal development of Th2 immune responses: role of dendritic cells. J Immunol 168:4524–4530, 2002.
122. Dakic A, Shao QX, D'Amico A, et al. Development of the dendritic cell system during mouse ontogeny. J Immunol 172:1018–1027, 2004.
123. Muthukkumar S, Goldstein J, Stein KE. The ability of B cells and dendritic cells to present antigen increases during ontogeny. J Immunol 165:4803–4813, 2000.
124. Siegrist CA. Neonatal and early life vaccinology. Vaccine 19:3331–3346, 2001.
125. Dadaglio G, Sun CM, Lo-Man R, et al. Efficient in vivo priming of specific cytotoxic T cell responses by neonatal dendritic cells. J Immunol 168:2219–2224, 2002.
126. Sun CM, Deriaud E, Leclerc C, et al. Upon TLR9 signaling, CD5+ B cells control the IL-12-dependent Th1-priming capacity of neonatal DCs. Immunity 22:467–477, 2005.
127. Mazmanian SK, Liu CH, Tzianabos AO, et al. An immunomodulatory molecule of symbiotic bacteria directs maturation of the host immune system. Cell 122:107–118, 2005.
128. Adkins B. T-cell function in newborn mice and humans. Immunol Today 20:330–335, 1999.
129. Wu CY, Demeure C, Kiniwa M, et al. IL-12 induces the production of IFN-gamma by neonatal human CD4 T cells. J Immunol 151:1938–1949, 1993.
130. Gasparoni A, Ciardelli L, Avanzini A, et al. Age-related changes in intracellular TH1/TH2 cytokine production, immunoproliferative T lymphocyte response and natural killer cell activity in newborns, children and adults. Biol Neonate 84:297–303, 2003.
131. Ehlers S, Smith KA. Differentiation of T cell lymphokine gene expression: the in vitro acquisition of T cell memory. J Exp Med 173:25–36, 1991.
132. Pirenne-Ansart H, Paillard F, De Groote D, et al. Defective cytokine expression but adult-type T-cell receptor, CD8, and p56lck modulation in CD3- or CD2-activated T cells from neonates. Pediatr Res 37:64–69, 1995.

133. Trivedi HN, HayGlass KT, Gangur V, et al. Analysis of neonatal T cell and antigen presenting cell functions. Hum Immunol 57:69–79, 1997.
134. Lewis DB, Prickett KS, Larsen A, et al. Restricted production of interleukin 4 by activated human T cells. Proc Natl Acad Sci USA 85:9743–9747, 1988.
135. Lewis DB, Yu CC, Meyer J, et al. Cellular and molecular mechanisms for reduced interleukin 4 and interferon-gamma production by neonatal T cells. J Clin Invest 87:194–202, 1991.
136. Chen L, Cohen AC, Lewis DB. Impaired allogeneic activation and T-helper 1 differentiation of human cord blood naive CD4 T cells. Biol Blood Marrow Transplant 12:160–171, 2006.
137. Ziegler SF. FOXP3: of mice and men. Annu Rev Immunol 24:209–226, 2006.
138. Melvin AJ, McGurn ME, Bort SJ, et al. Hypomethylation of the interferon-gamma gene correlates with its expression by primary T-lineage cells. Eur J Immunol 25:426–430, 1995.
139. White GP, Watt PM, Holt BJ, et al. Differential patterns of methylation of the IFN-gamma promoter at CpG and non-CpG sites underlie differences in IFN-gamma gene expression between human neonatal and adult CD45RO- T cells. J Immunol 168:2820–2827, 2002.
140. Tra J, Kondo T, Lu Q, et al. Infrequent occurrence of age-dependent changes in CpG island methylation as detected by restriction landmark genome scanning. Mech Ageing Dev 123:1487–1503, 2002.
141. Ameratunga R, Lederman HM, Sullivan KE, et al. Defective antigen-induced lymphocyte proliferation in the X-linked hyper-IgM syndrome. J Pediatr 131:147–150, 1997.
142. Jain A, Atkinson TP, Lipsky PE, et al. Defects of T-cell effector function and post-thymic maturation in X-linked hyper-IgM syndrome. J Clin Invest 103:1151–1158, 1999.
143. Jullien P, Cron RQ, Dabbagh K, et al. Decreased CD154 expression by neonatal CD4+ T cells is due to limitations in both proximal and distal events of T cell activation. Int Immunol 15:1461–1472, 2003.
144. Nonoyama S, Penix LA, Edwards CP, et al. Diminished expression of CD40 ligand by activated neonatal T cells. J Clin Invest 95:66–75, 1995.

Chapter 13

Breast Milk and Viral Infection

Marianne Forsgren, MD, PhD •
Björn Fischler, MD, PhD • Lars Navér, MD, PhD

HIV and Breastfeeding

HTLV-I and Breastfeeding

Hepatitis B Infection and Breastfeeding

Hepatitis C Infection and Breastfeeding

Cytomegalovirus and Breastfeeding

Breast milk is the most important nutrient to all newborn babies – preterm and full-term. Breast milk supplies the infant with not only essential nutrition but also factors for its immune defense (1).

The immune system of the newborn term child is developed but far from complete in its function. During the period while infants are building up their own immune system, immunity transferred from the mother protects the child by transplacental mechanisms and by immune modulating factors in breast milk. Active transport of maternal IgG via an Fcγ receptor in placenta cells starts slowly in the second trimester (2). At delivery the full-term child has in average 90% of the maternal total IgG level for its defense; certain antibodies, e.g., rubella, with high binding capacity, may even reach higher levels in the newborn than in the mother. The more preterm a child is born, the lower the level of maternal antibodies and passive protection. After birth there is a gradual decay of maternal antibodies, with a half-life of 25–30 days (2), but the protective effect lasts for the first 6–12 months until the infant's own IgG antibodies are produced. The IgG synthesis starts at about 3–4 months of life.

Transfer of immunity by breast milk occurs via transfer of many protective components such as secretory IgA, compensating for the inability of the fetus to produce IgA, and numerous other factors: cellular (e.g. lymphocytes) as well as a number of inhibitory substances. The protective role may, however, vary. For example, lactoferrin is reported to inhibit HIV in vitro but seems to stimulate the growth of HTLV-I (3).

The immune components that are transferred from the mother protect the child from many but not all microbial threats. Maternal breast milk may also be a source of infection.

In the acute phase of a primary generalized viral infection such as varicella, parvovirus, hepatitis A or rubella, the mother has no protection to transfer to the infant and the breast milk contains virus. Transfer by breast milk is probably of minor importance as the child in most instances is already exposed through the mother by other routes. Continuation of breastfeeding is probably in the best interests of both the infant and the mother. Also live vaccine may be transmitted to the child via breast milk to a low extent, e.g. after rubella vaccination given

Table 13-1   Pathogens

The most important pathogen transmitted by breast milk is **HIV**, human immunodeficiency virus, the causative agent of AIDS, a huge problem of global dimensions

A second retrovirus, **HTLV-I**, strongly associated with long-term risk of a special form of leukaemia and demyelinating disease, is transmitted from mother to child mainly by breastfeeding; an important problem in endemic areas

Hepatitis B and C are globally spread chronic infections of the liver. The role of transmission by breastfeeding seems low as compared to the highly effective transmission of hepatitis B through contact with infectious maternal blood at delivery

Cytomegalovirus (CMV) is the pathogen most commonly transmitted by breast milk CMV seems to have a potential pathogenic role as cofactor aggravating the clinical course of a pre-existing pulmonary, hematologic, or hepatic condition. CMV disease and symptoms are infrequent in the normal child – full-term or preterm

postpartum (4). This early neonatal exposure to rubella vaccine virus does not cause clinical symptoms or enhance or suppress responses to rubella vaccination in early childhood (5). Varicella vaccine virus, on the other hand, is not detected in breast milk and virus is transferred to the breastfed infant (6).

More important problems arise from viruses with capacity to evade the immune defense by different mechanisms and establish chronic infection with free and/or cellular viremia and infect cells or milk whey in breast milk.

The chronic infection in the mother is as a rule not disclosed by clinical signs. Identification of infected individuals is possible by large-scale testing, enabled by recent advances in microbiological technology. As there is currently no easily available and clinically useful tissue culture or animal model system to measure the degree of infectivity of the mother – CMV excepted – qualitative and quantitative analyses of viral nucleic acid are used as surrogate markers. The full potential of modern molecular biology is applied to research. See Table 13-1.

HIV AND BREASTFEEDING

HIV is transmitted through infected blood and body fluids. The routes of transmission are through sexual intercourse, blood products, needle sharing during intravenous drug use, unsterile health care procedures and mother-to-child transmission (MTCT). One of the most tragic aspects of the global epidemic is the vertical transmission of the virus to the next generation. UNAIDS estimated 2.9 million deaths of AIDS in 2006, whereof 380 000 were children under 15 years. Approximately 17.7 million women are infected worldwide, most of them young and poor – a population where breastfeeding is critical for the survival of their children. According to UNAIDS, over 300 000 children are infected with HIV through breastfeeding every year.

Once infection is established proviral DNA is integrated in the human genome. At present there is no cure and vaccine approaches have to date not been successful. Antiviral drugs targeting different steps in viral replication may suppress viral replication. Two types of HIV can be distinguished, HIV-1 and HIV-2, of which HIV-1 is by far the most important. There is not much information available about MTCT of HIV-2 by any route, but it appears to be rare (7, 8). This chapter will only deal with different aspects of breastfeeding and HIV-1 (referred to as HIV).

Diagnosis of HIV Infection

Detection of viral antibodies is the cornerstone in individuals over 18 months and widely available for screen test and also adapted to field conditions. Confirmatory tests and a set-up of analyses for proviral DNA and virus RNA for direct diagnosis of infant infection and determination of viral load, subtyping of virus, and resistance against antiviral drugs are available in the specialized laboratory and the full potential of molecular microbiology is applied to HIV research.

Mother-to-Child Transmission

Transmission of HIV from an infected mother to her child can occur before, during or after birth. Before the era of antiretroviral prophylaxis, the prevalence of MTCT was 15–25% in industrialized countries, provided the mother did not breast-feed (9, 10), but studies from breastfeeding settings in Africa have shown transmission rates as high as 30–42% (11).

Among children of non-breastfeeding women approximately 60–70% become infected during delivery, and the remaining 30–40% are thought to be infected in utero (12, 13) The vast majority of the children infected in utero are infected during the last months of pregnancy (14, 15). Transmission during the first trimester appears to be rare (16). The infection rate during the second trimester is reported to be 2–5% (17, 18).

Breast Milk: Transmission

HIV transmission through breastfeeding has been demonstrated in several clinical trials of formula feeding versus breastfeeding (19, 20), but only one randomized. In the randomized study from Kenya (19) the cumulative probability of HIV infection by 24 months was 20.5% among children who were bottle fed and 36.7% among those who were breastfed. The estimated risk of HIV transmission through breastfeeding was 16.2% by the age of 24 months (20). In a meta-analysis (21) the additional risk of MTCT through breastfeeding was similarly found to be 16% and the contribution of breastfeeding to the overall MTCT of HIV was estimated to 47% (21).

HIV in Breast Milk

HIV in breast milk is present as both free (22–24) and cell-associated virus (25, 26). Cell-free virus was detected in 34–63% of breast milk samples from HIV-infected women at different time-points after delivery. Median virus load in colostrum/early milk was significantly higher than that in more mature breast milk collected 14 days after delivery (24). The prevalence and mean cell-free viral load in breast milk collected more than 1 week after delivery were not affected by postnatal age (24, 27). Cell-free viral load in breast milk correlates positively with viral load in plasma (23), even though the plasma load is generally higher (24), and negatively with maternal CD4+ cell count (23, 27).

The prevalence of cell-associated virus in breast milk ranges from 21 to 70% in different studies (25, 26). The number of infected breast milk cells per million cells is associated with the level of cell-free HIV RNA in breast milk (26) and the concentration of infected cells was higher in colostrum and early milk than in more mature milk (26).

The origin of HIV in breast milk is not well-defined. No study has evaluated the occurrence of productive HIV infective cells in breast milk. Cells, including macrophages and lymphocytes, and cell-free virus may migrate from the systemic compartment to breast milk. HIV can infect and reproduce in mammary epithelial cells in vitro (28) but it is not known whether the ductal or alveolar cells contribute to local viral replication in vivo. In paired samples, the HIV populations in blood and breast milk have been found to be similar. No unique variants existed in either compartment, suggesting that viruses in the blood plasma and breast milk are well equilibrated (29).

HIV Transmission: Mechanisms

The mechanism for MTCT through breastfeeding is not well-described and it is unclear whether infection occurs through cell-free virus or through infected cells. The infant gut mucosal surface is the most likely site at which transmission occurs. Cell-free or cellular virus may penetrate to the submucosa in the setting of mucosal breaches or lesions, via trancytosis (30, 31). Oral transmission has been demonstrated in a macaque simian immunodeficiency model and this pathway probably exists in humans as well (32). In vitro models suggest that secretory IgA and IgM may inhibit trancytosis of HIV across enterocytes (30, 31) but HIV-specific secretory IgA in breast milk does not appear to be a protective factor against HIV transmission among breastfed infants (33).

A higher cell-free viral load in breast milk (23, 34) as well as a higher viral load in plasma (35, 36) is associated with a higher risk of MTCT. The presence of HIV-infected cells in the milk 15 days postpartum was strongly predictive of HIV infection in the child (25). Primary HIV infection is associated with high levels of virus in plasma and probably also in breast milk and a high risk of postnatal transmission (20). Another study demonstrated a 6-fold risk increase if the mother seroconverted while breastfeeding (37). A reduction in both cell-associated and cell-free virus in breast milk was recently shown to significantly reduce HIV transmission by breastfeeding (38).

Timing of Transmission

It has been suggested that the risk of HIV transmission through breast milk is higher in young infants than in older children (19, 39). In the Kenyan randomized study of breastfeeding vs. formula feeding the major breast milk transmission occurred early, with 75% of the risk difference between the two arms by 6 months, although transmission continued during the whole period of exposure (19). Possible risk factors for increased transmission early in life are an immature immune system and an increased permeability of the gut in combination with higher virus content in early breast milk (25). The high additional risk of even a few weeks of early postnatal breastfeeding do support the importance of the early risk factors (20, 40). Both cell-free viral load (35) and the concentration of infected cells (26) have been shown to be high in colostrum and early milk as previously mentioned. However, a study from Brazil did not show that intake of colostrum affected the transmission rate (40).

The risk of HIV transmission correlates with the duration of breastfeeding (35, 41–43) In a meta-analysis the risk for breast milk transmission was 21% among women who breastfed for 3 months or more compared to 13% among those who breastfed for less than 2 months (21). In another recently published meta-analysis of late postnatal transmission in breastfed children who were uninfected by 4 weeks of age the transmission rate through breast milk was 1.6% at 3 months and increased gradually to 9.3% at 18 months (44). The analysis demonstrated that the risk of late postnatal transmission was cumulative, and fairly constant throughout breastfeeding. The overall risk of late postnatal transmission was 8.9 transmissions/100 child years of breastfeeding, which is approximately 0.8% risk for each additional month throughout the breastfeeding period.

The overall probability of breast milk transmission of HIV has been estimated to be approximately one infected child/1500 L breast milk. The average breastfeeding infant in the studied cohort consumed 150 L of breast milk during the course of breastfeeding (45).

Exclusive Versus Mixed Breastfeeding

Exclusive breastfeeding during the first 6 months of age is associated with less morbidity and mortality from other infectious diseases than from HIV (46–48). In a study from Botswana, breastfeeding with zidovudine prophylaxis was not as effective as formula feeding in preventing postnatal HIV transmission but the cumulative all-cause infant mortality at 7 months was significantly higher in formula-fed infants than in those assigned to breastfeeding and zidovudine (49). It becomes indeed more and more evident that exclusive breastfeeding is advantageous over mixed feeding (breast milk and formula, cow's milk, tea, juice or water) also with regard to MTCT of HIV. In a randomized controlled study from Durban, South Africa, investigating the effect of vitamin A on the risk of MTCT, women self-selected to breastfeed or formula-feed after being counseled. The mode of feeding was not randomized and the study was retrospectively re-analyzed to evaluate the effect of feeding pattern on MTCT of HIV. The cumulative probability of MTCT at 6 months of age in never breastfed and exclusively breastfed was similar, 19.4% and 19.4%, respectively. The transmission in the mixed breastfed group was 26.1% (50). It is noteworthy that at 3 months the transmission rate in those exclusively breastfed was lower (14.6%) than in those never breastfed (18.8%), which could indicate a selection bias. Another trial of a vitamin A intervention showed that HIV postnatal transmission risk and mortality were higher in mixed breastfed infants than in those who were exclusively breastfed. Compared with exclusive breastfeeding, early mixed feeding was associated with 4.03, 3.79 and 2.6 greater risk of postnatal transmission at 6, 12 and 18 months, respectively (51). In a recently published non-randomized cohort study breastfed infants who received solid foods in addition to breast milk had an 11-fold increased risk of acquiring HIV than those exclusively breastfed, and infants who received both breast milk and formula doubled their risk of HIV acquisition. The mortality in the first 3 months of life was roughly doubled in the group receiving replacement feeding compared with the exclusively breastfeeding group (15% vs. 6%) (52). Although observational, this is the first study in which measurement of transmission by feeding method was the primary aim.

It has been hypothesized but not confirmed that mixed feeding (breast milk and solids, formula, cow's milk, tea, juice or water) might enhance the MTCT rate by introduction of contaminated fluids that predispose to gastrointestinal infection, inflammation and increased gut permeability (53). Breast milk viral load has recently been shown to be substantially higher after rapid weaning, so an increased risk of transmission may exist when breastfeeding is resumed after a period of cessation (54). The probable advantages of exclusive breastfeeding on MTCT of HIV have to be confirmed, and several prospective studies are in progress to examine this issue.

Antiretroviral Therapy and Transmission

Nevirapine, lamivudine and zidovudine administered during the last trimester of pregnancy and after delivery reached concentrations in breast milk similar to or higher than in plasma and significantly reduced HIV RNA levels in breast milk (55). It is likely that combination antiretroviral therapy to the mother during lactation could reduce transmission, but it is not clear whether infants of women on combination antiretroviral therapy with undetectable viral load are at risk for transmission of HIV through breast milk. A number of studies are ongoing or planned (56). Passage of antiretroviral drugs into breast milk has been evaluated for some antiretroviral drugs. ZDV, 3TC, and nevirapine can be detected in human breast milk, and ddI, d4T, abacavir, delavirdine, indinavir, ritonavir, saquinavir and amprenavir can be detected in the breast milk of lactating rats (57). If the infant becomes infected through breast milk during maternal antiretroviral therapy, resistant virus may emerge in the infant as a consequence of suboptimal infant drug levels.

Additional Risk Factors

The risk of MTCT is increased when maternal breast pathologies such as mastitis, breast abscess and nipple lesions are present (35, 37), and also if oral candidiasis of the infant is present (37).

Inactivation of HIV

HIV is heat-sensitive and is inactivated by boiling (58) and pasteurization at temperatures between 56 and 62.5°C (59, 60). HIV-infected milk was pasteurized at 62.5°C for 30 min (59) or by a simplified technique developed for low-income settings, the Pretoria pasteurization (60). No infective virus was recovered after the processing. On the other hand, HIV RNA levels were remarkably stable in whole milk after three freeze-thaw cycles (53) and 6–30 h at room temperature was inadequate to destroy HIV (58, 61). The conclusion in a review by Rollins et al. was that correctly applied heat treatment of expressed breast milk reliably inactivated HIV within the milk (62). However, freezing and inherited lipolytic activity of breast milk is inadequate for destruction of HIV (58, 61). The use of alkyl sulfate microbicides to treat HIV-infected breast milk may be a novel alternative to prevent/reduce transmission through breastfeeding (63). See Tables 13-2 and 13-3.

HTLV-I AND BREASTFEEDING

An infection with the retrovirus HTLV-I is followed by a latent period and 3–5% of the carriers develop after 30–60 years adult T-cell leukemia (ATL) or HTLV-associated progressive and spastic paresis in lower limbs (HAM) caused by demyelinating myelopathy (64, 65). HTLV-I enters the body inside infected CD4+ lymphocytes in breast milk, blood or semen and is transmitted by breastfeeding, sexual intercourse, blood transfusion and sharing contaminated needles and syringes. There is no curative therapy or vaccine.

Table 13-2   HIV: Recommendations

- HIV screening of pregnant women is crucial for effective MTCT prevention programmes, including counseling about feeding practices
- Appropriate strategies need to be developed to increase the number of pregnant women who are tested for HIV and who are able to accept the available interventions
- If possible, HIV-infected women are strongly recommended to avoid breastfeeding completely. This is only of interest if alternatives to breastfeeding are feasible, affordable, safe and available
- If complete avoidance is not possible, the current WHO recommendation is early weaning from breast milk (e.g., at 3–6 months of age), if feasible. This recommendation is under debate as the association between mixed breastfeeding and HIV transmission, together with evidence that exclusive breastfeeding can be successfully supported by HIV-infected women in resource-limited settings, warrants revision of the present UNICEF, WHO and UNAIDS infant feeding guidelines
- Antiretroviral therapy for the mother and/or infant during the period of breastfeeding is not an option at present but might become an alternative in the future
- Treatment of breast milk with heat or chemical agents is an option but the methodologies would be difficult to utilize in many affected settings

---

Table 13-3   HIV: Research Directions

There are several urgent research directions in the field of HIV and breastfeeding
- Among the most important topics are to further evaluate the possible benefits from exclusive breastfeeding

To study
- the effects and safety of antiretroviral therapy to the mother and/or child during breastfeeding
- the effect of early cessation of breastfeeding on HIV transmission, morbidity and mortality
- mechanisms by which HIV is transmitted through breast milk

More than a million people (even up to 15–20 million) are estimated to be infected (64). The infection is distributed across the world but is mainly concentrated in certain areas within countries in the Caribbean (66), southern Japan (67), equatorial Africa (64), Papua New Guinea (68) and parts of South America (64), where a combination of vertical and horizontal transmission can maintain 5–30% levels of infection from generation to generation. Highest figures are reported from areas of southwestern Japan, with up to 10% of the pregnant women being seropositive (69).

In the USA and Europe, ATL and HAM are found in immigrants from endemic areas, but the rate is very low in blood donors and the spread among drug users limited, although being reported in New York already in the early 1990s and in Brazil (64, 70, 71). A closely related virus, HTLV-II, spread in similar mode, is linked to HAM (72) but not to lymphoproliferative disease (73). The infection is more prevalent than HTLV-I among intravenous drug users in the USA and Europe and has been introduced at a low rate in the general population and blood donors.

Diagnosis of Infection

Antibody tests used for screen testing of HTLV cross-react between HTLV type I and II. Confirmatory tests and demonstration of type-specific HTLV proviral DNA are required to confirm true infection and HTLV type.

Mother-to-Child Transmission

Virus transmission in utero seems to be of minor importance. The major transmission route is through breast milk (69, 74–76).

Breast Milk: Transmission

About 1 out of 5 children breastfed by HTLV-I mothers become infected (69, 74, 75). Long-term breastfeeding (>6 months), high provirus load in milk and high antibody level in maternal blood are risk factors predicting infection (77, 78). Studies in Japan demonstrate that bottle-feeding reduces the infection rate in the child to a few percent (2.5; 5.6%) (69, 74, 75). The transmission risk after short-term breastfeeding (< 6 months) is of the same magnitude (3.9; 3.8%) but it is high after long-term breastfeeding (14.5–20.3%).

The virus is cell-associated, being present in CD4+ lymphocyte. Procedures inactivating cells in breast milk – heating, freeze-thawing – eliminate the infectivity and viral transmission. Feeding the infant with the mother's milk after freeze-thawing may thus be an alternative to bottle feeding (79). See Table 13-4.

Table 13-4   HTLV: Recommendations

- Prenatal screening of pregnant women from endemic areas and counseling of seropositive mothers regarding risk of transmission through breastfeeding has substantially reduced the transmission and infection rate (76)
- Also in other areas prenatal screening should be recommended to immigrants from endemic areas and encouraged in pregnant women from risk populations in which HTLV-I has emerged
- If possible, HTLV-I-infected women are strongly recommended to avoid breastfeeding completely. This is only of interest if alternatives to breastfeeding are feasible, affordable, safe and available
- If complete avoidance is not possible, early weaning from breast milk (e.g. at 3–6 months of age), if feasible, would limit exposure to HTLV-I-infected breast milk
- Feeding the infant with the mother's milk after freeze-thawing may be an alternative to bottle-feeding
- The prospective risk with maternal HTLV-II is not known. However, authorities recommend that HTLV-II-infected mothers refrain from breastfeeding when and where safe nutritional alternatives exist

HEPATITIS B INFECTION AND BREASTFEEDING

Chronic hepatitis B virus (HBV) infection is estimated to occur in 350 million people globally (80). HBV is transmitted via contaminated blood or blood products, but also through sexual contacts. There is currently no easily available and clinically useful tissue culture or animal model system to test infectivity of the virus.

Diagnosis of HBV Infection

The detection of the viral antigens HBsAg and HBeAg and their corresponding antibodies are the cornerstones in the diagnostic management of HBV infection. Thus, the presence of HBsAg in serum for 6 months or more is defined as a chronic infection. Furthermore, the concomitant detection of HBeAg denotes a high level of viremia, indicating infectivity. On the other hand, if HBeAg is not detected, but rather its antibody anti-HBe, a lower grade of viremia and infectivity has been assumed. In the 1990s, with the availability of new diagnostic tools of molecular virology, such as PCR, the latter assumption was proven to be right in most but not in all such situations. The exception, i.e., when high levels of viremia and infectivity occur despite the presence of anti-HBe and the absence of HBeAg, is associated with the presence of mutated HBV virus. Certain mutated viral strains do not produce HBeAg and can therefore avoid the immune system and replicate in high numbers despite the presence of anti-HBe.

Mother-to-Child Transmission

Pregnant women who are HBV-infected run a high risk of passing the virus on to the offspring. The most efficient route of infection seems to be the perinatal one. However, prenatal infection may also occur, although in a much lower proportion of cases. It is also well-established that HBV infection acquired early in life will become chronic in a majority of cases. In contrast, if the virus is acquired in adulthood the development of a chronic infection is uncommon.

The introduction of HBV immunization, in combination with the administration of HBV-specific immune globulins, has greatly decreased the risk of mother-to-infant transmission (81).

Breast milk: Transmission Mechanisms

Most available studies suggest that the virus can be found in breast milk from infected mothers. Thus, both HBsAg and HBeAg have been detected in the breast milk of a large proportion of infected mothers and later PCR studies have confirmed the presence of HBV-DNA as well (82–85). The virus has been detected in both the cellular and whey fractions of centrifuged colostrum. The level of viral antigens in breast milk is lower than in serum (84). The highest levels in breast milk were found in mothers with the highest levels of antigenemia (84). The failure of other investigators to detect viral antigens in breast milk may be due to differences in the sensitivity of the methods that were used or to differences in the levels of antigens in breast milk (86).

It is still unclear whether the presence of viral antigen in breast milk will influence the risk of the infant becoming infected. In a study from Taiwan 147 infants of HBsAg-positive mothers were studied. The study was performed before any preventive measures were available and the HBeAg status of the mothers was not reported. However, the rate of infection was high but not different in both breastfed (49% infected) and bottle-fed (53% infected) children, all of whom were followed for a mean of 11 months (86).

In studies performed in Italian infants of infected mothers, the effect of feeding habits on the vaccination effect was investigated. No difference in the risk of developing hepatitis B was seen when breastfed and bottle-fed infants were compared (87). The vaccine effect was similar in the two groups with regard to the rate of seroconversion. Interestingly, bottle-fed infants had transient but significantly higher antibody levels to HBs. In general, no or very few data are available on the possible HBV immune modulating effect of breast milk.

In practice, for HBV-vaccinated babies of infected mothers, breastfeeding is not looked upon as an additional risk factor. The rate of successful vaccinations is high (90–95%) and in those few, unfortunate cases where a chronic infection still develops it is thought to be associated with a prenatal transmission.

It is still unclear whether or not non-vaccinated babies of infected mothers should be breastfed. Indeed, some authors argue against such a practice, although we have no data supporting the possible risk of such feeding (84). Caution may also be suggested in the case of bleeding nipple lesions, if the mother has high levels of viremia.

Very few data are available on the risk of transferring the infection via banked breast milk. Considering the findings of the virus in colostrums, as discussed above, compulsory HBV testing of breast milk donors seems appropriate. In particular, it should be considered in areas of the world where universal HBV vaccination is not yet established.

In most centers pasteurization of banked breast milk is mandatory. Although there are no reports on the specific effect on the HBV content in breast milk, it is clear that this method is effective in order to achive viral safety when used for plasma related products (88). See Table 13-5.

HEPATITIS C INFECTION AND BREASTFEEDING

Chronic hepatitis C virus (HCV) infection, which is mainly transmitted via the blood-borne route, occurs in approximately 170 million people around the world (80). A majority of infected individuals develop a chronic infection.

Diagnosis of HCV Infection

No laboratory system for the detection or culture of the virus is currently available. Thus, the diagnosis relies on the detection of antibodies to the virus (anti-HCV)

Table 13-5   Hepatitis B: Recommendations

- In practice, for HBV vaccinated babies of infected mothers, breastfeeding is not looked upon as an additional risk factor. The rate of successful vaccinations is high (90–95%) and in those few, unfortunate cases where a chronic infection still develops, it is thought to be associated with a prenatal transmission
- It is still unclear whether or not non-vaccinated babies of infected mothers should be breastfed. Indeed, some authors argue against such practice, although we have no data supporting the possible risk of such feeding (84). Caution may also be suggested in the case of bleeding nipple lesions, if the mother has high levels of viremia
- Few data are available on the risk of transferring the infection via banked breast milk. Considering the findings of the virus in colostrum, as discussed in the text, compulsory HBV testing of breast milk donors seems appropriate. In particular, it should be considered in areas of the world where universal HBV vaccination is not yet established
- In most centers pasteurization of banked breast milk is mandatory. Although there are no reports on the specific effect on the HBV content in breast milk, it is clear that this method is effective in order to achieve viral safety when used for plasma related products (88)

in serum. Additionally, for information on the infectivity of the individual a PCR test to detect HCV-RNA, i.e. the viral genome, in serum is needed.

Mother-to-Child Transmission

The transmission rate from an HCV-infected mother to her infant is approximately 5% (89–91). To date, no preventive measures that could lower this figure have been defined. Thus, no vaccine or immune globulin is available and routine use of cesarean section does not seem to improve the situation (92, 93). The timing of viral transmission seems to be prenatal in one-third of infected cases, with perinatal transmission accounting for a majority of the remaining cases (94). The maternal level of HCV viremia has been suggested as a risk factor for transmission to the infant. However, no clear cut-off level of viremia between mothers transmitting and not transmitting the virus has been defined. Theoretically, antiviral treatment during the latter parts of pregnancy and at the time of birth to selected mothers with high levels of viremia could be of value. However, the positive effects in a rather low number of infants might not balance the possibly negative effect of such drugs to a large number of fetuses/infants.

Breast Milk: Transmission

Several studies have adressed the question of infection via breast milk. The data concerning viral content in breast milk are contradictory. Some authors report exclusively negative findings concerning HCV-RNA in breast milk, while others report positive findings in each studied sample (95–97). The reasons for this discrepancy could be differences in viremia levels of the study subjects, differences in sensitivity in PCR methods that were used, or the fact that different portions of breast milk were studied. In a Taiwanese study, all 15 mothers had HCV-RNA detected in the colostrum, at consistently lower levels than in the corresponding serum sample. Interestingly, none of the children was infected on follow-up (96). On the other hand, Kumar et al., who studied 65 infected mothers, all of whom had HCV-RNA in the breast milk, diagnosed HCV infection in three of the children. The authors noted that all three seemed to have been infected postnatally and had mothers with clinical signs of advanced HCV infection (95).

Utilizing larger cohorts of HCV-infected mothers and their exposed children, the rate of infection can be compared between breastfed and bottle-fed children. In a retrospective study of HCV-infected mothers performed by the European Paediatric Hepatitis C Network (EPHN), no difference in transmission rate between these two groups of infants was seen (98). An increased risk of HCV transmission in infants to mothers with HIV-HCV co-infection has been reported. When children whose mothers had such co-infection were analyzed separately, an increase in the risk of HCV transmission was seen in breastfed subjects (98). However, in a more recent, prospective study from EPHN, no such difference was seen, most probably due to the secondary effects of modern HIV therapy on the HCV viremia (99). The recommendations from EPHN and other authors are currently that breastfeeding need not be avoided in the case of maternal HCV. However, if the mother has HCV-HIV co-infection breastfeeding should be discouraged (100).

There is a shortage of data concerning HCV and banked breast milk, suggesting caution as described in the same setting for hepatitis B above, i.e., donor testing and pasteurization procedures are recommended (101). The latter seems efficient in reducing the risk of transmitting HCV via plasma-derived products (88). It should be noted that donated breast milk might often be used for premature babies. On theoretical grounds, extremely premature newborns may be more prone to viral infections than term babies, due to differences in the development of the immune system. See Table 13-6.

CYTOMEGALOVIRUS AND BREASTFEEDING

Cytomegalovirus (CMV) infections are ubiquitous and are rarely symptomatic in the immuno-competent individual. Primary infection is followed by life-long latency of virus in with intermittent activation and excretion of virus. Virus is spread vertically from mother to child and horizontally by close contact with body secretions from children, later by kissing, sexual intercourse, blood or organ transfusion. The epidemiology varies greatly in different populations and the range of susceptibility among women of fertile age varies from none in close-living societies to about half of the women living in highly hygienic surroundings. CMV infections may cause serious disease in the immuno-incompetent patient and in the fetus (102). A vaccine approach has so far been without success. Antiviral agents may suppress the viral replication but toxicity restricts their use in pregnant women and infants (103).

Diagnosis of Infection

The presence of CMV-specific IgG in maternal serum denotes past or present infection. If simultaneously CMV IgM is demonstrable and the CMV IgG is of low avidity the mother has an ongoing primary infection. If not, she has previous experience of CMV and her latent virus infection may be reactivated. If neither CMV IgG or IgM is found, the mother has no latent CMV infection and virus

---

Table 13-6   Hepatitis C: Recommendations

- The recommendations from EPHN and other authors are currently that breastfeeding need not be avoided in the case of maternal HCV. However, if the mother has HCV-HIV co-infection breastfeeding should be discouraged (100)
- There is a shortage of data concerning HCV and banked breast milk, suggesting caution as described in the same setting for hepatitis B, i.e., donor testing and pasteurization procedures are recommended (101). The latter seems efficient in reducing the risk of transmitting HCV via plasma-derived products (88)

---

cannot be reactivated. Viral DNA is used to demonstrate the presence of CMV virus in, for example, breast milk or the infant's throat or urine and may also be quantitated to measure viral load. Ongoing replication of virus is indicated by presence of viral RNA and infectious virus by culture isolation.

Mother-to-Child Transmission

CMV is a very common viral pathogen that may be transmitted in utero, at delivery by exposure to CMV in the birth canal or – in the majority of cases – from breastfeeding by mothers reactivating CMV in the mammary gland. Congenital infection has been reported in 0.2–2% of all children. Neonatal disease is seen in 10–15% and about 18% of all children with congenital CMV will have long-term sequelae such as neuro-developmental handicaps, including sensorineural hearing impairment and mental retardation. Severe handicap may result from infection in any period of fetal life although the highest risk is believed to be in the early phase.

Breast Milk: Transmission

During delivery the child may be infected by CMV in the birth canal. The major source of postnatal CMV infection is, however, viral excretion in maternal breast milk (102, 104). With sensitive analysis CMV reactivation may be found in breast milk from the majority of CMV seropositive individuals and is found in milk whey and cells (105, 106). Excretion time varies between individuals but seems low in the first week postpartum, reaches a maximum at about 4–8 weeks after delivery and ends at about 9–12 weeks (105, 106). The presence of virus is not equal to transmission. The risk of transmission is correlated to viral load in the milk whey and transmission occurs close to maximal excretion in the milk. Virus in breast milk is readily inactivated by pasteurization at 65 or 62.5°C for 30 min, a procedure destroying not only infectivity but also beneficial factors in the milk. More of these factors are preserved after freeze-thawing, a procedure previously reported to lower or abolish infectivity (104). However, new data indicate that although the virus load may be reduced transmission may still occur (104, 107).

An important question is whether breast-milk-transmitted CMV from a mother to her own child may cause disease in the infant. In term infants, subclinical infections are very common; morbidity from postnatal CMV is held to be very low and transitory although a potential role, e.g., in the development of neonatal cholestatic diseases has been suggested (108, 109). Protection of the infants from disease has been attributed to passively transferred maternal CMV IgG as well as nutritional and immunological factors in the breast milk (110). However, a very premature infant with an immature immune system who was born before the major transfer of immunoglobulin (at 28 weeks and later) may be more vulnerable. Significant disease, even with fatal outcome, was observed in preterm infants with CMV infection acquired by transfusion of blood from CMV-seropositive donors (see ref. 111). This problem is largely eliminated by the use of CMV-free blood products from CMV-negative donors and/or leukocyte-depleted blood. Disease in relation to breast-milk-transmitted CMV with risk of long-term neurologic but not auditory sequelae was also reported in the 1980s (112, 113).

Recently this question has been readdressed in several studies (see ref. 104). The transmission rate was with one exception higher when the infant was fed fresh breast milk (25–55%) than when fed frozen milk (10–15%). The reported rates of symptoms interpreted as CMV-related were divergent but severe sepsis-like illness at the time of onset of viral excretion was reported after feeding fresh milk, and in some cases also when frozen milk was fed. Risk factors for proposed CMV disease

Table 13-7   CMV: Conclusions

- Breast milk from a CMV-seronegative donor mother does not transmit CMV
- Breast milk from a CMV-seropositive mother transmitts CMV at a high rate to her child but symptoms appear only infrequently in a full-term healthy child
- In very preterm children (<1000 g and gestational age <30 weeks) serious disease has previously been attributed to breast-milk-acquired CMV (114)
- Now available data indicate, however, that CMV transmitted from the seropositive mother to her very preterm child
  - may induce mild transient symptoms in some children
  - does not seem to influence the outcome in the "normal" preterm child
  - at follow-up, auditory or mental retardation attributable to CMV infection have not been reported
  - CMV may be a cofactor aggravating the course of some pre-existing pulmonary, hematologic or hepatic conditions
  - CMV inactivating procedure may be beneficial for selected patient groups
  - freezing of the milk reduces but does not eliminate the risk of CMV transmission
  - short-term pasteurization may be used to abolish CMV infectivity
- Donated breast milk should be fully pasteurized according to present recommendations
- CMV-seronegative donor may be an alternative if available and other serious potential pathogens in the breast milk are excluded

were preterm infant below 1000 g and gestational age below 30 weeks. No cases were lethal and in available follow-up studies at 2–4 years and 6 months, respectively, no increased risk for delay in neuromotor development or sensorineural hearing loss was found (114–116).

These studies seemed to indicate that severe CMV disease may occur. However, the causative role of CMV infection in incidents of sepsis-like disease in these very preterm infants is difficult to evaluate as such incidents of unknown etiology are not uncommon. As the original study of serious CMV disease was not case-controlled the interpretation of the data has provoked a debate. In several subsequently published studies from other centers, serious CMV-like disease was only sporadically observed (107, 111, 116–119). A case-control analysis of the observations in the original report has now been undertaken (120) and it has become clear that also in this study most neonatal symptoms attributable to postnatal CMV were mild and transient and that the CMV infection had no effect on neonatal outcome of the normal preterm infant. However, from this and other reports (114, 120, 121) it is clear that CMV transmission through breast milk may be a factor aggravating the clinical course of some underlying pre-existing pulmonary, hematologic or hepatic conditions, and a mild pasteurization inactivating CMV infectivity (122) of a CMV-seropositive mother's milk might be of value for selected patients.

Donor milk from a seropositive mother should not be given without prior pasteurization to a vulnerable preterm or full-term child born by a seronegative mother.

See Table 13-7 for a summary.

REFERENCES

1. Hanson LA, Korotkova M, Lundin S, et al. The transfer of immunity from mother to child. Ann N Y Acad Sci 987:199–206, 2003.
2. Simister NE. Placental transport of immunoglobulin G. Vaccine 21:3365–3369, 2003.
3. Moriuchi M, Moriuchi H. A milk protein lactoferrin enhances human T cell leukemia virus type I and suppresses HIV-1 infection. J Immunol 166:4231–4236, 2001.
4. Losonsky GA, Fishaut JM, Strussenberg J, et al. Effect of immunization against rubella on lactation products. II. Maternal-neonatal interactions. J Infect Dis 145:661–666, 1982.
5. Krogh V, Duffy LC, Wong D, et al. Postpartum immunization with rubella virus vaccine and antibody response in breast-feeding infants. J Lab Clin Med 113:695–699, 1989.

6. Bohlke K, Galil K, Jackson LA, et al. Postpartum varicella vaccination: is the vaccine virus excreted in breast milk? Obstet Gynecol 102:970–977, 2003.

7. Andreasson PA, Dias F, Naucler A, et al. A prospective study of vertical transmission of HIV-2 in Bissau, Guinea-Bissau. AIDS 7:989–993, 1993.

8. European Collaborative Study. Risk factors for mother-to-child transmission of HIV-1. Lancet 339:1007–1012, 1992.

9. O'Donovan D, Ariyoshi K, Milligan P, et al. Maternal plasma viral RNA levels determine marked differences in mother-to-child transmission rates of HIV-1 and HIV-2 in The Gambia. MRC/Gambia Government/University College London Medical School working group on mother-child transmission of HIV. Aids 14:441–448, 2000.

10. The Working Group on Mother-To-Child Transmission of HIV. Rates of mother-to-child transmission of HIV-1 in Africa, America, and Europe: results from 13 perinatal studies. J Acquir Immune Defic Syndr Hum Retrovirol 8:506–510, 1995.

11. Read J. Prevention of mother-to-child transmission. In: Zeichner S, Read J, eds., Textbook of pediatric HIV care. New York: Cambridge University Press; 2005: 111–133.

12. Dunn DT, Brandt CD, Krivine A, et al. The sensitivity of HIV-1 DNA polymerase chain reaction in the neonatal period and the relative contributions of intra-uterine and intra-partum transmission. AIDS 9:F7–11, 1995.

13. Kuhn L, Steketee RW, Weedon J, et al. Distinct risk factors for intrauterine and intrapartum human immunodeficiency virus transmission and consequences for disease progression in infected children. Perinatal AIDS Collaborative Transmission Study. J Infect Dis 179:52–58, 1999.

14. Ehrnst A, Lindgren S, Dictor M, et al. HIV in pregnant women and their offspring: evidence for late transmission. Lancet 338:203–207, 1991.

15. Lallemant M, Jourdain G, Le Coeur S, et al. A trial of shortened zidovudine regimens to prevent mother-to-child transmission of human immunodeficiency virus type 1. Perinatal HIV Prevention Trial (Thailand) Investigators. N Engl J Med 343:982–991, 2000.

16. Sprecher S, Soumenkoff G, Puissant F, Degueldre M. Vertical transmission of HIV in 15-week fetus. Lancet 2:288–289, 1986.

17. Brossard Y, Aubin JT, Mandelbrot L, et al. Frequency of early in utero HIV-1 infection: a blind DNA polymerase chain reaction study on 100 fetal thymuses. AIDS 9:359–366, 1995.

18. Phuapradit W, Panburana P, Jaovisidha A, et al. Maternal viral load and vertical transmission of HIV-1 in mid-trimester gestation. AIDS 13:1927–1931, 1999.

19. Nduati R, John G, Mbori-Ngacha D, et al. Effect of breastfeeding and formula feeding on transmission of HIV-1: a randomized clinical trial. JAMA 283:1167–1174, 2000.

20. Dunn DT, Newell ML, Ades AE, et al. Risk of human immunodeficiency virus type 1 transmission through breastfeeding. Lancet 340:585–588, 1992.

21. John GC, Richardson BA, Nduati RW, et al. Timing of breast milk HIV-1 transmission: a meta-analysis. East Afr Med J 78:75–79, 2001.

22. Thiry L, Sprecher-Goldberger S, Jonckheer T, et al. Isolation of AIDS virus from cell-free breast milk of three healthy virus carriers. Lancet 2:891–892, 1985.

23. Pillay K, Coutsoudis A, York D, et al. Cell-free virus in breast milk of HIV-1-seropositive women. J Acquir Immune Defic Syndr 24:330–336, 2000.

24. Rousseau CM, Nduati RW, Richardson BA, et al. Longitudinal analysis of human immunodeficiency virus type 1 RNA in breast milk and of its relationship to infant infection and maternal disease. J Infect Dis 187:741–747, 2003.

25. Van de Perre P, Simonon A, Hitimana DG, et al. Infective and anti-infective properties of breastmilk from HIV-1-infected women. Lancet 341:914–918, 1993.

26. Rousseau CM, Nduati RW, Richardson BA, et al. Association of levels of HIV-1-infected breast milk cells and risk of mother-to-child transmission. J Infect Dis 190:1880–1888, 2004.

27. Willumsen JF, Filteau SM, Coutsoudis A, et al. Breastmilk RNA viral load in HIV-infected South African women: effects of subclinical mastitis and infant feeding. AIDS 17:407–414, 2003.

28. Toniolo A, Serra C, Conaldi PG, et al. Productive HIV-1 infection of normal human mammary epithelial cells. AIDS 9:859–866, 1995.

29. Henderson GJ, Hoffman NG, Ping LH, et al. HIV-1 populations in blood and breast milk are similar. Virology 330:295–303, 2004.

30. Bomsel M. Transcytosis of infectious human immunodeficiency virus across a tight human epithelial cell line barrier. Nat Med 3:42–47, 1997.

31. Bomsel M, Heyman M, Hocini H, et al. Intracellular neutralization of HIV transcytosis across tight epithelial barriers by anti-HIV envelope protein dIgA or IgM. Immunity 9:277–287, 1998.

32. Stahl-Hennig C, Steinman RM, Tenner-Racz K, et al. Rapid infection of oral mucosal-associated lymphoid tissue with simian immunodeficiency virus. Science 285:1261–1265, 1999.

33. Kuhn L, Trabattoni D, Kankasa C, et al. Hiv-specific secretory IgA in breast milk of HIV-positive mothers is not associated with protection against HIV transmission among breast-fed infants. J Pediatr 149:611–616, 2006.

34. Semba RD, Kumwenda N, Hoover DR, et al. Human immunodeficiency virus load in breast milk, mastitis, and mother-to-child transmission of human immunodeficiency virus type 1. J Infect Dis 180:93–98, 1999.

35. John GC, Nduati RW, Mbori-Ngacha DA, et al. Correlates of mother-to-child human immunodeficiency virus type 1 (HIV-1) transmission: association with maternal plasma HIV-1 RNA load, genital HIV-1 DNA shedding, and breast infections. J Infect Dis 183:206–212, 2001.

36. Fawzi W, Msamanga G, Spiegelman D, et al. Transmission of HIV-1 through breastfeeding among women in Dar es Salaam, Tanzania. J Acquir Immune Defic Syndr 31:331–338, 2002.
37. Embree JE, Njenga S, Datta P, et al. Risk factors for postnatal mother-child transmission of HIV-1. AIDS 14:2535–2541, 2000.
38. Koulinska IN, Villamor E, Chaplin B, et al. Transmission of cell-free and cell-associated HIV-1 through breast-feeding. J Acquir Immune Defic Syndr 41:93–99, 2006.
39. Miotti PG, Taha TE, Kumwenda NI, et al. HIV transmission through breastfeeding: a study in Malawi. JAMA 282:744–749, 1999.
40. Tess BH, Rodrigues LC, Newell ML, et al. Infant feeding and risk of mother-to-child transmission of HIV-1 in Sao Paulo State, Brazil. Sao Paulo Collaborative Study for Vertical Transmission of HIV-1. J Acquir Immune Defic Syndr Hum Retrovirol 19:189–194, 1998.
41. de Martino M, Tovo PA, Tozzi AE, et al. HIV-1 transmission through breast-milk: appraisal of risk according to duration of feeding. AIDS 6:991–997, 1992.
42. Bobat R, Moodley D, Coutsoudis A, et al. Breastfeeding by HIV-1-infected women and outcome in their infants: a cohort study from Durban, South Africa. AIDS 11:1627–1633, 1997.
43. Datta P, Embree JE, Kreiss JK, et al. Mother-to-child transmission of human immunodeficiency virus type 1: report from the Nairobi Study. J Infect Dis 170:1134–1140, 1994.
44. The Breastfeeding and HIV International Transmission Study Group. Late postnatal transmission of HIV-1 in breast-fed children: an individual patient data meta-analysis. J Infect Dis 189:2154–2166, 2004.
45. Richardson BA, John-Stewart GC, Hughes JP, et al. Breast-milk infectivity in human immunodeficiency virus type 1-infected mothers. J Infect Dis 187:736–740, 2003.
46. Brown KH, Black RE, Lopez de Romana G, et al. Infant-feeding practices and their relationship with diarrheal and other diseases in Huascar (Lima), Peru. Pediatrics 83:31–40, 1989.
47. Victora CG, Smith PG, Vaughan JP, et al. Evidence for protection by breast-feeding against infant deaths from infectious diseases in Brazil. Lancet 2:319–322, 1987.
48. Bahl R, Frost C, Kirkwood BR, et al. Infant feeding patterns and risks of death and hospitalization in the first half of infancy: multicentre cohort study. Bull World Health Organ 83:418–426, 2005.
49. Thior I, Lockman S, Smeaton LM, et al. Breastfeeding plus infant zidovudine prophylaxis for 6 months vs formula feeding plus infant zidovudine for 1 month to reduce mother-to-child HIV transmission in Botswana: a randomized trial: the Mashi Study. Jama 296:794–805, 2006.
50. Coutsoudis A, Pillay K, Kuhn L, et al. Method of feeding and transmission of HIV-1 from mothers to children by 15 months of age: prospective cohort study from Durban, South Africa. Aids 15:379–387, 2001.
51. Iliff PJ, Piwoz EG, Tavengwa NV, et al. Early exclusive breastfeeding reduces the risk of postnatal HIV-1 transmission and increases HIV-free survival. Aids 19:699–708, 2005.
52. Coovadia HM, Rollins NC, Bland RM, et al. Mother-to-child transmission of HIV-1 infection during exclusive breastfeeding in the first 6 months of life: an intervention cohort study. Lancet 369:1107–1116, 2007.
53. Rollins NC, Filteau SM, Coutsoudis A, et al. Feeding mode, intestinal permeability, and neopterin excretion: a longitudinal study in infants of HIV-infected South African women. J Acquir Immune Defic Syndr 28:132–139, 2001.
54. Thea DM, Aldrovandi G, Kankasa C, et al. Post-weaning breast milk HIV-1 viral load, blood prolactin levels and breast milk volume. Aids 20:1539–1547, 2006.
55. Giuliano M, Guidotti G, Andreotti M, et al. Triple antiretroviral prophylaxis administered during pregnancy and after delivery significantly reduces breast milk viral load: a study within the Drug Resource Enhancement Against AIDS and Malnutrition Program. J Acquir Immune Defic Syndr 44:286–291, 2007.
56. Gaillard P, Fowler MG, Dabis F, et al. Use of antiretroviral drugs to prevent HIV-1 transmission through breast-feeding: from animal studies to randomized clinical trials. J Acquir Immune Defic Syndr 35:178–187, 2004.
57. AidsInfo. Recommendations for Use of Antiretroviral Drugs in Pregnant HIV-1-Infected Women for Maternal Health and Interventions to Reduce Perinatal HIV-Transmission in the United States. http://aidsinfo.nih.gov/.
58. Chantry CJ, Morrison P, Panchula J, et al. Effects of lipolysis or heat treatment on HIV-1 provirus in breast milk. J Acquir Immune Defic Syndr 24:325–329, 2000.
59. Orloff SL, Wallingford JC, McDougal JS. Inactivation of human immunodeficiency virus type I in human milk: effects of intrinsic factors in human milk and of pasteurization. J Hum Lact 9:13–17, 1993.
60. Jeffery BS, Webber L, Mokhondo KR, et al. Determination of the effectiveness of inactivation of human immunodeficiency virus by Pretoria pasteurization. J Trop Pediatr 47:345–349, 2001.
61. Ghosh MK, Kuhn L, West J, et al. Quantitation of human immunodeficiency virus type 1 in breast milk. J Clin Microbiol 41:2465–2470, 2003.
62. Rollins N, Meda N, Becquet R, et al. Preventing postnatal transmission of HIV-1 through breast-feeding: modifying infant feeding practices. J Acquir Immune Defic Syndr 35:188–195, 2004.
63. Urdaneta S, Wigdahl B, Neely EB, et al. Inactivation of HIV-1 in breast milk by treatment with the alkyl sulfate microbicide sodium dodecyl sulfate (SDS). Retrovirology 2:28, 2005.
64. Proietti FA, Carneiro-Proietti AB, Catalan-Soares BC, et al. Global epidemiology of HTLV-I infection and associated diseases. Oncogene 24:6058–6068, 2005.
65. Yamaguchi K, Watanabe T. Human T lymphotropic virus type-I and adult T-cell leukemia in Japan. Int J Hematol 76 (Suppl 2):240–245, 2002.

66. Mortreux F, Gabet A-S, Wattel E. Molecular and cellular aspects of HTLV-1 associated leukemo-genesis in vivo. Leukemia 17:26–38, 2003.
67. Hanchard B. Adult T-cell leukemia/lymphoma in Jamaica: 1986–1995. J Acquir Immune Defic Syndr Hum Retrovirol Suppl 1:S20–S25, 1996.
68. Yanagihara R. Human T-cell lymphotropic virus type I infection and disease in the Pacific basin. Hum Biol 64:843–854, 1992.
69. Takezaki T, Tajima K, Ito M, et al. Short-term breast-feeding may reduce the risk of vertical trans-mission of HTLV-I. The Tsushima ATL Study Group. Leukemia 11 (Suppl. 3):60–62, 1997.
70. Trachtenberg AI, Gaudino JA, Hanson CV. Human T-cell lymphotrophic virus in California's injec-tion drug users. J Psychoactive Drugs 23:225–232, 1991.
71. de Araujo AC, Casseb JS, Neitzert E, et al. HTLV-I and HTLV-II infections among HIV-1 seropos-itive patients in Sao Paulo, Brazil. Eur J Epidemiol 10:165–171, 1994.
72. Black FL, Biggar RJ, Lal RB, et al. Twenty-five years of HTLV type II follow-up with a possible case of tropical spastic paraparesis in the Kayapo, a Brazilian Indian tribe. AIDS Res Hum Retroviruses 12:1623–1627, 1996.
73. Roucoux DF, Murphy EL. The epidemiology and disease outcomes of human T-lymphotropic virus type II. AIDS Rev 6:144–154, 2004.
74. Oki T, Yoshinaga M, Otsuka H, et al. A sero-epidemiological study on mother-to-child transmission of HTLV-I in southern Kyushu, Japan. Asia Oceania J Obstet Gynaecol 18:371–377, 1992.
75. Ando Y, Matsumoto Y, Nakano S, et al. Long-term follow-up study of HTLV-I infection in bottle-fed children born to seropositive mothers. J Infect 46:9–11, 2003.
76. Hino S, Katamine S, Miyata H, et al. Primary prevention of HTLV-I in Japan. J Acquir Immune Defic Syndr Hum Retrovirol 13 (Supp. 1):S199–S203, 1996.
77. Li HC, Biggar RJ, Miley WJ, et al. Provirus load in breast milk and risk of mother-to-child trans-mission of human T lymphotropic virus type I. J Infect Dis 190:1275–1278, 2004. Epub 2004 Aug 30. Comment in: J Infect Dis191:1780, 2005; author reply 1781.
78. Yoshinaga M, Yashiki S, Oki T, et al. A maternal risk factor for mother-to-child HTLV-I transmis-sion: viral antigen-producing capacities in culture of peripheral blood and breast milk cells. Jpn J Cancer Res 86:649–654, 1995.
79. Ando Y, Ekuni Y, Matsumoto Y, Nakano S, et al. Long-term serological outcome of infants who received frozen-thawed milk from human T-lymphotropic virus type-I positive mothers. J Obstet Gynaecol Res 30:436–438, 2004.
80. Slowik MK, Jhaveri R. Hepatitis B and C viruses in infants and young children. Semin Pediatr Infect Dis 16:296–305, 2005.
81. Chang MH, Chen CJ, Lai MS, et al. Universal hepatitis B vaccination in Taiwan and the incidence of hepatocellular carcinoma in children. Taiwan Childhood Hepatoma Study Group. N Engl J Med 336 (26):1855–1859, 1997.
82. Boxall EH, Flewett TH, Dane DS, et al. Letter: Hepatitis-B surface antigen in breast milk. Lancet 2:1007–1008, 1974.
83. Linnemann CC Jr, Goldberg S. Letter: HBAg in breast milk. Lancet 2:155, 1974.
84. Lin HH, Hsu HY, et al. Hepatitis B virus in the colostra of HBeAg-positive carrier mothers. J Pediatr Gastroenterol Nutr 17 (2):207–210, 1993.
85. Mitsuda T, Yokota S, Mori T, et al. Demonstration of mother-to-infant transmission of hepatitis B virus by means of polymerase chain reaction. Lancet 2:886–888, 1989.
86. Beasley RP, Stevens CE, Shiao IS, et al. Evidence against breast-feeding as a mechanism for vertical transmission of hepatitis B. Lancet 2:740–741, 1975.
87. de Martino M, Appendino C, Resti M, et al. Should hepatitis B surface antigen positive mothers breast feed? Arch Dis Child 60:972–974, 1985.
88. Hilfenhaus J, Groner A, Nowak T, et al. Analysis of human plasma products: polymerase chain reaction does not discriminate between live and inactivated viruses. Transfusion 37:935–940, 1997.
89. Fischler B, Lindh G, Lindgren S, et al. Vertical transmission of hepatitis C virus infection. Scand J Infect Dis 28:353–356, 1996.
90. Kelly D, Skidmore S. Hepatitis C-Z: recent advances. Arch Dis Child 86 (5):339–343, 2002.
91. Thomas SL, Newell ML, Peckham CS, et al. A review of hepatitis C virus (HCV) vertical transmis-sion: risks of transmission to infants born to mothers with and without HCV viraemia or human immunodeficiency virus infection. Int J Epidemiol 27:108–117, 1998.
92. Pembreya L, Newella ML, Tovo PA. The management of HCV infected pregnant women and their children European paediatric HCV network. J Hepatol 43:515–525, 2005.
93. England K, Pembrey L, Tovo PA, et al. Excluding hepatitis C virus (HCV) infection by serology in young infants of HCV-infected mothers. Acta Paediatr 94 (4):444–450, 2005.
94. Mok J, Pembrey L, Tovo PA, et al. When does mother to child transmission of hepatitis C virus occur? Arch Dis Child Fetal Neonatal Ed 90 (2):F156–160, 2005.
95. Kumar RM, Shahul S. Role of breast-feeding in transmission of hepatitis C virus to infants of HCV-infected mothers. J Hepatol 29:191–197, 1998.
96. Lin HH, Kao JH, Hsu HY, et al. Absence of infection in breast-fed infants born to hepatitis C virus-infected mothers. J Pediatr 126:589–591, 1995.
97. Polywka S, Schroter M, Feucht HH, et al. Low risk of vertical transmission of hepatitis C virus by breast milk. Clin Infect Dis 29:1327–1329, 1999.
98. European Paediatric Hepatitis C Virus Network. Effects of mode of delivery and infant feeding on the risk of mother- to- child transmission of hepatitis C virus. Brit J Obstetr Gynaecol 78:371–377, 2001.

99. European Paediatric Hepatitis C Virus Network. A significant sex - but not elective Cesarean section - effect on mother-to-child transmission of hepatitis C infection. J Infect Dis 192:1872–1879, 2005.

100. Pembrey L, Newell ML, Tovo PA, et al. The management of HCV infected pregnant women and their children. European paediatric HCV network. J Hepatol 43:515–525, 2005.

101. Lindemann PC, Foshaugen I, Lindemann R. Characteristics of breast milk and serology of women donating breast milk to a milk bank. Arch Dis Child Fetal Neonatal Ed 89:F440–441, 2004.

102. Stagno S. Cytomegalovirus. In: Remington JS, Klein JO, eds. Infectious diseases of the fetus and newbom infant, 5th edn. Philadelphia: WB Saunders; 2001: 389–424.

103. Schleiss MR. Antiviral therapy of congenital cytomegalovirus infection. Semin Pediatr Infect Dis 16:50–59, 2005.

104. Hamprecht K, Goelz R, Maschmann J. Breast milk and cytomegalovirus infection in preterm infants. Early Hum Dev 81:989-996, 2005. Epub 2005 Nov 7.

105. Yasuda A, Kimura H, Hayakawa M, et al. Evaluation of cytomegalovirus infections transmitted via breast milk in preterm infants with a real-time polymerase chain reaction assay. Pediatrics 111:1333–1336, 2003.

106. Hamprecht K, Witzel S, Maschman J, et al. Rapid detection and quantification of cell free cytomegalovirus by a high-speed centrifugation-based microculture assay: comparison to longitudinally analyzed viral DNA load and pp67 late transcript during lactation. J Clin Virol 28:303–316, 2003.

107. Curtis N, Chau L, Garland S, et al. Cytomegalovirus remains viable in naturally infected breast milk despite being frozen for 10 days. Arch Dis Child Fetal Neonatal Ed 90:F529–530, 2005.

108. Tarr PI, Haas JE, Christie DL. Biliary atresia, cytomegalovirus, and age at referral. Pediatricsa 97:828–831, 1996.

109. Fischler B, Woxenius S, Nemeth A, Papadogiannakis N. Immunoglobulin deposits in liver tissue from infants with biliary atresia and the correlation to cytomegalovirus infection. J Pediatr Surg 40:541–546, 2005.

110. Mussi-Pinhata MM, Pinto PC, Yamamoto AY, et al. Placental transfer of naturally acquired, maternal cytomegalovirus antibodies in term and preterm neonates. J Med Virol 69:232–239, 2003.

111. Forsgren M. Cytomegalovirus in breast milk: reassessment of pasteurization and freeze-thawing. Pediatr Res 56:526–528, 2004.

112. Paryani SG, Yeager AS, Hosford-Dunn H, et al. Sequelae of acquired cytomegalovirus infection in premature and sick term infants. J Pediatr 107:451–456, 1985.

113. Johnson SJ, Hosford-Dunn H, Paryani S, et al. Prevalence of sensorineural hearing loss in premature and sick term infants with perinatally acquired cytomegalovirus infection. Ear Hear 7:325–327, 1986.

114. Vollmer B, Seibold-Weiger K, Schmitz-Salue C, et al. Postnatally acquired cytomegalovirus infection via breast milk: effects on hearing and development in preterm infants. Pediatr Infect Dis J 23:322–327, 2004.

115. Jim WT, Shu CH, Chiu NC, et al. Transmission of cytomegalovirus from mothers to preterm infants by breast milk. Pediatr Infect Dis J 23:848–851, 2004.

116. Miron D, Brosilow S, Felszer K, et al. Incidence and clinical manifestations of breast milk-acquired Cytomegalovirus infection in low birth weight infants. J Perinatol 25:299–303, 2005.

117. Bryant P, Morley C, Garland S, Curtis N. Cytomegalovirus transmission from breast milk in premature babies: does it matter? Arch Dis Child Fetal Neonatal Ed 87:F75–77, 2002.

118. Willeitner A. Transmission of cytomegalovirus (CMV) through human milk: are new breastfeeding policies required for preterm infants?. Adv Exp Med Biol 554:489–494, 2004.

119. Schanler RJ. CMV acquisition in premature infants fed human milk: reason to worry? J Perinatol 25:297–298, 2005.

120. Neuberger P, Hamprecht K, Vochem M, et al. Case-control study of symptoms and neonatal outcome of human milk-transmitted cytomegalovirus infection in premature infants. J Pediatr 148:326–331, 2006.

121. Omarsdottir S, Casper C, Zweygberg Wirgart B, et al. Transmission of cytomegalovirus to extremely preterm infants through breast milk. Acta Paediatr 96:492–494, 2007.

122. Hamprecht K, Maschmann J, Muller D, et al. Cytomegalovirus (CMV) inactivation in breast milk: reassessment of pasteurization and freeze-thawing. Pediatr Res 56:529–535, 2004. Epub 2004 Aug 4.

Chapter 14

Control of Antibiotic-Resistant Bacteria in the Neonatal Intensive Care Unit

Philip Toltzis, MD

Epidemiology of MRSA in the NICU

Epidemiology of MDR-GNR in the NICU

Control Strategies for Non-Epidemic MRSA and MDR-GNR

Control Strategies for NICU Outbreaks of MRSA and MDR-GNR

The neonatal intensive care unit (NICU) harbors many microorganisms expressing antibiotic resistance. Three ICU-related resistance phenotypes have generated particular concern over the past decade, namely, methicillin-resistant *Staphylococcus aureus* (MRSA), vancomycin-resistant enterococci (VRE), and multiple-drug resistant Gram-negative rods (MDR-GNR). There is accumulating evidence in adult patients that infections by resistant organisms prolong hospitalization and increase health care costs, and that they are associated with a higher mortality compared with infection by susceptible bacteria (1). Mortality is increased in part because resistance limits the choice of antibiotics, forcing the use of agents that have poor tissue penetration (for example, vancomycin for MRSA) or that are bacteristatic rather than -cidal (for example, trimethoprim-sulfamethoxasole for multiple-drug resistant *Stenotrophomonas*). Furthermore, the expression of resistance may lead to delays in prescribing the most effective therapies for the first 2–3 days of illness, the time required to complete drug susceptibility testing (1). In the NICU, an additional consequence of antibiotic resistance is that it may obligate the clinician to use an antimicrobial agent for which there are few or no data regarding pharmacokinetics, distribution, or toxicity in premature infants.

Given the alarming consequences of infection by antibiotic-resistant organisms, it is imperative to understand and apply strategies to contain their spread, particularly among vulnerable populations such as those admitted to the NICU. VRE has only occasionally been problematic in the intensive care nursery, despite its high prevalence in non-neonatal ICUs over the past 15 years. This article, therefore, will review the epidemiology of MRSA and MDR-GNR in the NICU setting and will discuss strategies to contain them.

EPIDEMIOLOGY OF MRSA IN THE NICU

Recent surveys from the Centers for Disease Control and Prevention (CDC) indicate that over half of *S. aureus* isolated in American ICUs are methicillin-resistant (http://www.cdc.gov/ncidod/dhqp/pdf/nnis/2003NNISReport_AJIC.PDF).   MRSA appeared in NICUs beginning in the early 1980s soon after its discovery elsewhere, and it has persisted in intensive care nurseries ever since (2–9). This phenotype is mediated through the expression of an altered penicillin-binding protein, resulting in diminished affinity of all β-lactams for their target molecule on the bacterial cell wall (10). The abnormal penicillin-binding protein is encoded by the gene *mecA*, which is included on a cassette inserted into the bacterial chromosome. The de novo acquisition of *mecA* is an infrequent event, and the majority of MRSA isolates are derived from a finite number of international clones. Recently investigators at the CDC categorized American MRSA isolates based upon DNA restriction fragment polymorphisms as defined by pulsed field gel electrophoresis (PFGE) (11), a technique commonly used to establish clonal relationships between bacteria of the same species. Over 93% of their sample of 957 American isolates belonged to one of only eight major clones as defined by PFGE. These observations indicate that, in a given patient, MRSA is virtually never derived from a susceptible staphylococcus which emerges resistant under antibiotic pressure; rather, the organism is always acquired from an external source (particularly other patients via the hands of caregivers) (12). The key to control of MRSA therefore focuses on interrupting its spread from those external sources.

Almost all data regarding MRSA in the nursery are derived from outbreak reports (2–9). Little is known about endemic colonization and disease in the NICU, although certainly sporadic cases of MRSA occur. Once introduced into the NICU environment, however, MRSA may spread rapidly, and the identification of any case of MRSA in a hospitalized newborn should be considered a sentinel event of a potential outbreak. Once an epidemic is established, frequently 20–50% of all infants become colonized or infected (3–5, 13). MRSA characteristically is difficult to eradicate from the NICU using conventional infection-control measures after an outbreak has started (2–4, 7). Consequently, the duration of published MRSA nursery epidemics is long, ranging from 2 months to over 4 years (2–8, 13, 14).

As in older patients, infants become colonized with MRSA precedent to their infection. In newborns the organism most commonly colonizes the anterior nares, similar to patients outside the newborn period, but MRSA also may be isolated from the umbilicus, the axillary and groin skin folds, and the rectum. The duration of MRSA colonization in the neonate is variable. Some infants are colonized transiently, while in others colonization may persist for weeks or months, allowing spread of the organism to household contacts after the baby has been discharged from the hospital (4, 15).

MRSA colonization and infection in the newborn usually is a nosocomial event, appearing typically on day of life 15–30 (3, 5, 8, 9). The organism affects infants at high risk of a complicated NICU course, particularly those of low birth weight and gestation age requiring indwelling catheters and mechanical ventilation (5, 8, 9, 13). Other predisposing factors for MRSA colonization and infection include multiple gestation, prior surgery, and prolonged exposure to antibiotics (8, 13, 14), all confounders of a prolonged, complicated course.

Recently, two subtypes of MRSA have been identified in infants that may prove even more prone to spread rapidly once introduced into the NICU compared with current hospital-associated strains. The first is termed "community-acquired MRSA" (CA-MRSA), because these strains initially were identified outside the hospital. In 1998 several previously healthy children with no risk factors for acquisition of MRSA were infected with a methicillin-resistant organism. The strains implicated in these cases were molecularly unrelated to previously studied hospital-associated MRSA (16). In particular, the *mecA* gene was included on cassettes distinct from hospital-associated strains, and the organisms remained susceptible to many antibiotics, including clindamycin, to which hospital-associated MRSA were resistant (16). Moreover, they replicated very rapidly and frequently expressed exotoxins that were unusual in hospital-associated isolates. Chief among these is Panton-Valentine leukocidin (PVL), a molecule that lyses white blood cells and fosters the development of tissue necrosis (17). The past several years have witnessed the alarmingly rapid geographical dissemination of CA-MRSA throughout North America and Europe, presumably reflecting biological characteristics that especially promote person-to-person transmission.

Recently CA-MRSA has been implicated in infections affecting both the mother and her full-term newborn. Mother-to-child transmission of CA-MRSA may occur after maternal peripartum sepsis or maternal mastitis (5, 14, 18, 19). Most of the infants in these report suffered from bacteremia or skin and soft tissue infection (5, 14, 19, 20). More worrisome is the occurrence of nosocomially acquired CA-MRSA among premature NICU residents (21). A recent report from Houston, a metropolitan area with a particularly high prevalence of CA-MRSA, described six NICU infants within a year who acquired CA-MRSA after admission to the unit. Similar to the typical experience with hospital-associated MRSA, the patients were of low birth weight and onset of infection occurred several weeks after gestation. Unlike prior experience with hospital-associated strains, however, patients typically experienced fulminate septic shock, necrotizing pneumonia, and severe central nervous system infection (21), raising the concern that the PVL-positive CA-MRSA strains may be particularly virulent if introduced into the tertiary care nursery.

The second newly described subtype of MRSA produces a condition termed neonatal toxic-shock-syndrome-like exanthematous disease (NTED). Despite production of exotoxins not found in typical strains of hospital-associated MRSA, NTED strains produce relatively mild disease in the newborn (22, 23). Infants with NTED are uniformly colonized with a clone of MRSA that produces the superantigen exotoxins responsible for adult toxic shock syndrome, namely, Toxic Shock Syndrome Toxin-1 and Staphylococcal Enterotoxin C. NTED has occurred almost exclusively in Japan, but within a decade of its first description it is established as a nation-wide epidemic. Many of the affected infants are full-term, presenting on day of life 2–6 with a diffuse macular rash on the trunk that then coalesces as it spreads to the face and extremities. The infants usually demonstrate a moderate to severe thrombocytopenia. Except for elevated C-reactive protein, other elements of adult toxic shock syndrome are absent. Recovery usually occurs with supportive care, even without antibiotics (23).

EPIDEMIOLOGY OF MDR-GNR IN THE NICU

As with MRSA, the epidemiology of MDR-GNR can be best appreciated by reviewing the mechanisms of resistance (10). The phenotypes for MDR-GNR are varied, encompassing resistance to all classes of β-lactam agents, to the aminoglycosides, and to the quinolones. Many of the resistance determinants to the β-lactams and aminoglycosides, the phenotypes relevant to the NICU, are encoded on transmissible genetic elements such as integrons or plasmids. Those resistance genes that are encoded on the bacterial genome usually are controlled by upstream sequences that turn on production of the resistance molecule in the presence of antibiotic, or, alternatively, that spontaneously mutate to generate constitutively resistant subpopulations that then expand under antibiotic pressure. In all these cases, resistance is promoted by antibiotic exposure, so that the association between prior antibiotic administration and colonization or infection by MDR-GNR is much stronger than with MRSA. Once resistance is selected, the organisms primarily colonize the gastrointestinal tract and in most cases are asymptomatically excreted in the stool. Hand contamination by care-givers during routine care can result in transfer to the NICU environment or direct horizontal transmission

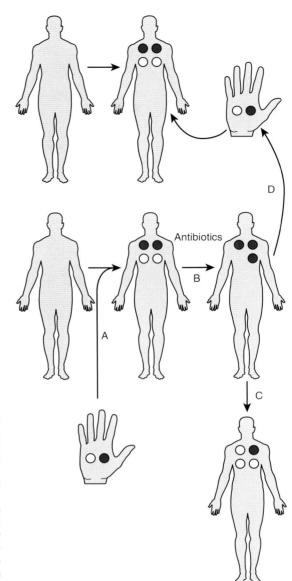

Fig. 14-1 Descriptive epidemiology of MDR-GNR in the NICU during a non-outbreak period. Infants are born uncolonized by Gram-negative bacilli and acquired their Gram-negative flora, both antibiotic-susceptible (open circles) and antibiotic-resistant (closed circles), from the NICU environment, largely through the hands of care-givers (A). Antibiotic exposure reduces susceptible bacilli while selecting resistant ones, increasing the density of the latter (B). In most infants the colonization by the resistant organism is transient and quickly replaced by susceptible and other resistant Gram-negative bacilli (C), but in some instances the resistant organism contaminates the hands of care-givers, who then transmit it to another infant (D).

to a non-colonized infant. In sum, then, the infant can acquire an MDR-GNR by several different mechanisms, namely, by exposure to an antibiotic which selects or induces a resistant subpopulation, or by acquisition from a contaminated external source, or both.

Epidemiology of MDR-GNR during Non-Outbreak Periods

Unlike MRSA, some aspects of the epidemiolo;gy of MDR-GNR during non-outbreak periods in the nursery have been defined (Fig. 14–1). Under normal circumstances fetal development occurs in the sterile intrauterine environment and the infant is born uncolonized. The gastrointestinal ecology of the healthy, non-hospitalized infant rapidly assumes great complexity, involving many different anaerobic and facultative species, including but not limited to *Bifidobacteria*, *Bacteroides*, *Clostridia*, enteric streptococci, *Veillonella*, *Bacillus* and *Lactobacillus*.

This gastrointestinal ecology is essentially established by the fifth day of life and remains stable over the next several months (24–27). It is likely that the normal flora at least partially prevents sustained colonization by pathogenic species such as those represented by MDR-GNRs.

Initial Colonization by Gram-negative Bacilli in the NICU (Figure 14–1, A and B)

The newborn admitted to the NICU does not have the opportunity to acquire normal colonizing flora from postnatal maternal contact and acquisition is not mediated by breast milk or formula in the newborn too ill to feed. The colonizing flora of the infant admitted to the NICU, therefore, is primarily influenced by the organisms present in that environment and by exposure to antibiotics. It is assumed that Gram-negative bacilli, both antibiotic-susceptible and resistant, initially are acquired by the patient via the contaminated hands of care-givers, since besides the mother's vaginal tract there are few other conceivable sources for these organisms. Studies performed decades ago indicated that hands of hospital care-givers frequently are positive for Gram-negative bacilli (28, 29). Hand cultures performed on NICU nurses in the early 1970s, for example, revealed bacillary contamination in over 86% of samples (29). The density of bacilli contaminating the hands of hospital care-givers tends to decrease during the course of the workday, lowered by repeated hand-washing, but increases in density outside the hospital as the permanent resident bacteria replicate (30). Not surprisingly, hand contamination by Gram-negative bacilli is especially associated with close patient contact or contact with bed linens, patient clothing, or body fluids, but Gram-negative bacteria can be isolated even from the hands of administrative staff who have limited patient contact (31, 32).

Goldmann and colleagues (33) were among the first to describe the ontogeny of bacterial colonization in the critically ill newborn. In their study approximately 50% of rectal and nasal swab specimens demonstrated no growth of any organism on admission to the NICU, and 16–30% of samples were still negative for growth by the third NICU day. The slow acquisition of a colonizing flora appeared to be the consequence of nearly uniform exposure to antibiotics upon admission to the NICU and to the relative paucity of contact with humans who were not hospital personnel (33). When colonization ultimately did occur, over half of the infants became colonized with *Klebsiella*, *Enterobacter*, or *Citrobacter* species, and once such organisms appeared they grew to high density (33). This abnormal ontogeny of stool flora among NICU residents compared with healthy infants has been confirmed by many subsequent studies (34–37).

Gain and Loss of MDR-GNR while in the NICU (Figure 14–1, C)

Once the NICU resident becomes colonized by a resistant Gram-negative organism, either by transmission directly from the environment or by selection of resistance after antibiotic exposure, usually colonization is inconsequential and short-lived. Recently we studied the acquisition of MDR-GNR in a tertiary care NICU in Cleveland, Ohio, over a 12-month period (38). Nasopharyngeal and rectal swab specimens were obtained three times a week and screened for Gram-negative bacilli resistant to gentamicin, piperacillin-tazobactam, or ceftazidime. A total of 8.6% of infants in the Cleveland NICU became colonized with a Gram-negative bacillus resistant to at least one of these agents before discharge. Antibiotic-resistant organisms were acquired from the first NICU day and acquisition then continued gradually and cumulatively throughout the infants' NICU course. When colonization with a resistant organism did occur it frequently was cleared rapidly, however, with the median duration less than a week (38), reflecting a particularly unstable microflora in this population.

Horizontal Transmission of MDR-GNR to other NICU Patients (Figure 14–1, D)

The degree of direct infant-to-infant transmission of Gram-negative bacilli during non-outbreak periods was addressed by two studies, our study in Cleveland (38) and a second conducted at Yale-New Haven Hospital (39). Both studies prospectively performed sequential rectal swab cultures on large numbers of NICU patients. The isolated organisms were subjected to PFGE analysis to determine the proportion of PFGE types that were present in more than one infant, suggesting person-to-person spread. Over 21% of infants colonized with an antibiotic-resistant Gram-negative bacterium in New Haven shared an organism with another NICU resident (39). In the Cleveland survey, approximately 12% of the 154 genetically distinct resistant bacilli were shared. In both studies horizontal transmission clustered among infants housed in the same room during overlapping periods but each cluster resolved without specific interventions. The clusters involved up to 11 infants at Yale but almost all cases of horizontal transmission in our institution involved only two infants (38, 39). These data suggest that undetected mini-epidemics of antibiotic-resistant Gram-negative bacilli probably occur routinely in busy referral NICUs but that they are small and self-limiting. The large majority of Gram-negative organisms acquired in the NICU are genetically unique, however, and are not acquired directly from another infant.

Epidemiology of MDR-GNR during Outbreaks

NICU outbreaks with antibiotic-resistant bacilli have been reported throughout the era of modern infant intensive care (40). Resistant organisms causing outbreaks have evolved over time, encompassing ever greater varieties of genera and resistance phenotypes. Recently reported NICU outbreaks have been caused primarily by *Enterobacter* (41–45), *Klebsiella* (46–48) and *Serratia* (49–52) that typically express resistance to one or more parenteral antibiotic commonly employed in the NICU. Over the past several years NICU outbreak reports have emphasized the importance of organisms expressing extended-spectrum β-lactamases (ESBLs) (45, 53–56). The plasmid-encoded ESBLs are most commonly found in *E. coli* and *Klebsiella*, although they are being increasingly identified in other genera as well. ESBL-producing organisms are particularly associated with therapeutic failures after treatment with recent generation ß-lactams, especially cephalosporins.

The epidemiologic characteristics of outbreaks of Gram-negative bacilli differ from those noted during endemic periods. After introduction of the epidemic strain into the unit, the clone spreads rapidly from infant to infant. Cross-sectional surveillance frequently reveals previously undetected colonization in a large proportion of infants. The strain characteristically persists, both in the individual patient but especially in the unit, over long periods; similar to MRSA, it is not unusual for colonization and infection by the epidemic strain to occur over months or even years. In outbreaks due to antibiotic-resistant organisms, acquisition of the epidemic clone is strongly associated with exposure to the antibiotic to which the bacillus is resistant.

Contrary to the endemic situation, where environmental contamination by Gram-negative bacilli is of low density, an outbreak clone frequently is readily cultured from one or more environmental sources that then serve to perpetuate the epidemic. Recent NICU outbreaks of Gram-negative bacilli have isolated the epidemic strain from rectal thermometers (44, 48), incubator doors (52), pulse oximeter probes (48), re-used suction catheters and laryngoscope blades (57, 58), breast pumps (57), and handwashing disinfectants (49). Additionally, outbreak clones have been identified from nutritional sources, including contaminated parenteral nutrition solutions (59) and formula (60).

CONTROL STRATEGIES FOR NON-EPIDEMIC MRSA AND MDR-GNR

There are few reports outside NICU outbreak descriptions that address the containment of MRSA and MDR-GNR in the NICU. Some potential strategies to control resistant organisms during endemic periods can be derived from expert opinion and experience in non-neonatal ICUs, however. Given the differences in their epidemiology, not all potential measures are applicable to both MRSA and MDR-GNR; each measure listed below (summarized in Table 14-1) is denoted accordingly.

(a) Prevent Infections (MRSA and MDR-GNR)

The key to preventing infections due to antibiotic-resistant organisms is to prevent all infections. Controlled studies in older populations indicate that the incidence of central catheter-related bloodstream infection is reduced by adequately training personnel in their insertion, for example (61). Furthermore, central catheter placement should be executed with the use of full sterile barrier protection and include sterile gloves and gowns and the use of a mask. Central catheters should be removed immediately when no longer required for care of the infant. Although few studies have examined ventilator-associated pneumonia in neonates (62), studies of other critically ill populations suggest that reducing aspiration events through supine positioning, limiting trips outside the intensive care unit while the baby is intubated, extubating as early as possible, and employing non-invasive ventilation when feasible, all reduce the risk of nosocomial pneumonia (63).

(b) Promote Regular Hand Hygiene (MRSA and MDR-GN)

In the absence of universal screening and prospective identification of all patients for antibiotic-resistant organisms (see below), an unrecognized reservoir of MRSA and MDR-GNR will virtually always exist in the NICU. Hand hygiene between all patient contacts, therefore, remains a principal component to the control of MRSA and MDR-GNR in the NICU. The organisms are sensitive to alcohol, and alcohol-based hand rubs have demonstrated efficacy in reducing the transmission of resistant bacteria outside the NICU. Pittet and colleagues (64), for example, introduced

---

Table 14-1   Measures to Reduce MRSA and MDR-GNR Colonization and Infection in the NICU

Endemic
Prevent infection
Promote hand hygiene
Apply barrier isolation to identified infants
Reserve equipment and decontaminate surfaces
Develop antibiotic policies
Perform pre-emptive surveillance

Epidemic
Strictly enforce and police hand hygiene
Cohort identified infants
Enforce strict barrier isolation
Assign all equipment to colonized versus non-colonized patients
Screen HCWs (MRSA)
Perform environmental cultures (MDR-GNR)
Restrict antibiotics (MDR-GNR)
Close the unit

alcohol hand rubs accompanied by an aggressive training and reinforcement campaign regarding their use in a hospital in Geneva, Switzerland. Overall compliance of hand hygiene increased from 48% to 66% over a 3-year observation period. During the same time, the hospital-wide incidence of all nosocomial infections decreased from 16.9% to 9.9% ($P < 0.04$) and MRSA infection in particular decreased from 2.16 to 0.93 infections/10 000 patient days ($P < 0.001$).

Recently the importance of diseased skin or long fingernails in promoting bacterial contamination of the hands of care-givers has been emphasized in NICUs. Studies by Hedderwick and colleagues (65) demonstrated that potentially pathogenic microorganisms are recovered more frequently and at higher density from artificial nails compared with short natural nails. Sometimes nail colonization can have frightening consequences in the NICU. A cluster of cases of *Pseudomonas* infection in the NICU at a tertiary care unit in New York City (66) led to investigations that uncovered three nurses with *Pseudomonas* hand colonization; one with onychomycosis harbored the same PFGE-type isolated from 17 different infants. An outbreak of *Pseudomonas aeruginosa* in an Oklahoma NICU identified colonization of long or artificial fingernails among nurses as an important source in a deadly epidemic (67).

(c) Instituting and Enforcing Maximal Barrier Protection

This includes gloves, gowns and, for MRSA, masks when caring for infants identified with colonization or infection by antibiotic-resistant organisms (MRSA and MDR-GNR). Most patient acquisition of MRSA in the hospital is the result of transmission from a colonized health care worker (HCW) and at least some acquisition of MDR-GNR is acquired in the same fashion. The hands and possibly the clothing of the HCW (68) are the likely culprits in most circumstances, underlining the requirement for glove and gown use when caring for a patient with established resistant-organism colonization or infection. In our hospital, barrier isolation is initiated for all patients colonized or infected with MRSA or Gram-negative bacteria resistant to two or more classes of antibiotic. It should be emphasized that hands frequently become contaminated when the gloves are removed. Therefore, hand hygiene must be applied upon de-gloving. MRSA colonization also may become established in the HCW's nares (3, 7, 8), which then serves as a reservoir for repeated hand contamination. This colonization can be prevented by the additional use of a mask.

(d) Decontamination of Environmental Surfaces (MRSA and MDR GNR)

The role of MRSA- and MDR-GNR-contaminated medical equipment and environmental surfaces in promoting transmission has not been well studied, but it is certain that such contamination occurs. Boyce and colleagues documented contamination of inanimate surfaces in over two-thirds of rooms occupied by MRSA-colonized adult patients (68). The HCW may acquire MRSA on his or her ungloved hand after contact with such contaminated surfaces, resulting in transmission to an unaffected patient. Even in the absence of clear evidence implicating contaminated fomites in the spread of MRSA and MDR-GNR in the nursery, it is prudent to assign medical equipment for exclusive use in the MRSA- and MDR-GNR-colonized infant and to thoroughly disinfect the immediate area once the patient has been discharged.

(e) Antibiotic Control (MDR-GNR)

There are no compelling data that antibiotic control limits the presence of MRSA. A portion of antibiotic resistance in MDR-GNR emerges under antibiotic pressure, however, suggesting that manipulation of antibiotics in the NICU may afford some benefit.

There are some data that document the relative propensity of different classes of antibiotics to promote bacillary resistance in the NICU. Many centers have used gentamicin in combination with ampicillin and vancomycin for well over a decade, for example, and have had few if any problems with resistance to aminoglycosides (69). Tullus and colleagues surveyed rectal swab samples from 22 Swedish nurseries through the late 1980s; (70) none of 1369 isolates of *E. coli*, *Klebsiella*, and *Enterobacter* screened during the course of this study was resistant to gentamicin, despite the routine use of this drug by many of the participating centers. The use of the third-generation cephalosporins, on the other hand, may be especially associated with the promotion of autologous resistance among Gram-negative species in the NICU. Indeed, it is well established that exposure to this class of antibiotics among seriously ill adults may rapidly select ß-lactam resistant Enterobacteriaceae, especially among *Enterobacters* (71) and ESBL-producing bacteria (55, 72). When cefotaxime was substituted for gentamicin in a NICU experiencing an outbreak of gentamicin-resistant *K. pneumoniae*, a high frequency of colonization with cephalosporin-resistant *E. cloacae* appeared after just 10 weeks (69). De Man and colleagues (73) studied the relative propensity of penicillin-tobramycin use and ampicillin-cefotaxime in promoting resistance in a Dutch NICU, employing a 6-month crossover design during which each regimen was used as the preferred first-line antibiotic choice in side-by-side nurseries. These investigators found a marked increase in colonization and infection by cephalosporin-resistant *E. cloacae* during the period of ampicillin-cefotaxime use, versus little aminoglycoside resistance during the penicillin-tobramycin periods. These experiences caution against routine sustained use of third-generation cephalosporins in the NICU during non-outbreak periods.

Stopping antibiotics in a patient in whom infection appears unlikely is probably effective in reducing colonization and infection with resistant organisms in all ICU settings. In the study by Singh and colleagues (74), adult ICU patients in whom a diagnosis of ventilator-associated pneumonia was suspected were evaluated by a pneumonia-infection score when therapy was initiated and again 3 days later. The investigators then used a persistently low score to identify patients in whom the diagnosis of pulmonary infection was unlikely, recognizing that in common practice such patients regularly are treated with a prolonged course of antibiotics anyway. This trial demonstrated that stopping antibiotics in low-risk patients at day 3 of therapy resulted in significantly lower acquisition of antibiotic-resistant organisms, without adversely affecting patient mortality and length of stay in the ICU, when compared with similar patients in whom antibiotic stoppage was not mandated (74).

Another strategy involving antibiotic control that has been proposed to reduce the prevalence of MDR-GNR in the ICU setting is "antibiotic cycling". This strategy mandates a regular, scheduled rotation in antibiotic preference within the ICU. We tested the benefit of antibiotic cycling in our NICU in Cleveland (75). A monthly rotation of gentamicin, piperacillin-tazobactam, and ceftazidime was compared with unrestricted antibiotic use in side-by-side NICU populations. Pharyngeal and rectal samples were obtained three times a week and tested for Gram-negative bacilli resistant to each of the antibiotics in the rotation schedule. Over a 1-year trial, cycling failed to reduce the prevalence of colonization by resistant Gram-negative rods: 10.7% infants in the population assigned to the antibiotic cycling schedule were colonized with an organism resistant to one or more of the rotation antibiotics, versus 7.7% of the control population ($P < 0.09$) (75). The incidences of nosocomial infection and mortality also were similar between study populations. While some trials of antibiotic cycling in adult ICUs have been more positive (76), more recent data in non-NICU patients have been less optimistic (77). Unfortunately, co-resistance to agents of different antibiotic classes is common in hospital-acquired Gram-negative bacilli and consequently changing from one broad-spectrum agent to another may not relieve antibiotic pressure. Additionally, some resistance determinants in MDR-GNRs are linked to other factors conferring survival advantage, such as those improving adherence to epithelial surfaces or resulting in resistance to disinfectants (78, 79), properties that will not be easily surrendered in the face of antibiotic cycling. As a result, it is unlikely that this strategy will have major impact in reducing the endemic presence of MDR-GNRs in the NICU.

(f) Pre-Emptive Surveillance and Isolation of all Patients for MRSA Colonization (MRSA)

Perhaps the most controversial potential strategy to control endemic MRSA currently debated among non-neonatologists is the routine performance of surveillance cultures in all patients upon hospital admission and at fixed intervals thereafter. Most authorities have estimated that the risk of MRSA transmission in adult ICUs is reduced 3–16-fold if the colonized subject is in isolation versus on the open ward (12, 80, 81). Recent mathematical models of MRSA transmission in the hospital have implicated the unidentified, and therefore non-isolated, MRSA-colonized patient as being the most influential factor in the spread of resistant staphylococci (80, 81).

In response to these observations, some European countries, most notably the Netherlands, have adapted a very aggressive national health institute-mandated policy for pre-emptive screening for MRSA that they have termed the "Search and Destroy" strategy. Hospital-wide, all patients are regularly screened for MRSA colonization upon admission, and those falling into pre-defined high-risk categories are isolated immediately with full barrier protection until proven MRSA-free. Patients at lesser risk similarly are isolated if colonization is subsequently identified. Identification of colonization in a patient who had not been isolated triggers immediate screening of all nearby patients and all exposed health care workers. The identification of secondary cases generates further screening. Identified health care workers are furloughed with pay until their colonization disappears. Infection control officers have the authority to close whole wards and even whole hospitals based upon surveillance data. The results are compelling: the incidence of nosocomial MRSA infections in Dutch facilities remains minuscule compared with that measured in North American hospitals.

The most pressing argument against implementing the Search and Destroy strategy in the NICU is that it is likely to have little impact unless the policy is applied hospital-wide. Without this universal application, a portion of the personnel who routinely work outside the NICU (for example, surgical staff and other non-neonatology consultants) may import the organism from other parts of the hospital where the control of MRSA is more lax (7). There perhaps is a stronger rationale to pre-emptively screen infants transferred from another hospital for MRSA colonization if they have been hospitalized at the referring unit for longer than a few hours. Indeed, in some circumstances pre-emptive screening of transferred infants for MDR-GNR has proved useful as well (50).

CONTROL STRATEGIES FOR NICU OUTBREAKS OF MRSA AND MDR-GNR

In many ways control of a nursery outbreak of an antibiotic-resistant organism is more straightforward than control of endemic disease. For both MRSA and

MDR-GNR, accumulated experience has recommended several maneuvers to contain an epidemic (Table 14-1) (40). These measures usually are instituted simultaneously or in rapid succession, so the independent contribution of each is unknown. It may be that no one intervention can succeed on its own and that successful containment requires application of a package of measures, including the following.

(a) Reinforce strict hand hygiene practices, including presentation of in-services and policing of adherence through overt and covert observation. Use of alcohol hand rubs is acceptable unless the hands are visibly soiled.

(b) Cohort colonized and infected patients. This measure usually requires that cross-sectional prevalence of colonization be defined by culturing at frequent and regular intervals (for example, once or twice a week). Culture-positive subjects then are moved to a geographically distinct area of the nursery. When staffing allows, nursing should be segregated so that each person cares only for colonized infants or for non-colonized infants. Segregation of physician and ancillary staff may be required as well.

(c) Establish and enforce strict barrier isolation precautions for all contact with a colonized or infected patient. This includes wearing gowns and gloves and, for MRSA, a mask, and changing protective gear with each new patient contact. Hand hygiene should be applied between each patient contact; that is, gloving and gowning does not preclude hand washing or use of alcohol-based hand gels. In the face of a rapidly progressive outbreak, barrier isolation may need to be applied to every infant in the NICU, regardless of colonization status, because cross-sectional prevalence audits may miss a small proportion of colonized infants.

(d) Assign medical equipment to individual colonized or infected patients or, if sharing cannot be avoided, segregate equipment to colonized versus non-colonized groups.

(e) If the above measures fail, close the unit to new admissions until the outbreak is contained.

Additional measures may be applied specifically to MRSA and MRD-GNR outbreaks, respectively. For MRSA epidemics:

(f) Screen HCWs for nasal colonization with MRSA and decontaminate when possible. The role of HCW MRSA nares colonization in sustaining an outbreak is uncertain, but there is growing opinion that it is important (12). In the ideal situation colonized HCWs are relieved of duties until colonization either spontaneously disappears or is eradicated. There has been anecdotal success using the following regimen for MRSA decontamination in the adult: mupirocin ointment to the nares 2–3 times/day for 5–7 days, chlorhexidine baths once a day for 3–5 successive days, and a course of systemic antibiotics including rifampin and another agent to which the isolate is susceptible (12).

For MDR-GNR epidemics:

(g) Perform environmental cultures to determine whether there is a common source for the outbreak strain. The need for these cultures depends to some extent on the organism. *Serratia marcesans* in particular has frequently been implicated in common-source epidemics.

(h) Restrict the use of antibiotics to which the outbreak strain is resistant.

REFERENCES

1. Cosgrove SE. The relationship between antimicrobial resistance and patient outcomes: mortality, length of hospital stay, and health care costs. Clin Infect Dis 42(Suppl 2):S82–89, 2006.
2. Back NA, Linnemann CC Jr, Staneck JL, Kotagal UR. Control of methicillin-resistant Staphylococcus aureus in a neonatal intensive-care unit: use of intensive microbiologic surveillance and mupirocin. Infect Control Hosp Epidemiol 17(4):227–231, 1996.
3. Haley RW, Cushion NB, Tenover FC, et al. Eradication of endemic methicillin-resistant Staphylococcus aureus infections from a neonatal intensive care unit. J Infect Dis 171(3):614–624, 1995.

4. Haddad Q, Sobayo EI, Basit OB, Rotimi VO. Outbreak of methicillin-resistant Staphylococcus aureus in a neonatal intensive care unit. J Hosp Infect 23(3):211–222, 1993.

5. Regev-Yochay G, Rubinstein E, Barzilai A, et al. Methicillin-resistant Staphylococcus aureus in neonatal intensive care unit. Emerg Infect Dis 11(3):453–456, 2005.

6. Karchmer TB, Durbin LJ, Simonton BM, Farr BM. Cost-effectiveness of active surveillance cultures and contact/droplet precautions for control of methicillin-resistant Staphylococcus aureus. J Hosp Infect 51(2):126–132, 2002.

7. Saiman L, Cronquist A, Wu F, et al. An outbreak of methicillin-resistant Staphylococcus aureus in a neonatal intensive care unit. Infect Control Hosp Epidemiol 24(5):317–321, 2003.

8. Graham DR, Correa-Villasenor A, Anderson RL, Vollman JH, Baine WB. Epidemic neonatal gentamicin-methicillin–resistant Staphylococcus aureus infection associated with nonspecific topical use of gentamicin. J Pediatr 97(6):972–978, 1980.

9. Campbell JR, Zaccaria E, Mason EO Jr, Baker CJ. Epidemiological analysis defining concurrent outbreaks of Serratia marcescens and methicillin-resistant Staphylococcus aureus in a neonatal intensive-care unit. Infect Control Hosp Epidemiol 19(12):924–928, 1998.

10. Toltzis P, Blumer JL. Antibiotic resistance. In: Feigin RD, Cherry JD, Demmler GL, Kaplan SL, eds. Textbook of pediatric infectious disease. Phildelphia: Saunders; 2004:2944-2964.

11. McDougal LK, Steward CD, Killgore GE, et al. Pulsed-field gel electrophoresis typing of oxacillin-resistant Staphylococcus aureus isolates from the United States: establishing a national database. J Clin Microbiol 41(11):5113–5120, 2003.

12. Muto CA, Jernigan JA, Ostrowsky BE, et al. SHEA guideline for preventing nosocomial transmission of multidrug-resistant strains of Staphylococcus aureus and enterococcus. Infect Control Hosp Epidemiol 24(5):362–386, 2003.

13. Khoury J, Jones M, Grim A, Dunne WM Jr, Fraser V. Eradication of methicillin-resistant Staphylococcus aureus from a neonatal intensive care unit by active surveillance and aggressive infection control measures. Infect Control Hosp Epidemiol 26(7):616–621, 2005.

14. Bratu S, Eramo A, Kopec R, et al. Community-associated methicillin-resistant Staphylococcus aureus in hospital nursery and maternity units. Emerg Infect Dis 11(6):808–813, 2005.

15. Hollis RJ, Barr JL, Doebbeling BN, et al. Familial carriage of methicillin-resistant Staphylococcus aureus and subsequent infection in a premature neonate. Clin Infect Dis 21(2):328–332, 1995.

16. Deresinski S. Methicillin-resistant Staphylococcus aureus: an evolutionary, epidemiologic, and therapeutic odyssey. Clin Infect Dis 40(4):562–573, 2005.

17. Lina G, Piemont Y, Godail-Gamot F, et al. Involvement of Panton-Valentine leukocidin-producing Staphylococcus aureus in primary skin infections and pneumonia. Clin Infect Dis 29(5):1128–1132, 1999.

18. Behari P, Englund J, Alcasid G, et al. Transmission of methicillin-resistant Staphylococcus aureus to preterm infants through breast milk. Infect Control Hosp Epidemiol 25(9):778–780, 2004.

19. Eckhardt C, Halvosa JS, Ray SM, Blumberg HM. Transmission of methicillin-resistant Staphylococcus aureus in the neonatal intensive care unit from a patient with community-acquired disease. Infect Control Hosp Epidemiol 24(6):460–461, 2003.

20. Saiman L, O'Keefe M, Graham PL 3rd, et al. Hospital transmission of community-acquired methicillin-resistant Staphylococcus aureus among postpartum women. Clin Infect Dis 37(10):1313–1319, 2003.

21. Healy CM, Hulten KG, Palazzi DL, et al. Emergence of new strains of methicillin-resistant Staphylococcus aureus in a neonatal intensive care unit. Clin Infect Dis 39(10): 1460–1466, 2004.

22. Kikuchi K, Takahashi N, Piao C, et al. Molecular epidemiology of methicillin-resistant Staphylococcus aureus strains causing neonatal toxic shock syndrome-like exanthematous disease in neonatal and perinatal wards. J Clin Microbiol 41(7):3001–3006, 2003.

23. Takahashi N, Nishida H, Kato H, et al. Exanthematous disease induced by toxic shock syndrome toxin 1 in the early neonatal period. Lancet 351(9116):1614–1619, 1998.

24. Hokama T, Imamura T. Members of the throat microflora among infants with different feeding methods. J Trop Pediatr 44(2):84–86, 1998.

25. Balmer SE, Scott PH, Wharton BA. Diet and faecal flora in the newborn: lactoferrin. Arch Dis Child 64(12):1685–1690, 1989.

26. Balmer SE, Wharton BA. Diet and faecal flora in the newborn: breast milk and infant formula. Arch Dis Child 64(12):1672–1677, 1989.

27. Benno Y, Sawada K, Mitsuoka T. The intestinal microflora of infants: composition of fecal flora in breast-fed and bottle-fed infants. Microbiol Immunol 28(9):975–986, 1984.

28. Casewell M, Phillips I. Hands as route of transmission for Klebsiella species. Br Med J 2(6098):1315–1317, 1977.

29. Knittle MA, Eitzman DV, Baer H. Role of hand contamination of personnel in the epidemiology of gram-negative nosocomial infections. J Pediatr 86(3):433–437, 1975.

30. Guenthner SH, Hendley JO, Wenzel RP. Gram-negative bacilli as nontransient flora on the hands of hospital personnel. J Clin Microbiol 25(3):488–490, 1987.

31. Pittet D, Dharan S, Touveneau S, et al. Bacterial contamination of the hands of hospital staff during routine patient care. Arch Intern Med 159(8):821–826, 1999.

32. Sanderson PJ, Weissler S. Recovery of coliforms from the hands of nurses and patients: activities leading to contamination. J Hosp Infect 21(2):85–93, 1992.

33. Goldmann DA, Leclair J, Macone A. Bacterial colonization of neonates admitted to an intensive care environment. J Pediatr 93(2):288–293, 1978.

34. Savey A, Fleurette J, Salle BL. An analysis of the microbial flora of premature neonates. J Hosp Infect 21(4):275–289, 1992.

35. Tullus K, Fryklund B, Berglund B, et al. Influence of age on faecal carriage of P-fimbriated Escherichia coli and other gram-negative bacteria in hospitalized neonates. J Hosp Infect 11(4):349–356, 1988.

36. Finelli L, Livengood JR, Saiman L. Surveillance of pharyngeal colonization: detection and control of serious bacterial illness in low birth weight infants. Pediatr Infect Dis J 13(10):854–859, 1994.

37. Eriksson M, Melen B, Myrback KE, et al. Bacterial colonization of newborn infants in a neonatal intensive care unit. Acta Paediatr Scand 71(5):779–783, 1982.

38. Toltzis P, Dul MJ, Hoyen C, et al. Molecular epidemiology of antibiotic-resistant gram-negative bacilli in a neonatal intensive care unit during a nonoutbreak period. Pediatrics 108(5):1143–1148, 2001.

39. Almuneef MA, Baltimore RS, Farrel PA, et al. Molecular typing demonstrating transmission of gram-negative rods in a neonatal intensive care unit in the absence of a recognized epidemic. Clin Infect Dis 32(2):220–227, 2001.

40. Toltzis P, Blumer JL. Antibiotic-resistant gram-negative bacteria in the critical care setting. Pediatr Clin North Am 42(3):687–702, 1995.

41. Fernandez-Baca V, Ballesteros F, Hervas JA, et al. Molecular epidemiological typing of Enterobacter cloacae isolates from a neonatal intensive care unit: three-year prospective study. J Hosp Infect 49(3):173–182, 2001.

42. Liu SC, Leu HS, Yen MY, et al. Study of an outbreak of Enterobacter cloacae sepsis in a neonatal intensive care unit: the application of epidemiologic chromosome profiling by pulsed-field gel electrophoresis. Am J Infect Control 30(7):381–385, 2002.

43. Kartali G, Tzelepi E, Pournaras S, et al. Outbreak of infections caused by Enterobacter cloacae producing the integron-associated beta-lactamase IBC-1 in a neonatal intensive care unit of a Greek hospital. Antimicrob Agents Chemother 46(5):1577–1580, 2002.

44. van Dijk Y, Bik EM, Hochstenbach-Vernooij S, et al. Management of an outbreak of Enterobacter cloacae in a neonatal unit using simple preventive measures. J Hosp Infect 51(1):21–26, 2002.

45. Talon D, Menget P, Thouverez M, et al. Emergence of Enterobacter cloacae as a common pathogen in neonatal units: pulsed-field gel electrophoresis analysis. J Hosp Infect 57(2):119–125, 2004.

46. Berthelot P, Grattard F, Patural H, et al. Nosocomial colonization of premature babies with Klebsiella oxytoca: probable role of enteral feeding procedure in transmission and control of the outbreak with the use of gloves. Infect Control Hosp Epidemiol 22(3):148–151, 2001.

47. Jeong SH, Kim WM, Chang CL, et al. Neonatal intensive care unit outbreak caused by a strain of Klebsiella oxytoca resistant to aztreonam due to overproduction of chromosomal beta-lactamase. J Hosp Infect 48(4):281–288, 2001.

48. Macrae MB, Shannon KP, Rayner DM, et al. A simultaneous outbreak on a neonatal unit of two strains of multiply antibiotic resistant Klebsiella pneumoniae controllable only by ward closure. J Hosp Infect 49(3):183–192, 2001.

49. Villari P, Crispino M, Salvadori A, Scarcella A. Molecular epidemiology of an outbreak of Serratia marcescens in a neonatal intensive care unit. Infect Control Hosp Epidemiol 22(10):630–634, 2001.

50. Fleisch F, Zimmermann-Baer U, Zbinden R, et al. Three consecutive outbreaks of Serratia marcescens in a neonatal intensive care unit. Clin Infect Dis 34(6):767–773, 2002.

51. Assadian O, Berger A, Aspock C, et al. Nosocomial outbreak of Serratia marcescens in a neonatal intensive care unit. Infect Control Hosp Epidemiol 23(8):457–461, 2002.

52. Jang TN, Fung CP, Yang TL, et al. Use of pulsed-field gel electrophoresis to investigate an outbreak of Serratia marcescens infection in a neonatal intensive care unit. J Hosp Infect 48(1):13–19, 2001.

53. Otman J, Cavassin ED, Perugini ME, Vidotto MC. An outbreak of extended-spectrum beta-lactamase-producing Klebsiella species in a neonatal intensive care unit in Brazil. Infect Control Hosp Epidemiol 23(1):8–9, 2002.

54. Lebessi E, Dellagrammaticas H, Tassios PT, et al. Extended-spectrum beta-lactamase-producing Klebsiella pneumoniae in a neonatal intensive care unit in the high-prevalence area of Athens, Greece. J Clin Microbiol 40(3):799–804, 2002.

55. Linkin DR, Fishman NO, Patel JB, et al. Risk factors for extended-spectrum beta-lactamase-producing Enterobacteriaceae in a neonatal intensive care unit. Infect Control Hosp Epidemiol 25(9):781–783, 2004.

56. Conte MP, Venditti M, Chiarini F, et al. Extended Spectrum Beta-Lactamase-producing Klebsiella pneumoniae outbreaks during a third generation cephalosporin restriction policy. J Chemother 17(1):66–73, 2005.

57. Jones BL, Gorman LJ, Simpson J, et al. An outbreak of Serratia marcescens in two neonatal intensive care units. J Hosp Infect 46(4):314–319, 2000.

58. Pillay T, Pillay DG, Adhikari M, et al. An outbreak of neonatal infection with Acinetobacter linked to contaminated suction catheters. J Hosp Infect 43(4):299–304, 1999.

59. Tresoldi AT, Padoveze MC, Trabasso P, et al. Enterobacter cloacae sepsis outbreak in a newborn unit caused by contaminated total parenteral nutrition solution. Am J Infect Control 28(3):258–261, 2000.

60. van Acker J, de Smet F, Muyldermans G, et al. Outbreak of necrotizing enterocolitis associated with Enterobacter sakazakii in powdered milk formula. J Clin Microbiol 39(1):293–297, 2001.

61. O'Grady NP, Alexander M, Dellinger EP, et al. Guidelines for the prevention of intravascular catheter-related infections. The Hospital Infection Control Practices Advisory Committee, Center for Disease Control and Prevention. Pediatrics 110(5):e51, 2002.

62. Apisarnthanarak A, Holzmann-Pazgal G, Hamvas A, et al. Ventilator-associated pneumonia in extremely preterm neonates in a neonatal intensive care unit: characteristics, risk factors, and outcomes. Pediatrics 112(6 Pt 1):1283–1289, 2003.

63. Chastre J, Fagon JY. Ventilator-associated pneumonia. Am J Respir Crit Care Med 165(7):867–903, 2002.

64. Pittet D, Hugonnet S, Harbarth S, et al. Effectiveness of a hospital-wide programme to improve compliance with hand hygiene. Infection Control Programme. Lancet 356(9238):1307–1312, 2000.

65. Hedderwick SA, McNeil SA, Lyons MJ, Kauffman CA. Pathogenic organisms associated with artificial fingernails worn by healthcare workers. Infect Control Hosp Epidemiol 21(8):505–509, 2000.

66. Foca M, Jakob K, Whittier S, et al. Endemic Pseudomonas aeruginosa infection in a neonatal intensive care unit. N Engl J Med 343(10):695–700, 2000.

67. Moolenaar RL, Crutcher JM, San Joaquin VH, et al. A prolonged outbreak of Pseudomonas aeruginosa in a neonatal intensive care unit: did staff fingernails play a role in disease transmission? Infect Control Hosp Epidemiol 21(2):80–85, 2000.

68. Boyce JM, Potter-Bynoe G, Chenevert C, King T. Environmental contamination due to methicillin-resistant Staphylococcus aureus: possible infection control implications. Infect Control Hosp Epidemiol 18(9):622–627, 1997.

69. Bryan CS, John JF Jr, Pai MS, Austin TL. Gentamicin vs cefotaxime for therapy of neonatal sepsis. Relationship to drug resistance. Am J Dis Child 139(11):1086–1089, 1985.

70. Tullus K, Burman LG. Ecological impact of ampicillin and cefuroxime in neonatal units. Lancet 1(8652):1405–1407, 1989.

71. Chow JW, Fine MJ, Shlaes DM, et al. Enterobacter bacteremia: clinical features and emergence of antibiotic resistance during therapy. Ann Intern Med 115(8):585–590, 1991.

72. Zaoutis TE, Goyal M, Chu JH, et al. Risk factors for and outcomes of bloodstream infection caused by extended-spectrum beta-lactamase-producing Escherichia coli and Klebsiella species in children. Pediatrics 115(4):942–949, 2005.

73. de Man P, Verhoeven BA, Verbrugh HA, et al. An antibiotic policy to prevent emergence of resistant bacilli. Lancet 355(9208):973–978, 2000.

74. Singh N, Rogers P, Atwood CW, et al. Short-course empiric antibiotic therapy for patients with pulmonary infiltrates in the intensive care unit. A proposed solution for indiscriminate antibiotic prescription. Am J Respir Crit Care Med 162(2 Pt 1):505–511, 2000.

75. Toltzis P, Dul MJ, Hoyen C, et al. The effect of antibiotic rotation on colonization with antibiotic-resistant bacilli in a neonatal intensive care unit. Pediatrics 110(4):707–711, 2002.

76. Gruson D, Hilbert G, Vargas F, et al. Strategy of antibiotic rotation: long-term effect on incidence and susceptibilities of Gram-negative bacilli responsible for ventilator-associated pneumonia. Crit Care Med 31(7):1908–1914, 2003.

77. Warren DK, Hill HA, Merz LR, et al. Cycling empirical antimicrobial agents to prevent emergence of antimicrobial-resistant Gram-negative bacteria among intensive care unit patients. Crit Care Med 32(12):2450–2456, 2004.

78. Fierer J, Guiney D. Extended-spectrum beta-lactamases: a plague of plasmids. JAMA 281(6):563–564, 1999.

79. Timmis KN, Gonzalez-Carrero MI, Sekizaki T, Rojo F. Biological activities specified by antibiotic resistance plasmids. J Antimicrob Chemother 18(Suppl C):1–12, 1986.

80. Raboud J, Saskin R, Simor A, et al. Modeling transmission of methicillin-resistant Staphylococcus aureus among patients admitted to a hospital. Infect Control Hosp Epidemiol 26(7):607–615, 2005.

81. Forrester M, Pettitt AN. Use of stochastic epidemic modeling to quantify transmission rates of colonization with methicillin-resistant Staphylococcus aureus in an intensive care unit. Infect Control Hosp Epidemiol 26(7):598–606, 2005.

Chapter 15

Neonatal Fungal Infections

Charles R. Sims, MD • Luis Ostrosky-Zeichner, MD, FACP

Candidiasis

Aspergillosis

Zygomycosis (Mucormycosis)

Other Fungi

Summary

Fungal infections are common in the neonate and present with a variety of clinical syndromes ranging from trivial mucocutaneous infection to life-threatening fungemia and deeply invasive mycoses. Fungi are ubiquitous environmental organisms which can be found free-living in the soil, on bird and mammalian feces, and in decaying organic matter. They are also frequently found in the hospital environment. Some species, such as *Candida*, are commensal organisms in the human oral cavity, gastrointestinal tract, genitourinary tract, and moist intertriginous skin folds. Neonates most often acquire the organisms from their mother during passage through the birth canal and in utero from hematogenous spread or ascending vaginal infection. They can also acquire the infections post-partum through inhalation, ingestion, direct inoculation into the skin, and exposure to the hospital environment. Most of the specific defects in the immune response allowing susceptibility to fungal infections in certain individual are unknown and are under investigation. Risk factors, clinical presentation, diagnosis, therapy, and prognosis vary with each species of fungus and will be discussed below. There are limited data for neonates and so some conclusions are drawn from adult and pediatric data.

CANDIDIASIS

Epidemiology

The reported frequency of *Candida* infections has increased, and candidemia now represents the fourth most common cause of nosocomial bloodstream infection in adults in the USA (1). The reported incidence of neonatal sepsis due to *Candida* varies between 0.57 and 1.28% of all neonatal intensive care admission and between 4.8 and 7.0% of neonates <1500 g (2–5).

The cost of candidemia is enormous in terms of loss of life and monetary loss. Attributable mortality in neonates <1500 g varies from 10.2 to 43% (3, 6). The specific species causing the infection appears to affect mortality, as demonstrated in a recent study of adult candidemia showing an attributable mortality rate of 44% in all patients and an increased mortality in *C. glabrata* (60%) and *C. tropicalis* (75%) infections (7). The estimated costs in the USA of treating a single adult episode of nosocomial candidemia are $34 123 per Medicare patient and $44 536 per private insurance patient (8). The current annual monetary cost of candidemia in the USA may be approaching $1 billion (9) taking into account that the above figures were calculated just after the introduction of fluconazole and prior to the widespread use of lipid preparations of amphotericin or the echinocandins.

Candida colonization may be acquired by the fetus during gestational development or at delivery while passing through the birth canal (10). Although as many as 25% of pregnant women experience vaginal candidiasis late in gestation, congenital candidiasis is rare. The literature contains many case reports and short series of congenitally acquired candidiasis (cutaneous and disseminated) with intact or ruptured membranes, placental involvement, and umbilical cord involvement (11–13). Many of these cases are associated with uterine foreign bodies, including intrauterine contraceptive devices and cervical cerclage sutures (14). Although maternal candidemia has been described, hematogenous spread to the fetus has not. In addition to the maternal–fetal transmission, *Candida* species are also found in the hospital environment in the air, on food, floors and other surfaces and objects, and on the hands of hospital personnel (15). Nosocomial spread among patients has been traced to hand carriage and to artificial nails (16–18). General risk factors for candidiasis are related to the specific site of infection and to the disease process and are summarized in Table 15-1.

Of the greater than 100 species of *Candida*, seven are well-known pathogens in humans, and many other species are described infrequently in epidemiological surveys, case reports, or short case series. Table 15-2 summarizes the overall frequency distribution of *Candida* species causing fungemia in neonates. Most neonatal series note a higher percentage of *C. parapsilosis* (up to 36% (19)) than adult series. Although *Candida albicans* remains the most common isolate, non-*albicans Candida* have greatly increased in frequency as the cause of invasive disease (20–22). Studies in neonates have shown a non-*albicans* rate between 35 and 79% (4, 23).

Diagnosis

There are currently multiple direct and indirect methods of diagnosing *Candida* infections (24). The indirect methods, unfortunately, have not yet been widely accepted for clinical use, and current direct diagnostic methods have sub-standard performance. Although *Candida* will grow in standard blood-culture bottles, detection and growth can be enhanced by pre-treating blood specimens by lysis and centrifugation (25, 26). Still, in the best of circumstances, cultures are negative in the presence of disseminated candidiasis in at least one-quarter to one-third of

Table 15-1	Risk Factors and Conditions Associated with Invasive Candidiasis	
Primary risk factors	**Associated conditions**
Prolonged antibiotic use	Birth weight less than 1000 g
Central venous catheter	Gestational age less than 32 weeks
ICU stay longer than 7 days	5 min Apgar < 5
Abdominal surgery	Gastrointestinal *Candida* colonization
Hyperalimentation	Nasogastric tubes
Acid-suppressing medications	Vaginal birth

From Saiman et al. (5) and Shetty et al. (139).

Table 15-2 Species Distribution (%) of Candida Bloodstream Isolates in Neonates and General Susceptibility of *Candida* Species to Antifungal Agents

Species	Frequency (%)	Fluc	Itra	Vori	5FC	Ampho	Caspo
C. albicans	53–70	S	S	S	S	S	S
C. parapsilosis	15–39	S	S	S	S	S	S (to I?)
C. glabrata	0–14	S-DD to R	S-DD to R	S to S-DD	S	S to I	S
C. tropicalis	0–16	S	S	S	S	S	S
C. krusei	0–3	R	S-DD to R	S to S-DD	I to R	S to I	S
Other *Candida* spp.	0–3	V	V	V	V	V	V

Frequency data from different surveillance studies (3–5, 139, 140–142). Fluc, fluconazole; Itra, itraconazole; Vori, voriconazole; 5FC, flucytosine; Ampho, amphotericin-B; Caspo, caspofungin; S, susceptible; S-DD, susceptible dose-dependent; I, intermediate; R, resistant; V, variable. Adapted from Pappas. PG, Rex JH, Sobel JD, et al. Guidelines for treatment of candidiasis. Clin Infect Dis 38(2):161–189, 2004.

cases (25). Once isolated, *C. albicans* can be presumptively identified in 90 min by germ tube formation. Other species may require 72 h to be identified by morphology and carbohydrate metabolism using many available commercial kits. Indirect methods for diagnosing *Candida* infections include detection of serologic markers and DNA (27). In adults, the most promising methods involve measuring serum mannan (28) and 1–3-beta-D-glucan (two cell-wall components) (29), enolase (a cytoplasmic enzyme) (30), antibodies against enolase and hsp90 (a stress protein) (31), and fungal metabolites such as D-arabinitol (32). Methods for detecting candidal DNA are also being investigated, but have not yet reached the clinical stage (33).

The clinician may be forced to treat empirically for candidiasis based on clinical suspicion and risk factors. The gold standard for the diagnosis of *Candida* infection is a positive culture from normally sterile body sites such as the blood, cerebrospinal fluid, joint aspirate, sterilely drained abscess or other sterile surgical specimen. Culture from tracheal aspirates, bronchoalveolar lavage fluid, exposed wounds, abdominal drains, epithelium, or other mucocutaneous sources are not diagnostic and cannot differentiate colonization from infection (34, 35). Heavy colonization is an important risk factor for development of deep candidiasis (36), but it must be interpreted with the rest of the clinical information in the individual patient and should not be the sole reason for treating with antifungal agents. Likewise, urine culture may be significant in the right clinical situation, but antibiotic administration and the presence of an indwelling urinary catheter are associated with asymptomatic urinary colonization with *Candida* (37), which does not require therapy.

Clinical Manifestations

Congenital Candidiasis

Congenital candidiasis is a rare complication caused by intrauterine *Candida* infection and presents with a spectrum of diseases depending on the maturity of the infant. In neonates >1000 g, the disease usually presents solely with cutaneous manifestation of erythematous macules, papules, and pustules that occasionally can form vesicles and bullae. Mortality is low (8%) in isolated cutaneous disease. Systemic disease, characterized by respiratory distress, leukocytosis, and positive blood, urine, or CSF culture, will occur in 10% of these infants and carries a high associated mortality. In neonates <1000 g, the disease presents with widespread desquamation, systemic disease is common (67%), and mortality is high (11). Risk factors include intrauterine foreign bodies such as intrauterine contraceptive devices and cervical cerclage sutures, as well as *Candida* chorioamnionitis, funisitis, or placental infection (13, 38). Congenital candidiasis develops in 16% of cases where examination of the placenta of infants shows evidence of *Candida* infection. These placental findings should prompt close neonatal evaluation.

Hematogenous Candidiasis

Hematogenous candidiasis may occur at the time of delivery or over the first few days of life in severe congenital candidiasis, or it may develop later as an acquired infection. The clinical presentation of hematogenous candidiasis is similar to that of bacterial sepsis, with respiratory distress and apnea being the prominent clinical signs. Fever, hypotension, and thrombocytopenia are also common. Hematogenous spread to multiple organs is commonly seen, with the skin (66%), CNS (64%), and retina (54%) being the most frequent areas affected (39). Persistence of candidemia greater than 24 h after achieving adequate antifungal dosing is associated with higher rates of end-organ disease and with higher mortality (40).

The routes of invasion of *Candida* can be divided into endogenous and exogenous. The endogenous route is the most important, as *Candida* infections originate predominantly from the patient's own colonizing organisms from the gastrointestinal tract and skin (22, 41). Infection, however, requires some defect in the normal host immunity. Breakdowns in mucosal barriers related to surgery, gastrointestinal injury in enterocolitis, and total parenteral nutrition (42) are examples. Cutaneous barriers are not well established in the fetus, allowing translocation (the likely mechanism in congenital candidiasis) and are disrupted in the neonate by central venous catheters, surgical wounds, and trauma. Cell-mediated immunity is not well developed in the neonatal period and is further inhibited by hyperglycemia and corticosteroids. Overgrowth of *Candida* in the gastrointestinal and genitourinary tracts occurs with antibiotic use and urinary catheterization. Critically ill neonates may have several of these defects at any given time.

There are two main theories regarding the mechanism responsible for candidemia. The first is translocation of colonizing *Candida* organisms across the gut epithelium. This theory is supported by multiple adult studies showing a relationship between the presence and density of colonization and increased rates of candidemia and correlation between the colonizing *Candida* strain and the strain isolated from the blood (41, 43–45). The second mechanism relates to the presence of intravenous catheters (46). Infection could be initiated by contamination of the catheter hub at the skin resulting in catheter infection or by transient candidemia from another source resulting in secondary catheter colonization/infection (41, 47). There is less evidence for catheters than for gut translocation being the primary source of candidemia, and the presence of central venous catheters may only serve as a marker for severity of illness. However, whether via primary or secondary infection, venous catheters are the prominent final site of *Candida* infection and can lead to longer candidemia, thrombophlebitis with seeding of organisms into the clot, and increased risk of disseminated disease (48, 49). Failure to promptly remove lines in candidemic neonates has been shown to lead to significantly higher mortality (50).

Exogenous routes of infection are infrequent but can be important depending on the site of contamination. Multiple related diseases have been described, including candidemia resulting from contaminated blood-pressure transducers, contaminated parenteral nutrition solutions and fluids (51, 52), and from healthcare workers' hands (16, 53).

Urinary Candidiasis

Although the urinary tract is normally a sterile site, asymptomatic colonization with *Candida* and other organisms is common, and culturing these from the urine may not have any clinical significance. Treatment of asymptomatic candiduria even in the presence of pyuria may hasten clearance of the candiduria, but does not change the overall natural history of the condition (54, 55). In candidemic neonates, secondary candiduria is seen in 40–70% and renal abscess in 0–14% (56). Primary urinary candidiasis is related to the presence of indwelling catheters, urinary tract instrumentation, diabetes, and steroid and antibiotic use. Clinical manifestations are varied, with a spectrum including benign colonization, urethritis, cystitis, pyelitis, fungus ball from papillary necrosis and sloughing, and perinephric or renal abscess (57). In the setting of urinary obstruction, instrumentation, or surgery, primary urinary candidiasis may rarely lead to disseminated infection (37).

Abdominal Candidiasis

Candida peritonitis is caused by two distinct clinical entities in the neonate, focal intestinal perforation and necrotizing enterocolitis. Although the clinical presentations may be similar, focal perforation lacks the X-ray findings and extensive bowel disease of necrotizing enterocolitis and is associated with lower birth weight infants. *Candida* is isolated from 44% of focal perforation cases as opposed to only 15% of necrotizing enterocolitis cases (58). *Candida* accounts for 8% of dialysis-related peritonitis in adults and is reported in infants undergoing peritoneal dialysis. *C. albicans* is the most commonly isolated species (59). Patients with dialysis-related *Candida* peritonitis usually present with fever, abdominal tenderness, cloudy dialysate, and peritoneal fluid neutrophil count >100 cells/mL and, if left untreated, may develop candidemia (60).

Endocarditis

Endocarditis involving the vena cava or cardiac valves occurs in approximately 5% of cases of candidemia (56), with reports as high as 13% (61). *C. albicans* accounts for one half of the *Candida* species (62). The mortality rate is lower than with other fungal causes of endocarditis, but it is still reported at up to 60%. Patients usually present with fever, respiratory distress, thrombocytopenia and a cardiac murmur (61). Risk factors include presence of a central venous catheter and prior antibiotic therapy (63) although cases without risk factors are described (64). Late development after fungemia has been described in adults after 22 months and has recently been described in neonatal endocarditis as well (65). Embolization is more common in *Candida* endocarditis than bacterial disease, occurring in two-thirds of cases (62).

Ocular Candidiasis

Ocular *Candida* infection can present as keratoconjuctivitis due to topical steroids or local trauma (66) or more importantly as chorioretinitis and endophthalmitis due to hematogenous seeding. Although retina involvement in candidemia is reported in 10–45% of adults (67–69) and 50% of neonates in older studies (70), more recent, large series have reported much lower rates of 0–17% in neonates (56, 71, 72). The lower rate may be due to earlier, more aggressive treatment of candidemia as end-organ involvement is associated with more prolonged candidemia (73). Ocular presentations may be the first manifestations of hematogenous disease or may develop after the diagnosis of candidemia (74, 75) and may lead to permanent blindness if not identified (76). The most common signs and symptoms are eye redness, hazy vitreous, pain, and diminished or blurry vision. Premature infants may be at higher risk of developing complicated ocular candidiasis (such as lens abscess) if candidemia occurs around 29 weeks post-conception as the lens structures lose their developmental arterial supply and become avascular and less likely to respond to systemic treatment (77). Endophthalmitis can present up to 2 weeks after the diagnosis of candidemia, and some authors have suggested that patients should have a dilated retinal exam at baseline and 2 weeks after the documentation of candidemia (74, 78). A recent consensus document, however, recommends that all patients with candidemia should have at least one careful retinal examination (79).

Central Nervous System Candidiasis

Candida infection of the CNS is usually secondary to hematogenous disease and presents as meningitis or brain abscess (80). Primary CNS disease is most commonly due to iatrogenic causes, including ventriculoperitoneal shunt placement (81). The rate of secondary *Candida* meningitis during candidemia is approximately 15%, with a range of 3–23% in the literature (56) and an overall rate of 0.4% of all neonatal ICU admissions (82). Symptoms of *Candida* meningitis are similar to bacterial meningitis and include fever, confusion, nuchal rigidity, and respiratory distress (83). CSF analysis generally shows hypoglycorrhachia. Pleocytosis and protein elevation is often mild or absent, and in one series, only 25% of patients any abnormality on CSF analysis (84). Another series confirms the lack of CSF abnormalities and further reported a negative Gram stain in 100% of cases and culture positive for *Candida* in only 74% (82). *Candida* brain abscess and ventriculitis is reported in 4% of neonates with candidemia (56). In adult patients who died of disseminated candidiasis, 50% were found to have *Candida* brain microabscesses at autopsy (85). These abscesses were not generally symptomatic, so the rate of brain microabscesses may be significantly higher than diagnosed.

Bone and Joint Candidiasis

Osteomyelitis and septic arthritis caused by *Candida* are usually the result of hematogenous spread, with primary disease being extremely rare and occurring in adults with inoculation of organisms into the area by trauma, during steroid injection into the joint, and during surgery (i.e. sternotomy or arthrotomy) (86–88). *Candida* accounts for 7–17% of cases of septic arthritis and osteomyelitis in neonates (89, 90). The literature consists of mostly case reports and small series showing *C. albicans* followed by *C. tropicalis* as the main isolates involved (91, 92). The most common symptom is localized pain, but soft tissue swelling with erythema, adjacent abscess and arthritis are also described. Fever and leukocytosis are usually absent. Large joints are most commonly affected, with at least one knee joint being involved in 71% of cases of polyarticular disease. In adults, synovial fluid microscopic analysis shows high white blood cells (15 000 to 100 000/mm^3) with polymorphonuclear cell predominance and visualization of the organisms in 20% of cases (24). Synovial fluid culture is positive in nearly 100% of cases (89). No data exist for neonates. The onset of symptoms of osteomyelitis may be concurrent with the candidemia or may present many months later. One case of neonatal *C. albicans* osteomyelitis is described 1 year after completion of presumed adequate therapy for candidemia (93).

Pulmonary Candidiasis

Although *Candida* is frequently isolated from multiple respiratory specimens, including sputum, bronchoalveolar lavage fluid, and endotracheal tube secretions, it is more commonly a colonizer than a pathogen in the seriously ill patient.

Definitive diagnosis is made by demonstrating fungal element invading the lung tissue. An adult study comparing various sampling modalities to autopsy in ICU patients showed a 40% colonization rate with only an 8% rate of *Candida* bronchopneumonia. The study also found no correlation between the type of sampling and the diagnosis of true pneumonia (34). The vast majority of true infection results from disseminated candidiasis causing seeding of the lungs. Notable exceptions are the rare cases of severe congenital candidiasis in which alveolitis is common (12) and direct lung exposure to *Candida*-infected amniotic fluid (94).

Mucocutaneous Candidiasis

Candida colonization occurs in 27% of neonates within the first week of life and approximately 8% will develop mucocutaneous candidiasis (10). Oropharyngeal infection (thrush) and axillary, intertriginous, perineal, and periumbilical dermatitis are the most common presentations. These diseases are usually self-limited and do not require therapy. Topical therapy is effective at clearing these sites of infection within 1 week; however, the infection commonly recurs after cessation of therapy. The importance of these mild forms of candidiasis lies in the fact that the rate of invasive candidiasis (of any type) is significantly higher in neonates with mucocutaneous disease. Rates may be as high as 32% in neonates <1000 g and do not decrease with topical treatment (39).

One severe form of mucocutaneous disease is invasive fungal dermatitis, which occurs in the smallest, most premature infants. Presentation occurs from 6–14 days of life with erosive, crusting lesions demonstrating fungal invasion beyond the stratum corneum on pathology. *C. albicans* is the most common etiology, but other *Candida* species, as well as other fungi, can cause the disease. Risk factors include prematurity, post-natal steroid administration, and hyperglycemia, and dissemination occurs in 69% of *Candida* cases (95).

Treatment

The decision on whether or not to treat candidiasis and with what agent depends on multiple factors, including the site of the infection, the clinical status of the patient, the toxicity of the medications, and the species of *Candida* isolated. Empiric therapy is warranted in some situations, while identification to the species level is critical in others. The Infectious Disease Society of America (IDSA) has recently issued guidelines based on the supporting evidence for the treatment of candidemia and invasive candidiasis (79), but only a small number of recommendations involve neonates as only a few small trials exist in this population. The most commonly used therapy is amphotericin B due to its long history of use and relative safety in the neonatal population. A significant number of data are accumulating for fluconazole, and most recently studies involving the echinocandins and lipid preparations of amphotericin B are being reported. Table 15-3 presents specific treatment recommendations for forms of invasive candidiasis.

As discussed earlier, the emergence of non-*albicans* species and the developing of acquired resistance may change the selection of antifungal agents for empiric treatment. Antifungal susceptibility testing is now an important piece of microbiological data to guide therapy. Clinical interpretive breakpoint MICs are available for fluconazole, itraconazole, voriconazole, and flucytosine (79). No interpretive breakpoints have been established for amphotericin B and its lipid preparations, the echinocandins, or the newer triazoles (posaconazole), but MIC data are available for these compounds for the pathologic *Candida* species (96). Table 15-2 summarizes the general susceptibility patterns of the most common pathologic species of *Candida*. Although susceptibility can usually be predicted knowing the species of the organism,

Table 15-3 Recommended Treatment for Specific Forms of Invasive Candidiasis

Condition	Specific comments
Candidemia and disseminated candidiasis	Candidemia and disseminated diseases are treated in a similar manner and options include: amphotericin B deoxycholate (0.6–1.0 mg/kg/day), lipid preparations of amphotericin B (3–5 mg/kg/day), fluconazole (6–12 mg/kg/day) (143), caspofungin (2 mg/kg/day) (100), micafungin (3 mg/kg/day) (144), or a combination of fluconazole and amphotericin B. Treatment should continue for 14 days after sterilization of blood cultures in candidemia. All central venous catheters should be removed
Abdominal candidiasis	*Candida* peritonitis should be treated with surgical drainage and intravenous amphotericin B or oral/intravenous fluconazole (6–12 mg/kg/day) (145, 146) for 2–6 weeks or until resolution of abscesses. The use of intraperitoneal amphotericin B is not recommended due to chemical peritonitis, pain, and fibrosis (147, 148). Most authorities recommend the removal of peritoneal dialysis catheters (149)
Endocarditis	*Candida* endocarditis requires a combination of surgery and systemic antifungal therapy. The recommended antifungal regimen is amphotericin B (deoxycholate or lipid formulation) for 1–2 weeks prior to and 6–8 weeks after surgery followed by fluconazole suppression for up to 2 years, although the doses and duration have not yet been established. Long-term flucytosine may be added to the regimen. Removal of pacemakers is almost always required.
Endophthalmitis	Ocular candidiasis requires immediate treatment to prevent blindness. Treatment option include: systemic amphotericin B (0.7–1.0 mg/kg/day) with or without flucytosine, and intravitreal amphotericin B (0.005 mg/0.01 mL) with or without pars plana vitrectomy (76, 150, 151), and fluconazole at 12 mg/kg/day until clinical response, then 6 mg/kg/day until 2 weeks after resolution of all signs and symptoms of infection (24). Experiences with voriconazole and caspofungin are encouraging (152). Patients with artificial lens implants may require these to be removed to achieve a cure (153)
Osteomyelitis and arthritis	*Candida* osteomyelitis requires surgical drainage and debridement of devitalized bone (90). Therapy with fluconazole (6–12 mg/kg/day) or amphotericin B with or without flucytosine for 6 weeks to 6 months (88, 92, 154, 155)
Central nervous system	The recommended treatment for *Candida* meningitis is systemic amphotericin B (0.5–1.0 mg/kg/day) plus flucytosine (100–200 mg/kg/day) (80, 156). An alternate therapeutic regimen consists of fluconazole (6–12 mg/kg/day) plus flucytosine. Case reports exist of refractory meningitis treated successfully with caspofungin (157). Treatment should continue until resolution of all signs and symptoms of meningitis. Brain abscess is associated with hematogenous disease and should be treated in a similar manner. If the brain abscess is large and causing focal symptoms, drainage may be indicated
Urinary candidiasis	Asymptomatic candiduria in a catheterized patient is usually a transient, benign condition that does not require antifungal therapy. Clearance of candiduria can be seen in 40% of patients simply by removing the urinary catheter and stopping antibiotics (55). The risk of invasive candidiasis is low in this setting with the exception of candiduria after renal transplantation (37) and patients in whom urologic instrumentation or surgery is planned. These patients can be treated with amphotericin B bladder irrigation or with systemic amphotericin B, flucytosine, or fluconazole (158). Also keep in mind that in a high-risk host, candiduria may be the only manifestation of disseminated candidiasis

one recent study has recommended susceptibility testing for *Candida* bloodstream isolates in the setting of prior azole use, recurrent mucosal disease, in deep infections requiring prolonged therapy (i.e., osteomyelitis, endocarditis, abscess), and in establishing local antibiograms to guide therapy in specific institutions (97).

Candidemia and General Guidelines

Initial management options in candidemia include amphotericin B deoxycholate (0.6–1.0 mg/kg/day), lipid preparations of amphotericin B (3–5 mg/kg/day), fluconazole (5–12 mg/kg/day), caspofungin (2 mg/kg/day), micafungin (3 mg/kg/day), or a combination of fluconazole and amphotericin B. The selection of therapy should depend on the presence of organ dysfunction affecting drug clearance, relative drug toxicity, the prior exposure to antifungal agents for therapy or prophylaxis, and the physician's knowledge of the species and potential susceptibility pattern of the isolate.

For a clinically unstable patient with an unknown isolate, many authorities recommend amphotericin B deoxycholate (98, 99) or lipid preparation (3), or an echinocandin in this setting as these agents are rapidly fungicidal. Caspofungin has been safe and effective in clearing fungemia in amphotericin-refractory disease from multiple sources (100). Although caspofungin is a good first-line agent in this setting, chronic use has resulted in resistance in *C. parapsilosis* (101). This should be considered if patients have been heavily pretreated with caspofungin and are at risk for this species. Neonates have been shown to clear echinocandins more quickly than children and adults (102, 103) and so the doses used must be higher for neonates. High-dose fluconazole has also been shown to be effective in this clinical setting (104), although it is a fungistatic agent. For those neonates with prior azole treatment or prophylaxis or for those patients whose mother received azoles for vaginal candidiasis in pregnancy, another class of agents should be considered. Voriconazole has been recently approved by the FDA for the treatment of candidemia in non-immunocompromised adults after a large clinical trial using amphotericin B as the comparator showed similar efficacy (105). A single case report exists for successfully using voriconazole (6 mg/kg every 8 h) in combination with liposomal amphotericin for a neonate with refractory candidemia (106). No pharmacodynamic information exists for voriconazole in neonates, but the increased frequency of dosing resulted in levels similar to those used to treat adult infection.

Refractory candidemia should prompt clinicians to evaluate several possibilities. Ensuring the accuracy of the diagnosis is the critical first step in evaluating refractory disease. Next, the dose of medication should be examined, as underdosing, particularly with azoles, is responsible for refractory disease and the development of resistance. Few data exist for pharmacokinetics of antifungals other than fluconazole in neonates, but what data are available generally show shorter half-lives as compared to adults given traditional doses. Once the above factors have been considered, a new drug regimen can be developed. Combination therapy with agents with different mechanisms of activity can also be considered in patients refractory to monotherapy. Combinations with flucytosine-amphotericin, flucytosine-azole, amphotericin-azole, and azole-echinocandin have been tried in adults with varying results (107). The only large-scale trial of combination therapy showed that fluconazole (12 mg/kg/day) plus amphotericin B (0.7 mg/kg/day) was not antagonistic compared to fluconazole alone. The combination showed a trend toward more rapid clearance of candidemia and successful treatment ($P = 0.043$), particularly in patients who were not at the extremes of the severity scores (108). All neonatal data on combination therapy come from single case reports.

In addition to antifungal chemotherapy, several other issues should be considered in the management of fungemia. Removal of any intravenous catheters or other implants should occur as soon as clinically possible, as this has been associated with lower mortality (50). A dilated ophthalmologic exam should be performed after resolution of candidemia to exclude endophthalmitis (74, 75) as this diagnosis would alter the length of therapy.

Prevention

Infection Control

Candida colonization of the hands and fingernails of health care workers, transmission of *Candida* from health care worker to patients, and transmission from patient to patient via health care workers' hands have all been documented, as discussed above. Hand hygiene, either via washing with soap and water (109) or use of alcohol gels, can reduce health care worker carriage and transmission to patients. Furthermore, outbreaks have been linked to the use of artificial nails (110), and the wearing of artificial nails should be restricted in the neonatal ICU. Transmission of *Candida* to patients has also been described via infusion of intravenous fluids and total parenteral nutrition solutions and via intravascular devices and surgical instruments. Proper handling of instruments and proper techniques in sterilizing and preparing these instruments and fluids can reduce nosocomial infection.

Chemoprophylaxis

Antifungal prophylaxis with intravenous fluconazole (6 mg/kg/day) starting during the first 5 days of life and continuing for f4–6 weeks has been shown to reduce *Candida* colonization and the rate of invasive candidiasis in neonates <1000 g (2, 111) and <1500 g (112). Colonization and invasive infection still occurred, but at lower rates. A significant lowering of mortality was demonstrated in infants <1000 g receiving prophylaxis, and a trend toward lower mortality was seen in those <1500 g. No increase in development of resistant strains of *Candida* was noted and no adverse events or toxicity was reported.

In the neonatal ICU, antifungal chemoprophylaxis should be administered to premature infants (<32 weeks) with any additional risk factor for invasive candidiasis, including central venous catheter, broad-spectrum antibiotics (especially third-generation cephalosporins), post-natal steroids, abdominal surgery, enterocolitis, total parenteral nutrition, and skin/mucosal defects (113). Alternative clinical prediction rules are under development in adults (114).

ASPERGILLOSIS

Epidemiology

Aspergillosis is a rare infection of the neonate but appears to be an emerging clinical entity as medical advances allow for the survival of more immature neonates (115). The organism is found throughout the world in grains and decaying organic matter. Many species exist but only eight have been found to be pathogens in humans. *A. fumigatus* and *A. flavus* are the most common. The disease ranges from isolated cutaneous disease to invasive pulmonary disease to disseminated aspergillosis. Most cases appear to be nosocomial in origin, with contact with contaminated medical equipment (116) and inhalation of spores (117) being identified sources. Risk factors include prematurity, chronic granulomatous disease, post-natal steroid administration, neutropenia, and environmental exposure (such as construction in the NICU) (118).

Clinical Manifestations

Primary cutaneous aspergillosis can develop as a maculopapular rash at the site of inoculation or contamination which later becomes scaling and pustular. Neonates with invasive pulmonary disease may have nasal sinusitis or have nodular infiltrates on chest radiographs and a clinical picture of pneumonia which does not respond to antibiotic therapy. Hepatosplenomegaly, jaundice, and skin lesions are common findings in disseminated disease. These skin lesions tend to be nodular, hyperpigmented to purple, and tend to ulcerate.

Diagnosis

Diagnosis is made by culturing the organism from a sterile site or by demonstrating invading fungal elements on tissue biopsy. Simply culturing *Aspergillus* from the skin or a pulmonary sample is not diagnostic as this is a common environmental pathogen. Blood cultures are usually negative. In adults, serologic test for galacto-mannan can be helpful in diagnosis, but data in neonates show an extremely high false-positive rate, making this test useless for diagnosis (119, 120).

Treatment

Treatment for primary cutaneous disease is surgical debridement along with systemic antifungal therapy, and the prognosis is good. There are case reports of cure with medical therapy alone (121). Invasive pulmonary aspergillosis and disseminated aspergillosis require systemic antifungal therapy. The prognosis in adults is poor, with survival between 14 and 71% depending on the underlying co-morbidity. Prognosis in neonates may be better as the largest review reports a survival of 73–88% (118, 122). Traditionally amphotericin B deoxycholate has been the treatment of choice. There are few neonatal data with lipid preparations of amphotericin in neonates, but some pediatric data showing lower toxicity (122). Presumably they should be as effective and potentially more effective due to the lower toxicity and ability to treat at higher doses and for longer duration in this severe, refractory disease. Recently, voriconazole and caspofungin have been approved for treatment of aspergillosis in adults for primary and salvage therapy. Voriconazole was found to be superior to amphotericin B in one study in immunocompromised patients (123) and has been used in combination with amphotericin successfully in the pediatric population (124). There are no data for the use of caspofungin in neonates with aspergillosis.

Currently, there are no controlled clinical trials to support combination therapy in invasive aspergillosis.

ZYGOMYCOSIS (MUCORMYCOSIS)

Epidemiology

Infections caused by the zygomycetes are another rare but emerging infection in the neonate (115). The organisms are found throughout the world in the soil, on animal feces, and on fruits. Most infections in the neonate are nosocomial and arise from ingestion or contact with contaminated objects. Cutaneous cases have been described from elastic tape used to secure umbilical catheters and monitoring devices (125) and wooden tongue depressors used as arm boards (126), and disseminated cases described from infusion of contaminated fluids (127). Other sporadic cases of neonatal cutaneous zygomycosis have been reported without a specific cause. In addition to traumatic inoculation or contact with contaminated materials, risk factors include prematurity, diabetes mellitus especially with ketoacidosis, immunosuppression, and neutropenia. Cases have been seen in neonates with acidosis due to conditions other than diabetes (128, 129).

Clinical Manifestations

Cutaneous zygomycosis manifests itself as a rapidly progressing cellulitis with black, necrotic ulceration. Destruction of deep tissue is rapid and sepsis can develop if not treated aggressively. Another disease manifestation in neonates is colonic zygomycosis, in which infants present with sepsis and peritonitis. Necrotic colon with perforation is found on surgery with fungal elements invading the tissues on histopathology. The diagnosis is difficult to make preoperatively, and mortality is very high (130). Disseminated disease occurs in neonates, but the rhinocerebral presentation most often associated with zygomycosis in adults is not reported in any patients younger than 8 months old (131).

Treatment

Aggressive surgical debridement is the cornerstone of therapy for isolated cutaneous disease. Systemic amphotericin in combination with surgery has shown the highest survival rates for this disease in adults (132), but there are case reports of successful treatment of cutaneous disease in the neonate with medical management alone (133). Colonic and disseminated infections require systemic antifungal therapy. Recent literature in adults shows lipid formulations of amphotericin to be successful for treatment. With less toxicity than amphotericin B, these preparations can be used for the longer periods of time (up to 6 weeks) and with the higher doses (up to 12 mg/kg/day) (134). Voriconazole should not be used in this infection as it has little activity against the zygomycetes and the disease has been repeatedly described in adult patients as a breakthrough mycosis on voriconazole prophylaxis (135).

OTHER FUNGI

Several other fungi have been described in a few case reports in neonates, including *Cryptococcus*, *Blastomycetes*, Histoplasma. Of these, *Cryptococcus* most frequently caused severe infections in pregnant women. In these cases of pneumonia and meningitis, there was no evidence of transplacental spread to the neonate (136). Although less common, cases of transplacental spread have been reported during maternal histoplasmosis (137) and blastomycosis (138).

SUMMARY

The incidence of neonatal mycoses is rising and will continue to rise as advances in medical therapies lead to an increased number of surviving premature infants requiring prolonged ICU care and increased use of invasive devices and catheters. There are several agents available to treat mycoses, including amphotericin B deoxycholate and its lipid preparations, caspofungin, micafungin, fluconazole, itraconazole, and voriconazole, and each will probably have a role in specific scenarios. The role of combination drug therapy is still being evaluated but may improve the outcome especially in breakthrough and refractory infections. The increased use of prophylaxis will prevent the more common types of mycoses but may increase selection for more resistant species in the future. The role of serologic markers for earlier diagnosis will lead to development of pre-emptive rather than prophylactic treatment strategies, resulting in lower utilization of drugs, lower toxicity, and less resistance.

REFERENCES

1. Pfaller MA, Jones RN, Messer SA, et al. National surveillance of nosocomial blood stream infection due to Candida albicans: frequency of occurrence and antifungal susceptibility in the SCOPE Program. Diagn Microbiol Infect Dis 31 (1):327–332, 1998.
2. Healy CM, Baker CJ, Zaccaria E, Campbell JR. Impact of fluconazole prophylaxis on incidence and outcome of invasive candidiasis in a neonatal intensive care unit. J Pediatr 147 (2):166–171, 2005.
3. Lopez Sastre JB, Coto GD, Cotallo, Fernandez Colomer B. Neonatal invasive candidiasis: a prospective multicenter study of 118 cases. Am J Perinatol 20 (3):153–163, 2003.

4. Roilides E, Farmaki E, Evdoridou J, et al. Neonatal candidiasis: analysis of epidemiology, drug susceptibility, and molecular typing of causative isolates. Eur J Clin Microbiol Infect Dis 23 (10):745–750, 2004.

5. Saiman L, Ludington E, Pfaller M, et al. Risk factors for candidemia in Neonatal Intensive Care Unit patients. The National Epidemiology of Mycosis Survey study group. Pediatr Infect Dis J 19 (4):319–324, 2000.

6. Ronnestad A, Abrahamsen TG, Medbo S, et al. Late-onset septicemia in a Norwegian national cohort of extremely premature infants receiving very early full human milk feeding. Pediatrics 115 (3):e269–e276, 2005.

7. Safdar A, Bannister TW, Safdar Z. The predictors of outcome in immunocompetent patients with hematogenous candidiasis. Int J Infect Dis 8 (3):180–186, 2004.

8. Rentz AM, Halpern MT, Bowden R. The impact of candidemia on length of hospital stay, outcome, and overall cost of illness. Clin Infect Dis 27 (4):781–788, 1998.

9. Miller LG, Hajjeh RA, Edwards JE Jr. Estimating the cost of nosocomial candidemia in the united states. Clin Infect Dis 32 (7):1110, 2001.

10. Baley JE, Kliegman RM, Boxerbaum B, Fanaroff AA. Fungal colonization in the very low birth weight infant. Pediatrics 78 (2):225–232, 1986.

11. Darmstadt GL, Dinulos JG, Miller Z. Congenital cutaneous candidiasis: clinical presentation, pathogenesis, and management guidelines. Pediatrics 105 (2):438–444, 2000.

12. Baud O, Boithias C, Lacaze-Masmonteil T, et al. (Maternofetal disseminated candidiasis and high-grade prematurity). Arch Pediatr 4 (4):331–334, 1997.

13. Qureshi F, Jacques SM, Bendon RW, et al. Candida funisitis: A clinicopathologic study of 32 cases. Pediatr Dev Pathol 1 (2):118–124, 1998.

14. Baley JE, Silverman RA. Systemic candidiasis: cutaneous manifestations in low birth weight infants. Pediatrics 82 (2):211–215, 1988.

15. Saiman L, Ludington E, Dawson JD, et al. Risk factors for Candida species colonization of neonatal intensive care unit patients. Pediatr Infect Dis J 20 (12):1119–1124, 2001.

16. Finkelstein R, Reinhertz G, Hashman N, Merzbach D. Outbreak of Candida tropicalis fungemia in a neonatal intensive care unit. Infect Control Hosp Epidemiol 14 (10):587–590, 1993.

17. Saxen H, Virtanen M, Carlson P, et al. Neonatal Candida parapsilosis outbreak with a high case fatality rate. Pediatr Infect Dis J 14 (9):776–781, 1995.

18. Huang YC, Lin TY, Leu HS, et al. Outbreak of Candida parapsilosis fungemia in neonatal intensive care units: clinical implications and genotyping analysis. Infection 27 (2):97–102, 1999.

19. Giusiano GE, Mangiaterra M, Rojas F, Gomez V. Yeasts species distribution in Neonatal Intensive Care Units in northeast Argentina. Mycoses 47 (7):300–303, 2004.

20. Abi-Said D, Anaissie E, Uzun O, et al. The epidemiology of hematogenous candidiasis caused by different Candida species. Clin Infect Dis 24 (6):1122–1128, 1997.

21. Krcmery V, Barnes AJ. Non-albicans Candida spp. causing fungaemia: pathogenicity and antifungal resistance. J Hosp Infect 50 (4):243–260, 2002.

22. Pfaller MA. Epidemiology of candidiasis. J Hosp Infect 30 (Suppl):329–338, 1995.

23. Gupta N, Mittal N, Sood P, et al. Candidemia in neonatal intensive care unit. Indian J Pathol Microbiol 44 (1):45–48, 2001.

24. Anaissie E, McGinnis MR, MA Pfaller, eds. Clinical Mycology, 1st edn. Philadelphia: Elsevier Science :195-239, 2003.

25. Berenguer J, Buck M, Witebsky F, et al., Lysis-centrifugation blood cultures in the detection of tissue-proven invasive candidiasis. Disseminated versus single-organ infection. Diagn Microbiol Infect Dis 17(2):103-109, 1993.

26. Noda T, Kohno S, Mitsutake K, et al. (Basic and clinical evaluation of lysis centrifugation in candidemia). Kansenshogaku Zasshi 69 (2):145–150, 1995.

27. Yamaguchi H. (Advances in serological systems for diagnosis of systemic fungal infections, particularly those caused by Candida and Aspergillus). Nippon Ishinkin Gakkai Zasshi 43 (4):215–231, 2002.

28. Rimek D, Redetzke K, Singh J, et al. (Performance of the Candida mannan antigen detection in patients with fungemia.). Mycoses 47 (Suppl 1):23–26, 2004.

29. Miyazaki T, Kohno S, Mitsutake K, et al. Plasma (1–>3)-beta-D-glucan and fungal antigenemia in patients with candidemia, aspergillosis, and cryptococcosis. J Clin Microbiol 33 (12):3115–3118, 1995.

30. Walsh TJ, Hathorn JW, Sobel JD, et al. Detection of circulating candida enolase by immunoassay in patients with cancer and invasive candidiasis. N Engl J Med 324 (15):1026–1031, 1991.

31. Reiss E, Obayashi T, Orle K, et al. Non-culture based diagnostic tests for mycotic infections. Med Mycol 38 (Suppl 1):147–159, 2000.

32. Walsh TJ, Merz WG, Lee JW, et al. Diagnosis and therapeutic monitoring of invasive candidiasis by rapid enzymatic detection of serum D-arabinitol. Am J Med 99 (2):164–172, 1995.

33. Alexander BD. Diagnosis of fungal infection: new technologies for the mycology laboratory. Transpl Infect Dis 4 (Suppl 3):32–37, 2002.

34. el-Ebiary M, Torres A, Fabregas N, et al. Significance of the isolation of Candida species from respiratory samples in critically ill, non-neutropenic patients. An immediate postmortem histologic study. Am J Respir Crit Care Med 156 (2 Pt 1):583–590, 1997.

35. Cornwell EE 3rd, Belzberg H, Offne TV, et al. The pattern of fungal infections in critically ill surgical patients. Am Surg 61 (10):847–850, 1995.

36. Safdar A, Armstrong D. Prospective evaluation of Candida species colonization in hospitalized cancer patients: impact on short-term survival in recipients of marrow transplantation and patients with hematological malignancies. Bone Marrow Transplant 30 (12):931–935, 2002.

37. Ang BS, Telenti A, King B, et al. Candidemia from a urinary tract source: microbiological aspects and clinical significance. Clin Infect Dis 17 (4):662–666, 1993.

38. Delprado WJ, Baird PJ, Russell P. Placental candidiasis: report of three cases with a review of the literature. Pathology 14 (2):191–195, 1982.

39. Faix RG, Kovarik SM, Shaw TR, Johnson RV. Mucocutaneous and invasive candidiasis among very low birth weight (less than 1,500 grams) infants in intensive care nurseries: a prospective study. Pediatrics 83 (1):101–107, 1989.

40. Chapman RL, Faix RG. Persistently positive cultures and outcome in invasive neonatal candidiasis. Pediatr Infect Dis J 19 (9):822–827, 2000.

41. Krause W, Matheis H, Wulf K. Fungaemia and funguria after oral administration of Candida albicans. Lancet 1 (7595):598–599, 1969.

42. Pappo I, Polacheck I, Zmora O, et al. Altered gut barrier function to Candida during parenteral nutrition. Nutrition 10 (2):151–154, 1994.

43. Uzun O, Anaissie EJ. Antifungal prophylaxis in patients with hematologic malignancies: a reappraisal. Blood 86 (6):2063–2072, 1995.

44. Voss A, Hollis RJ, Pfaller MA, et al. Investigation of the sequence of colonization and candidemia in nonneutropenic patients. J Clin Microbiol 32 (4):975–980, 1994.

45. Pfaller M, Cabezudo I, Koontz F, et al. Predictive value of surveillance cultures for systemic infection due to Candida species. Eur J Clin Microbiol 6 (6):628–633, 1987.

46. Wey SB, Mori M, Pfaller MA, et al. Risk factors for hospital-acquired candidemia. A matched case-control study. Arch Intern Med 149 (10):2349–2353, 1989.

47. Anaissie EJ, Rex JH, Uzun O, Vartivarian S. Predictors of adverse outcome in cancer patients with candidemia. Am J Med 104 (3):238–245, 1998.

48. Rex JH, Bennett JE, Sugar AM, et al. Intravascular catheter exchange and duration of candidemia. NIAID Mycoses Study Group and the Candidemia Study Group. Clin Infect Dis 21 (4):994–996, 1995.

49. Benoit D, Decruyenaere J, Vandewoude K, et al. Management of candidal thrombophlebitis of the central veins: case report and review. Clin Infect Dis 26 (2):393–397, 1998.

50. Karlowicz MG, Hashimoto LN, Kelly RE Jr, Buescher ES. Should central venous catheters be removed as soon as candidemia is detected in neonates? Pediatrics 106 (5):E63, 2000.

51. Weems JJ Jr, Chamberland ME, Ward J, et al. Candida parapsilosis fungemia associated with parenteral nutrition and contaminated blood pressure transducers. J Clin Microbiol 25 (6):1029–1032, 1987.

52. Plouffe JF, Brown DG, Silva J Jr, et al. Nosocomial outbreak of Candida parapsilosis fungemia related to intravenous infusions. Arch Intern Med 137 (12):1686–1689, 1977.

53. Voss A, Pfaller MA, Hollis RJ, et al. Investigation of Candida albicans transmission in a surgical intensive care unit cluster by using genomic DNA typing methods. J Clin Microbiol 33 (3):576–580, 1995.

54. Kauffman CA, Vazquez JA, Sobel JD, et al. Prospective multicenter surveillance study of funguria in hospitalized patients. The National Institute for Allergy and Infectious Diseases (NIAID) Mycoses Study Group. Clin Infect Dis 30 (1):14–18, 2000.

55. Sobel JD, Kauffman CA, McKinsey D, et al. Candiduria: a randomized, double-blind study of treatment with fluconazole and placebo. The National Institute of Allergy and Infectious Diseases (NIAID) Mycoses Study Group. Clin Infect Dis 30 (1):19–24, 2000.

56. Benjamin DK Jr, Poole C, Steinbach WJ, et al. Neonatal candidemia and end-organ damage: a critical appraisal of the literature using meta-analytic techniques. Pediatrics 112 (3 Pt 1):634–640, 2003.

57. Fisher JF, Chew WH, Shadomy S, et al. Urinary tract infections due to Candida albicans. Rev Infect Dis 4 (6):1107–1118, 1982.

58. Coates EW, Karlowicz MG, Croitoru DP, Buescher ES. Distinctive distribution of pathogens associated with peritonitis in neonates with focal intestinal perforation compared with necrotizing enterocolitis. Pediatrics 116 (2):e241–e246, 2005.

59. Echeverria MJ, Ayarza R, Lopez de Goicoechea MJ, Montenegro J. (Microbiological diagnosis of peritonitis in patients undergoing continuous ambulatory peritoneal dialysis. Review of 5 years at the Hospital de Galdakao). Enferm Infecc Microbiol Clin 11 (4):178–181, 1993.

60. Solomkin JS, Flohr AB, Quie PG, Simmons RL. The role of Candida in intraperitoneal infections. Surgery 88 (4):524–530, 1980.

61. Pacheco-Rios A, Araujo-Hernandez L, Cashat-Cruz M, et al. (Candida endocarditis in the first year of life). Bol Med Hosp Infant Mex 50 (3):157–161, 1993.

62. Ellis ME, Al-Abdely H, Sandridge A, et al. Fungal endocarditis: evidence in the world literature, 1965–1995. Clin Infect Dis 32 (1):50–62, 2001.

63. Tissieres P, Jaeggi ET, Beghetti M, Gervaix A. Increase of fungal endocarditis in children. Infection 33 (4):267–272, 2005.

64. Mogyorosy G, Soos G, Nagy A. Candida endocarditis in a premature infant. J Perinat Med 28 (5):407–411, 2000.

65. Divekar A, Rebekya IM, Soni R. Late onset Candida parapsilosis endocarditis after surviving nosocomial candidemia in an infant with structural heart disease. Pediatr Infect Dis J 23 (5):472–475, 2004.

66. Ainbinder DJ, Parmley VC, Mader TH, Nelson ML. Infectious crystalline keratopathy caused by Candida guilliermondii. Am J Ophthalmol 125 (5):723–725, 1998.

67. Parke DW 2nd, Jones DB, Gentry LO. Endogenous endophthalmitis among patients with candidemia. Ophthalmology 89 (7):789–796, 1982.

68. Brooks RG. Prospective study of Candida endophthalmitis in hospitalized patients with candidemia. Arch Intern Med 149 (10):2226–2228, 1989.

69. Henderson DK, Edwards JE Jr, Montgomerie JZ. Hematogenous candida endophthalmitis in patients receiving parenteral hyperalimentation fluids. J Infect Dis 143 (5):655–661, 1981.

70. Baley JE, Annable WL, Kliegman RM. Candida endophthalmitis in the premature infant. J Pediatr 98 (3):458–461, 1981.

71. Fisher RG, Karlowicz MG, Lall-Trail J. Very low prevalence of endophthalmitis in very low birth-weight infants who survive candidemia. J Perinatol 25 (6):408–411, 2005.

72. Donahue SP, Hein E, Sinatra RB. Ocular involvement in children with candidemia. Am J Ophthalmol 135 (6):886–887, 2003.

73. Baley JE, Ellis FJ. Neonatal candidiasis: ophthalmologic infection. Semin Perinatol 27 (5):401–405, 2003.

74. Krishna R, Amuh D, Lowder CY, et al. Should all patients with candidaemia have an ophthalmic examination to rule out ocular candidiasis? Eye 14 (Pt 1):30–34, 2000.

75. Rodriguez-Adrian LJ, King RT, Tamayo-Derat LG, et al. Retinal lesions as clues to disseminated bacterial and candidal infections: frequency, natural history, and etiology. Medicine (Baltimore) 82 (3):187–202, 2003.

76. Edwards JE Jr, Foos RY, Montgomerie JZ, Guze LB. Ocular manifestations of Candida septicemia: review of seventy-six cases of hematogenous Candida endophthalmitis. Medicine (Baltimore) 53 (1):47–75, 1974.

77. Drohan L, Colby CE, Brindle ME, et al. Candida (amphotericin-sensitive) lens abscess associated with decreasing arterial blood flow in a very low birth weight preterm infant. Pediatrics 110 (5):e65, 2002.

78. Arroyo JG, Bula DV, Grant CA, Murtha T. Bilateral Candida albicans endophthalmitis associated with an infected deep venous thrombus. Jpn J Ophthalmol 48 (1):30–33, 2004.

79. Pappas PG, Rex JH, Sobel JD, et al. Guidelines for treatment of candidiasis. Clin Infect Dis 38 (2):161–189, 2004.

80. Sanchez-Portocarrero J, Perez-Cecilia E, Corral O, et al. The central nervous system and infection by Candida species. Diagn Microbiol Infect Dis 37 (3):169–179, 2000.

81. Montero A, Romero J, Vargas JA, et al. Candida infection of cerebrospinal fluid shunt devices: report of two cases and review of the literature. Acta Neurochir (Wien) 142 (1):67–74, 2000.

82. Fernandez M, Moylett EH, Noyola DE, Baker CJ. Candidal meningitis in neonates: a 10-year review. Clin Infect Dis 31 (2):458–463, 2000.

83. Moylett EH. Neonatal Candida meningitis. Semin Pediatr Infect Dis 14 (2):115–122, 2003.

84. Doctor BA, Newman N, Minich NM, et al. Clinical outcomes of neonatal meningitis in very-low birth-weight infants. Clin Pediatr (Phila) 40 (9):473–480, 2001.

85. Salaki JS, Louria DB, Chmel H. Fungal and yeast infections of the central nervous system. A clinical review. Medicine (Baltimore) 63 (2):108–132, 1984.

86. Gathe JC Jr, Harris RL, Garland B, et al. Candida osteomyelitis. Report of five cases and review of the literature. Am J Med 82 (5):927–937, 1987.

87. Campen DH, Kaufman RL, Beardmore TD. Candida septic arthritis in rheumatoid arthritis. J Rheumatol 17 (1):86–88, 1990.

88. Malani PN, McNeil SA, Bradley SF, Kauffman CA. Candida albicans sternal wound infections: a chronic and recurrent complication of median sternotomy. Clin Infect Dis 35 (11):1316–1320, 2002.

89. Dan M. Neonatal septic arthritis. Isr J Med Sci 19 (11):967–971, 1983.

90. Deshpande SS, Taral N, Modi N, Singrakhia M. Changing epidemiology of neonatal septic arthritis. J Orthop Surg (Hong Kong) 12 (1):10–13, 2004.

91. Evdoridou J, Roilides E, Bibashi E, Kremenopoulos G. Multifocal osteoarthritis due to Candida albicans in a neonate: serum level monitoring of liposomal amphotericin B and literature review. Infection 25 (2):112–116, 1997.

92. Weisse ME, Person DA, Berkenbaugh JT Jr.. Treatment of Candida arthritis with flucytosine and amphotericin B. J Perinatol 13 (5):402–404, 1993.

93. Swanson H, Hughes PA, Messer SA, et al. Candida albicans arthritis one year after successful treatment of fungemia in a healthy infant. J Pediatr 129 (5):688–694, 1996.

94. Mamlok RJ, Richardson CJ, Mamlok V, et al. A case of intrauterine pulmonary candidiasis. Pediatr Infect Dis 4 (6):692–693, 1985.

95. Rowen JL, Atkins JT, Levy ML, et al. Invasive fungal dermatitis in the < or = 1000-gram neonate. Pediatrics 95 (5):682–687, 1995.

96. Ostrosky-Zeichner L, Rex JH, Pappas PG, et al. Antifungal susceptibility survey of 2,000 bloodstream Candida isolates in the United States. Antimicrob Agents Chemother 47 (10):3149–3154, 2003.

97. Hospenthal DR, Murray CK, Rinaldi MG. The role of antifungal susceptibility testing in the therapy of candidiasis. Diagn Microbiol Infect Dis 48 (3):153–160, 2004.

98. Edwards JE Jr, Bodey GP, Bowden RA, et al. International Conference for the Development of a Consensus on the Management and Prevention of Severe Candidal Infections. Clin Infect Dis 25 (1):43–59, 1997.

99. Buchner T, Fegeler W, Bernhardt H, et al. Treatment of severe Candida infections in high-risk patients in Germany: consensus formed by a panel of interdisciplinary investigators. Eur J Clin Microbiol Infect Dis 21 (5):337–352, 2002.

100. Odio CM, Araya R, Pinto LE, et al. Caspofungin therapy of neonates with invasive candidiasis. Pediatr Infect Dis J 23 (12):1093–1097, 2004.

101. Moudgal V, Little T, Boikov D, Vazquez JA. Multiechinocandin- and multiazole-resistant Candida parapsilosis isolates serially obtained during therapy for prosthetic valve endocarditis. Antimicrob Agents Chemother 49 (2):767–769, 2005.

102. Steinbach WJ, Benjamin DK. New antifungal agents under development in children and neonates. Curr Opin Infect Dis 18 (6):484–489, 2005.

103. Heresi G, Gerstmann DR, Blumer JL. Pharmacokinetic, safety, and tolerance study of micafungin (FK463) in premature infants. Pediatric Academic Society Annual Meeting, Abstract 1808. Seattle, WA: 2003..

104. Driessen M, Ellis JB, Cooper PA, et al. Fluconazole vs. amphotericin B for the treatment of neonatal fungal septicemia: a prospective randomized trial. Pediatr Infect Dis J 15 (12):1107–1112, 1996.

105. Kullberg BJ. Voriconazole compared with a strategy of amphotericin B followed by flucona- zole for treatment of candidaemia in non-neutropenic patients. Abstract No. O245. in 14th European Conference of Clinical Microbiology and Infectious Diseases. Prague, Czech Republic: 2004.

106. Muldrew KM, Maples HD, Stowe CD, Jacobs RF. Intravenous voriconazole therapy in a preterm infant. Pharmacotherapy 25 (6):893–898, 2005.

107. Johnson MD, C. MacDougall, Ostrosky-Zeichner L, et al. Combination antifungal therapy. Antimicrob Agents Chemother 48 (3):693–715, 2004.

108. Rex JH, Pappas PG, Karchmer AW, et al. A randomized and blinded multicenter trial of high-dose fluconazole plus placebo versus fluconazole plus amphotericin B as therapy for candidemia and its consequences in nonneutropenic subjects. Clin Infect Dis 36 (10):1221–1228, 2003.

109. Albert RK, Condie F. Hand-washing patterns in medical intensive-care units. N Engl J Med 304 (24):1465–1466, 1981.

110. Parry MF, Grant B, Yukna M, et al. Candida osteomyelitis and diskitis after spinal surgery: an outbreak that implicates artificial nail use. Clin Infect Dis 32 (3):352–357, 2001.

111. Kaufman D, Boyle R, Hazen KC, et al. Fluconazole prophylaxis against fungal colonization and infection in preterm infants. N Engl J Med 345 (23):1660–1666, 2001.

112. Bertini G, Perugi S, Dani C, et al. Fluconazole prophylaxis prevents invasive fungal infection in high-risk, very low birth weight infants. J Pediatr 147 (2):162–165, 2005.

113. Kaufman D. Strategies for prevention of neonatal invasive candidiasis. Semin Perinatol 27 (5):414–424, 2003.

114. Ostrosky-Zeichner L. New approaches to the risk of Candida in the intensive care unit. Curr Opin Infect Dis 16 (6):533–537, 2003.

115. Smolinski KN, Shah SS, Honig PJ, Yan AC. Neonatal cutaneous fungal infections. Curr Opin Pediatr 17 (4):486–493, 2005.

116. James MJ, Lasker BA, McNeil MM, et al. Use of a repetitive DNA probe to type clinical and environmental isolates of Aspergillus flavus from a cluster of cutaneous infections in a neonatal intensive care unit. J Clin Microbiol 38 (10):3612–3618, 2000.

117. Mahieu LM, De Dooy JJ, Van Laer FA, et al. A prospective study on factors influencing aspergillus spore load in the air during renovation works in a neonatal intensive care unit. J Hosp Infect 45 (3):191–197, 2000.

118. Groll AH, Jaeger G, Allendorf A, et al. Invasive pulmonary aspergillosis in a critically ill neonate: case report and review of invasive aspergillosis during the first 3 months of life. Clin Infect Dis 27 (3):437–452, 1998.

119. Mennink-Kersten MA, Klont RR, Warris A, et al. Bifidobacterium lipoteichoic acid and false ELISA reactivity in aspergillus antigen detection. Lancet 363 (9405):325–327, 2004.

120. Siemann M, Koch-Dorfler M, Gaude M. False-positive results in premature infants with the Platelia Aspergillus sandwich enzyme-linked immunosorbent assay. Mycoses 41 (9–10):373–377, 1998.

121. Perzigian RW, Faix RG. Primary cutaneous aspergillosis in a preterm infant. Am J Perinatol 10 (4):269–271, 1993.

122. Walsh TJ, Seibel NL, Arndt C, et al. Amphotericin B lipid complex in pediatric patients with invasive fungal infections. Pediatr Infect Dis J 18 (8):702–708, 1999.

123. Herbrecht R, Denning DW, Patterson TF, et al. Voriconazole versus amphotericin B for primary therapy of invasive aspergillosis. N Engl J Med 347 (6):408–415, 2002.

124. Shouldice E, Fernandez C, McCully B, et al. Voriconazole treatment of presumptive disseminated Aspergillus infection in a child with acute leukemia. J Pediatr Hematol Oncol 25 (9):732–734, 2003.

125. Dennis JE, Rhodes KH, Cooney DR, Roberts GD. Nosocomical Rhizopus infection (zygomycosis) in children. J Pediatr 96 (5):824–828, 1980.

126. Mitchell SJ, Gray J, Morgan ME, et al. Nosocomial infection with Rhizopus microsporus in pre- term infants: association with wooden tongue depressors. Lancet 348 (9025):441–443, 1996.

127. Todd NJ, Millar MR, Dealler SR, Wilkins S. Inadvertent intravenous infusion of Mucor during parenteral feeding of a neonate. J Hosp Infect 15 (3):295–297, 1990.

128. Lewis LL, Hawkins HK, Edwards MS. Disseminated mucormycosis in an infant with methylma- lonicaciduria. Pediatr Infect Dis J 9 (11):851–854, 1990.

129. Ng PC, Dear PR. Phycomycotic abscesses in a preterm infant. Arch Dis Child 64 (6):862–864, 1989.

130. Alexander P, Alladi A, Correa M, D'Cruz AJ. Neonatal colonic mucormycosis–a tropical perspec- tive. J Trop Pediatr 51 (1):54–59, 2005.

131. Butugan O, Sanchez TG, Goncalez F, et al. Rhinocerebral mucormycosis: predisposing factors, diagnosis, therapy, complications and survival. Rev Laryngol Otol Rhinol (Bord) 117 (1):53–55, 1996.

132. Roden MM, Zaoutis TE, Buchanan WL, et al. Epidemiology and outcome of zygomycosis: a review of 929 reported cases. Clin Infect Dis 41 (5):634–653, 2005.

133. Linder N, Keller N, Huri C, et al. Primary cutaneous mucormycosis in a premature infant: case report and review of the literature. Am J Perinatol 15 (1):35–38, 1998.

134. Herbrecht R, V. Letscher-Bru V, Bowden RA, et al. Treatment of 21 cases of invasive mucormycosis with amphotericin B colloidal dispersion. Eur J Clin Microbiol Infect Dis 20 (7):460–466, 2001.

135. Kontoyiannis DP, Lionakis MS, Lewis RE, et al. Zygomycosis in a tertiary-care cancer center in the era of Aspergillus-active antifungal therapy: a case-control observational study of 27 recent cases. J Infect Dis 191 (8):1350–1360, 2005.

136. Ely EW, Peacock JE Jr, Haponik EF, Washburn RG. Cryptococcal pneumonia complicating pregnancy. Medicine (Baltimore) 77 (3):153–167, 1998.

137. Whitt SP, Koch GA, Fender B, et al. Histoplasmosis in pregnancy: case series and report of transplacental transmission. Arch Intern Med 164 (4):454–458, 2004.

138. Watts EA, Gard PD Jr, Tuthill SW. First reported case of intrauterine transmission of blastomycosis. Pediatr Infect Dis 2 (4):308–310, 1983.

139. Shetty SS, Harrison LH, Hajjeh RA, et al. Determining risk factors for candidemia among newborn infants from population-based surveillance: Baltimore, Maryland, 1998–2000. Pediatr Infect Dis J 24 (7):601–604, 2005.

140. Rangel-Frausto MS, Wiblin T, Blumberg HM, et al. National epidemiology of mycoses survey (NEMIS): variations in rates of bloodstream infections due to Candida species in seven surgical intensive care units and six neonatal intensive care units. Clin Infect Dis 29 (2):253–258, 1999.

141. Stamos JK, Rowley AH. Candidemia in a pediatric population. Clin Infect Dis 20 (3):571–575, 1995.

142. Feja KN, Wu F, Roberts K, et al. Risk factors for candidemia in critically ill infants: a matched case-control study. J Pediatr 147 (2):156–161, 2005.

143. Huttova M, Hartmanova I, Kralinsky K, et al. Candida fungemia in neonates treated with fluconazole: report of forty cases, including eight with meningitis. Pediatr Infect Dis J 17 (11):1012–1015, 1998.

144. Ostrosky-Zeichner L, Kontoyiannis D, Raffalli J, et al. International, open-label, noncomparative, clinical trial of micafungin alone and in combination for treatment of newly diagnosed and refractory candidemia. Eur J Clin Microbiol Infect Dis 24 (10):654–661, 2005.

145. Levine J, Bernard DB, Idelson BA, et al. Fungal peritonitis complicating continuous ambulatory peritoneal dialysis: successful treatment with fluconazole, a new orally active antifungal agent. Am J Med 86 (6 Pt 2):825–827, 1989.

146. Salvaggio MR, Pappas PG. Current concepts in the management of fungal peritonitis. Curr Infect Dis Rep 5 (2):120–124, 2003.

147. Arfania D, Everett ED, Nolph KD, Rubin J. Uncommon causes of peritonitis in patients undergoing peritoneal dialysis. Arch Intern Med 141 (1):61–64, 1981.

148. Corbella X, Sirvent JM, Carratala J. Fluconazole treatment without catheter removal in Candida albicans peritonitis complicating peritoneal dialysis. Am J Med 90 (2):277, 1991.

149. Bren A. Fungal peritonitis in patients on continuous ambulatory peritoneal dialysis. Eur J Clin Microbiol Infect Dis 17 (12):839–843, 1998.

150. Stern WH, Tamura E, Jacobs RA, et al. Epidemic postsurgical Candida parapsilosis endophthalmitis. Clinical findings and management of 15 consecutive cases. Ophthalmology 92 (12):1701–1709, 1985.

151. Perraut LE Jr, Perraut LE, Bleiman B, Lyons J. Successful treatment of Candida albicans endophthalmitis with intravitreal amphotericin B. Arch Ophthalmol 99 (9):1565–1567, 1981.

152. Breit SM, Hariprasad SM, Mieler WF, et al. Management of endogenous fungal endophthalmitis with voriconazole and caspofungin. Am J Ophthalmol 139 (1):135–140, 2005.

153. Kauffman CA, Bradley SF, Vine AK. Candida endophthalmitis associated with intraocular lens implantation: efficacy of fluconazole therapy. Mycoses 36 (1–2):13–17, 1993.

154. Fitzgerald E, Lloyd-Still J, Gordon SL. Candida arthritis. A case report and review of the literature. Clin Orthop. 1975(106):143–7..

155. Petrikkos G, Skiada A, Sabatakou H, et al. Case report. Successful treatment of two cases of postsurgical sternal osteomyelitis, due to Candida krusei and Candida albicans, respectively, with high doses of triazoles (fluconazole, itraconazole). Mycoses 44 (9–10):422–425, 2001.

156. Smego RA Jr, Perfect JR, Durack DT. Combined therapy with amphotericin B and 5-fluorocytosine for Candida meningitis. Rev Infect Dis 6 (6):791–801, 1984.

157. Liu KH, Wu CJ, Chou CH, et al. Refractory candidal meningitis in an immunocompromised patient cured by caspofungin. J Clin Microbiol 42 (12):5950–5953, 2004.

158. Fan-Havard P, O'Donovan C, Smith SM, et al. Oral fluconazole versus amphotericin B bladder irrigation for treatment of candidal funguria. Clin Infect Dis 21 (4):960–965, 1995.

Chapter 16

Effects of Chemoprophylaxis for Neonatal Group B Streptococcal Infections on the Incidence of Gram-negative Infections and Antibiotic Resistance in Neonatal Pathogens

Gary D. Overturf, MD

Background on Intrapartum Antibiotic Prophylaxis

Effects of IAP on the Etiology of Early Neonatal Sepsis and Antibiotic Susceptibility

Summary and Conclusions

Intrapartum antibiotic prophylaxis (IAP) for group B streptococcal infections is now a widely accepted standard of practice. Since its inception, it has led to a striking decrease in the incidence of early-onset sepsis (EOS) in neonates caused by all serotypes of group B streptocci. However, concerns have been raised regarding the possible adverse influence of IAP as a cause of an increasing incidence of Gram-negative infection in early-onset sepsis and the possible increase in antibiotic-resistant pathogens causing these infections. In addition, there has been concern that the clinical presentation of infants with group B streptococcal infection or sepsis caused by other pathogens may have a modified clinical presentation due to the use of intrapartum antibiotics.

BACKGROUND ON INTRAPARTUM ANTIBIOTIC PROPHYLAXIS

Antepartum Treatment of Colonized Mothers or Sexual Partners

The potential use of prophylaxis for group B streptococcal (GBS) infection was conceived in the early 1970s, with hopes of targeting the eradication of high rates of early-onset disease occurring prior to the 7th day of life, most frequently in the first 72 h of life. Initial attempts to eradicate group B streptococcal carriers by administration of oral antimicrobial agents were unsuccessful because of persistent vaginal carriage. This occurred in as many as one-quarter of pregnant mothers following the end of antimicrobial administration (1). In addition, resumption of carriage occurred by the time of delivery in approximately three-quarters of mothers who had been "cleared" of their carriage. The addition of a co-treatment regimen of potential sources for persistent carriage by treatment of sexual partners was also associated with high failure rates (2, 3). These studies demonstrate that because group B streptococci are normal constituents of the normal flora, it was unlikely that treatment would successfully eradicate these organisms, which are essential components of the flora of the colon and the adjacent vagina.

Intrapartum Treatment of Colonized Mothers

In contrast to eradication of group B streptococci in the mother or her sexual contacts prior to delivery, early attempts at using either penicillin or ampicillin in the neonate were found to be effective in interrupting the transmission of group B streptococci to infants or preventing the onset of early disease. Yow and colleagues treated 34 women colonized with GBS at admission for delivery with single doses of 500 mg of ampicillin intravenously (4). Ampicillin treatment uniformly interrupted vertical transmission to the neonates, compared to an expected transmission rate of 50%. Subsequently, the sentinel study by Boyer and Gotoff provided strong evidence that intravenous ampicillin given to women with high risk for early onset GBS infection (delivery at <37 weeks, membrane rupture at 12 h before delivery or earlier, or intrapartum fever) would reduce subsequent infection rates. GBS sepsis developed in 5 of 79 (6.3%) neonates born to untreated mothers compared to 0 of 85 infants born to treated mothers (5). Many subsequent studies confirmed these results (see reviews in ref. 6). Thus, these early studies convincingly provided the rationale and led to the current algorithm for intrapartum antimicrobial prophylaxis (IAP) for GBS infections in infants born to mothers known to be colonized with the organism.

Current Recommended Regimen for IAP

The current algorithm and rationale for IAP and recommendations for screening are provided in other references, and a more complete discussion is beyond the scope of this chapter (7). However, the current prophylaxis regimen for group B streptococci focuses on the identification of known carrier mothers, rather than the use of IAP in defined high-risk mothers who have not been identified as carriers. This policy minimizes the wider exposure to antibiotics for mothers who are not colonized and, in part, minimizes the potential adverse microbiologic epidemiologic consequences (e.g., antibiotic resistance) of antibiotic administration to large numbers of mothers who are not carriers of group B streptococci. The current recommendations are summarized in Table 16-1. Penicillin G (5 million units initially, then 2.5 million units every 4 h until delivery) is the preferred agent for prophylaxis. Because of an increasingly common shortage of penicillin G, intravenous ampicillin (2 g initially, then 1 g every 4 h until delivery) has been the preferred alternative agent.

EFFECTS OF IAP ON THE ETIOLOGY OF EARLY NEONATAL SEPSIS AND ANTIBIOTIC SUSCEPTIBILITY

Effects of IAP on the Incidence of EOS due to Group B Streptococci and Non-Streptococcal Organisms

Although the efficacy of IAP in preventing early-onset group B streptococcal infection in numerous US and international studies is well established, the potential

Table 16-1   **Indications for Intrapartum Antimicrobial Prophylaxis (IAP) to Prevent Early-Onset Group B Streptococcal (GBS) Disease with the use of a Universal Prenatal Culture of Women At 35–37 Weeks of Gestation**

VAGINAL AND RECTAL GBS CULTURE OR MOLECULAR SCREEN AT 5–37 WEEKS GESTATION FOR ALL PREGNANT WOMEN	
IAP indicated	**IAP not indicated**
• Previous infant with invasive GBS disease • Positive GBS culture or molecular screen during current pregnancy (unless a planned C-section delivery is performed in the absence of labor or membrane rupture) • GBS bacteriuria during current pregnancy • Unknown GBS status and any of the following: delivery at <37 weeks gestation membrane rupture for ≥18 h intrapartum fever (temperature ≥38°C (≥100.4°F)	• Previous pregnancy with a positive GBS screening culture (unless a culture also was positive during the current pregnancy or previous infant with invasive GBS disease) • Planned C-section delivery performed in the absence of labor or membrane rupture (regardless of GBS current status) • Negative vaginal or rectal GBS screening culture in late gestation, regardless of intrapartum risk factors

impact of the increased use of IAP on the occurrence of sepsis caused by other bacteria, particularly Gram-negative organisms, and the possible emergence of greater antibiotic resistance in the causative organisms, has been debated. Most reports which have found an increase in the proportion of causative Gram-negative infections and increased antibiotic resistance have been studies restricted to preterm or low-birth-weight infants. Thus, multi-center studies which have demonstrated an increase in sepsis caused by *E. coli* have included only low-birth-weight infants or very-low-birth-weight infants. The impact of increased use of IAP on the occurrence of sepsis caused by organisms other than GBS has been an ongoing concern and subject of considerable evaluation. Concern has centered on the issue of a possible decline in GBS sepsis, but an increase in the incidence of infection caused by other non-GBS organisms, which have an increased resistance to ampicillin and, perhaps, to other beta-lactam antibiotics.

A relationship between neonatal death caused by ampicillin-resistant *E. coli* and prolonged antepartum exposure to ampicillin has been noted in one investigation (8). Although other studies designed to examine Enterobacteriaceae susceptibility to ampicillin following maternal exposure to antibiotics have had mixed or indeterminate results, at least one study has found no difference before and after the use of IAP utilizing either penicillin or ampicillin (9). Further, studies examining the effect of antibiotics on the antibiotic susceptibility of isolates in cultures at 6 weeks post-partum have revealed no increase in antibiotic resistance in either GBS or *E. coli* in women who had received antibiotics in labor (10).

In 2002, the Centers for Disease Control's Active Bacterial Core surveillance (ABCs) of the Emerging Infections Program Network provided data on 408 cases of early-onset infections occurring in 1998–2000 (11). GBS caused 166 (40.7%) of the cases, whereas other bacterial pathogens were identified in 242 cases, with an incidence of 0.62–0.76/100 live births for GBS sepsis and 0.95–0.99/100 live births for non-GBS cases. *E. coli* specifically caused 70 cases, with an incidence ranging from 0.25 to 0.31/100 live births. The proportion of *E. coli* infections that were resistant to ampicillin increased significantly, but only among preterm infants (from 29% to

84%) and not in full-term infants. Term infants experienced a decreased incidence of *E. coli* sepsis during this time, declining from 50% to 25% of cases. These rates are similar to earlier studies which have documented an increase in the rate or proportion of infants with early-onset sepsis caused by *E. coli*, but only in very-low-birth-weight infants (12). However, in some earlier studies such as those by Baltimore and colleagues, the rate of GBS EOS declined from 0.61/1000 live births to 0.23/1000 live births in the period from 1996 to 1999, whereas the annual rate of non-GBS sepsis remained steady at 0.65/1000 live births (13). In studies by the National Institute of Child Health and Human Development of early-onset neonatal sepsis (as defined by an onset within 72 h of birth) during the past 13 years in low–birth-weight infants (14), more than half the infections (53%) were caused by Gram-negative organisms in 2002–2003, with *E. coli* the most common organism (41%). Between 1991–1993 and 1998–2000, there was a significant increase in rates of *E. coli* infections, but in 2002–2003 there was no significant change, suggesting a leveling-off of the incidence.

Collectively, these studies suggest that the widespread use of IAP in recent years has not been associated with increased rate of Gram-negative or *E. coli* infections but rather a stabilized rate of Gram-negative infections with continuing declines of Gram-positive (e.g. GBS) in EOS. That is, the absolute rate of Gram-negative infections has not changed or increased, but rather the proportion of infections now caused by Gram-negative infections has increased due to the continued decline of EOS caused by Gram-positive bacteria.

Effect of IAP on Clinical Presentation of EOS in Infants

In addition to the possible changing rate of Gram-negative infections and possible emergence of antibiotic resistance among neonatal pathogens, the effect of IAP on the clinical presentation and implications for management of the infant exposed to antibiotics with possible sepsis has been studied. In studies at the Kaiser Permanente Southern California group, neither the clinical spectrum of EOS nor the time to onset of EOS was affected by the use of IAP assessed in 277 912 live births (15) in which 172 term infants with EOS were evaluated. In addition, the effect of IAP has been examined in relation to the possible effect on late-onset sepsis (LOS). Multi-institutional evaluations of late-onset sepsis have found that the vast majority of infants who survive beyond 3 days are infected by Gram-positive organisms (70%), in which coagulase-negative staphylococci account for 48% of all infections (16). However, mortality rates with infection caused by Gram-negative organisms or fungi were much higher than coagulase-negative staphylococci (36% and 32%, respectively). IAP has been associated with increased rates of late-onset serious infections in only a single study (17). In this study, more infants exposed to IAP (41%; $n = 90$) than those infants not exposed to IAP (27%; $n = 92$) had late-onset sepsis (OR 1.96, CI 1.05–3.66). The association was stronger when broad-spectrum antibiotics were used for IAP (adjusted OR 4.95, CI 2.04–11.98) as opposed to narrow-spectrum antibiotics, such as penicillin G. Bacteria that were isolated from infected infants who had been exposed to IAP were more likely to exhibit ampicillin resistance (OR 5.7, CI 2.3–14.3).

SUMMARY AND CONCLUSIONS

A summary of the findings in studies of the relationship of IAP for GBS EOS to the incidence, etiology and antibiotic resistance is provided in Table 16-2. To date, no clear causal link has been demonstrated between IAP and increasing rates of infections caused by *E. coli* or other Gram-negative bacteria, nor higher rates of infections caused by ampicillin-resistant Gram-negative bacteria. Although the

Table 16-2	Summary of Findings in Studies of the Effect of IAP on the Incidence of GBS EOS and LOS, the Frequency of Gram-negative Bacteria and the Effect on Antibiotic Resistance or Susceptibility

- The incidence of GBS sepsis has declined and the incidence of Gram-negative EOS and LOS has remained the same
- The proportion of Gram-negative bacteria causing EOS has increased with the concomitant reduction of neonatal EOS caused by group B streptococci
- Although the antibiotic resistance of *E. coli* and other Gram-negative bacteria isolated in neonatal units has increased, it is likely that factors unrelated to IAP have promoted the expansion of antibiotic resistance in neonatal units

proportion of infections caused by Gram-negative organisms causing EOS has increased, there is little evidence of increasing rate of Gram-negative infection in either EOS or LOS. In part this may be due to the many other factors affecting current evaluations, including the increased numbers of surviving very-low-birth-weight infants, the increasing effects of broad-spectrum antibiotic pressure in neonatal intensive care units with use of broad- or very broad-spectrum antibiotics (e.g. extended-spectrum cephalosporins and carbepenems) in the treatment of suspected or proven infections of the newborn infant and the recent change from a focus of risk-based IAP to the application of IAP to culture-confirmed carrier mothers. However, continuing surveillance for a shift in the etiology or the emergence of antibiotic resistance promoted by IAP is a reasonable and prudent recommendation.

REFERENCES

1. Gardner SE, Yow MD, Leeds LJ, et al. Failure of penicillin to eradicate the group B streptococcal colonization in the pregnant women. Am J Obstet Gynecol 135:1062–1065, 1977.
2. Hall RT, Barnes W, Krishnan L, et al. Antibiotic treatment of parturient women with group B streptococci. Am J Obstet Gynecol 124:630–634, 1976.
3. Lewin EB, Amstey MS. Natural history of group B streptococcus colonization and its therapy during pregnancy. Am J Obstet Gynecol 139:512–515, 1981.
4. Yow MD, Mason EO, Leeds LJ, et al. Ampicillin prevents intrapartum transmission of group B streptococcus. JAMA 241:1245–1247, 1979.
5. Boyer KM, Gotoff SP. Prevention of early-onset neonatal group B streptococcal disease with selective intrapartum chemoprophylaxis. N Engl J Med 314:1665–1669, 1986.
6. Remington JS, Klein JO, Wilson CB, Baker CJ. Infectious Diseases of the Fetus and Newborn Infant, 6th Edition, Elsevier Saunders, Philadelphia, PA, 2006.
7. American Academy of Pediatrics, Committee on Infectious Diseases. Report of the Committee on Infectious Diseases, 27th edn. Group B Streptococcal Infections. 620–626, 2006..
8. Terrone DA, Rinehart BK, Einstein MH, et al. Neonatal sepsis and death caused by resistant *Escherichia coli*: possible consequences of extended maternal ampicillin administration. Am J Obstet Gynecol 180:1345–3148, 1999.
9. Edwards RK, Clark P, Sistrom CL, et al. Intrapartum antibiotic prophylaxis1: relative effects of recommended antibiotics on gram negative pathogens. Obstetrics Gynecol 100:534–539, 2002.
10. Spaetgen R, DeBella K, Ma D, et al. Perinatal antibiotic usage and changes in colonization and resistance rates of group B streptococcus and other pathogens. Obstetrics Gynecol 100:525–533, 2002.
11. Hyde TB, Hilger MS, Reingold A, et al. Trends in the incidence and antimicrobial resistance of early-onset sepsis: Population–based surveillance in San Francisco and Atlanta. Pediatrics 110:690–695, 2002.
12. Levine EM, Ghai V, Barton JJ, et al. Intrapartum antibiotic prophylaxis increases the incidence of gram-negative neonatal sepsis. Infect Dis Obstet Gynecol 7:210–213, 1999.
13. Baltimore RS, Huie SM, Meek JI, et al. Early–onset neonatal sepsis in the era of group B streptococcal prevention. Pediatrics 108:1094–1099, 2001.
14. Stoll BJ, Hansen NI, Higgins RD, et al. Very low birth weight preterm infants with early onset neonatal sepsis. The predominance of gram-negative infections continues in the National Institute

of Child Health and Human Development Neonatal Research Network, 2002–2003. Pediatr Infect Dis J 24:635–644, 2005.

15. Bromberger P, Lawrence JM, Braun D, et al. The influence of intrapartum antibiotics on the clinical spectrum of early-onset Group B streptococcal infection in term infants. Pediatrics 106:244–250, 2000.

16. Glasgow TS, Young PC, Wallin J, et al. Association of intrapartum antibiotic exposure and late-onset serious bacterial infections in infants. Pediatrics 116:696–702, 2005.

Index

Page numbers for figures have suffix **f**, those for tables have suffix **t**